Sensations, Thoughts, and Emotions

Essays on Reality and Mental Health, 2013 – 2023

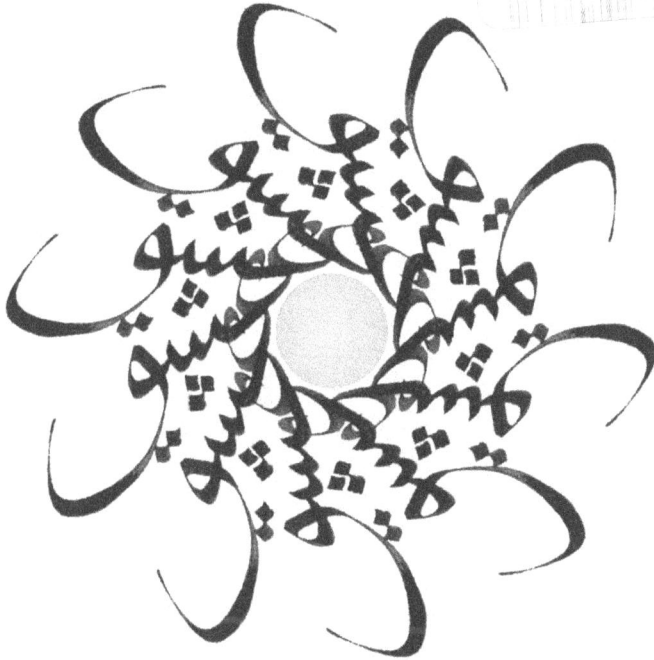

Lincoln Stoller

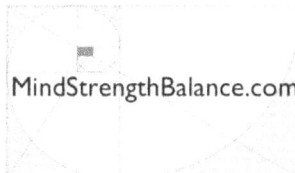

MindStrengthBalance.com

First Edition.
Published 2024 by Mind Strength Books, Victoria, British Columbia, Canada
http://www.mindstrengthbooks.com

Names: Stoller, Lincoln, 1956- author.
Title: Sensations, Thoughts, and Emotions: Essays on Reality and Mental Health, 2013 – 2023 / Lincoln Stoller.

Identifiers:
ISBN (paper) 978-1-7381399-0-3 | ISBN (hard cover) 978-1-7381399-2-7
ISBN (audio) 978-1-7381399-3-4 | ISBN (epub) 978-1-7381399-1-0

Subjects:
LCSH: Psychology, Applied. | Existential psychology. | Emotional intelligence. | Thought and thinking. | Mental health | LCGFT: Blogs. | Anthology.

BISAC:
SEL 016000 Self-Help/Personal Growth/General
PSY 051000 Cognitive Neuroscience & Cognitive Neuropsychology
PSY 055000 Psychology/Essays

Classification:
LCC BF637.S4 .S76 2023 (print) | LCC BF637.S4 (ebook) | DDC 158.1

Publisher's Cataloging-In-Publication Data
Library of Congress Control Number: 2023924190

Front cover illustration: Yamaji Shogen Masakuni, by Kuniyoshi.
Back cover illustration: Bamboo, by Lin Zexu

Praise for Sensations, Thoughts, and Emotions

"*Sensations, Thoughts and Emotions* takes readers on an odyssey that challenges our preconceptions, navigates the intersections of philosophy, psychology, and neuroscience, and invite us to grapple with the workings of our minds."
— **Allison Feduccia**, PhD, psychedelic scientist, co-founder of Psychedelic Support

"*Sensations, Thoughts and Emotions* invites us to excavate and resurrect the emotional, embodied, and subconscious aspects of our lives. This book is written for anyone remotely interested in self understanding and human change."
— **Lee Diener**, psychiatric mental health nurse practitioner

"Mr Stoller's excellent mind is at its best in this collection of wisdom of what it is to be. Digest one a day, like a fine meal. Many of these subjects are not addressed outside of books of Zen teachings horrible to read, or try the Upanishads."
— **Reverend Bill McCarter**, engineer and computer programmer

"The essay 'Developing Emotional Intelligence,' explores how our relationships create harmony. 'Fostering Empathy' takes us into the world of mirror neurons and empathetic responses. Every essay could expand into a captivating book."
— **Matthew McMillion**, researcher and writer

"That Stoller can make complex, subtle subjects a pleasure is a trick. That these writings are useful in our lives is miraculous. Bridging ancient Chinese ideas with Adler's organ dialects, everything is within reach of this self-effacing, well-tempered mind. A beautiful book."
— **Nikolaos Katranis**, filmmaker, painter, musician

"With an exceptional acerbic sense of humor, Dr. Stoller relentlessly dives into the depths of our human psyche, examining, questioning and challenging our very existence. This book is NOT for the small-minded."
— **Anneli Driessen** PhD, Metaphysics, Life Coaching, and Master Certified Coach

"An exploration, experience and an exposition; delightful, playful, and emotive. Agree or disagree, the analogies make you more conscious, and how delicious is that? A fantastic book I highly recommend, especially for inquiring into yourself."
— **James Hayes**, Founder of Collective Intelligence Group, and a serious nobody

"Stoller explores how paying attention to your body and mind's drive to action develops a truer reality of yourself. Get ready to dig into yourself, to become more aware, and enjoy a journey of self discovery that empowers you."
— **Arno Ilgner**, mountaineer and author of *The Rock Warrior's Way*

"The tone is powerful and the approach is never lazy. Stoller says that as a therapist he always assumes the client is lying. I rarely hear it put so directly. I am struck by it."
— **Raymond C. Russ**, PhD and editor of *The Journal of Mind and Behavior*

Also by Lincoln Stoller

The Learning Project; Rites of Passage

The Path To Sleep, Exercises for an Ancient Skill

Becoming Lucid, Self-Awareness in Sleeping & Waking Life

COVID-19: Illness & Illumination, A Hypnotic Exploration

Becoming Supergenius, Part I: The Outside World

Becoming Supergenius, Part II: The Inside World

For an updated book list, goto https://www.mindstrengthbooks.com

Table of Contents

Table of Figures

Table of Hypnotic Inductions

Prologue

Passion is essential. It is a personal commitment to act with meaning. We should passionately engage with all things that have essential meaning for us.

I've placed an `Ishq motif on the title page and at the start of each of the book's three sections: sensation, thought, and emotion. Each should be considered with equal passion.

`Ishq, a word for passion in Persian and other Semitic languages (Wikipedia 2023), "refers to a transcendental, all-encompassing Love with a capitalized "L" for the divine Beloved, Allah" (Ghazi 2022). Each of the attitudes explored here—sensate, thoughtful, and emotional —are aspects of the passionate experience. Keep this in mind.

To follow these ideas as I advance them further, subscribe to my blog at https://www.mindstrengthbalance.com/subscribe_msb.

References

Ghazi, G. (2022). Unraveling 'Ishq, Library of Congress. https://www.loc.gov/ghe/cascade/index.html?appid=ad7341e261ed4d9ea29e9be58c0590d4
Wikipedia (2023 Aug 22). "Ishq," Wikipedia.com. https://en.wikipedia.org/wiki/Ishq

Introduction

As humans, we have distinguished ourselves through the use of our hands and brains—in particular, our intellect. The intellect has become the source of our greatest strength and weakness. We are manipulators, but we are far from experts. We are poorly aware of our role in the world.

Much as medicine sees differences as abnormal, humans see the world through a lens of opportunity. If we better understood our spirits and emotions, we would be in greater touch with the consequences of our actions.

Before modern times, when we were more involved in the natural world, our intellects were more integrated with our emotions. Our knowledge was limited, but we were more deeply informed of those subjects in which we were involved. Our modern success and the global scale of our manipulations have given predominance to our impersonal, separate, and mechanistic inclinations.

We have developed the intellectual ability to fail and correct ourselves, but we have lost emotional stability and spiritual perception. Our isolation as individuals has led to us being emotionally out of touch with the social and environmental consequences of our actions. Our emotions have been buried beneath the intellectual demands of our modern world.

These essays do not cover all the territory of these topics. They are my reflections on issues that have come up in my role as a counselor. Some are specific, such as the essays on trauma and addiction. Others, like those on wisdom and imagination, address issues more broadly.

Sensations

We think with our bodies, emotions, and intellects. These three layers underlie our perception and cognition. Sensations are our most overlooked mode of thought, which we demote to the level of insensate perception, but senses have thoughts. They are our most fundamental level of awareness and ability.

Our primary sensation is sight, with sound and touch subordinate to it. In addition to

Introduction

perceptions from outside, a host of sensations come from within our bodies. Inner sensations include awareness of comfort, metabolism, health, and fitness. We're vaguely aware of many internal signals we cannot accurately resolve.

I see people through the lenses of sensations, thoughts, and emotions, and I work to regain a balance between these aspects of experience. Like all three-part structures—and unlike structures with more legs—three-legged structures can rest their feet on unlevel ground. I extend this metaphor to self-awareness: if we see ourselves as having three parts, then we can develop ourselves so that each part is grounded and stable.

Ten years ago I went on a dark, psychedelic trip with the help of a small plant of the mint family called Salvia divinorum. The world that unfolded was short-lived—it only lasted 10 minutes—but it was the darkest of possible worlds.

The experience was based on what I could sense of myself and what was around me, and it gave me first-hand knowledge of the desire to kill oneself. I was thinking clearly, but my sensations created a lifeless world. This proved to me that sensations can create reality.

Because our bodies take care of themselves, we believe our organs perceive the world without judgment. Besides attending to our needs, our bodies know how we understand and react. We may think our intellects are making all the decisions, but our bodies determine what we see and play a role in what we recognize.

The human intellect is both our crowning achievement and a tool for self-destruction. We can barely behave morally as individuals, and we're wholly unable to do so as a species. Ethical behavior must become innate through an integration of our neural structures. This is far beyond our current state.

This is sad because it ignores truth, which is rooted in feeling, and it's pathetic because, rather than being secondary, emotions rule the intellect. Our motivation to do anything is rooted in emotions of self, purpose, and survival. Yet we believe our intellects are fully informed and in complete control.

Thoughts

When we reflect, we are predominantly intellectual. In the project of gaining control of one's thoughts, it's critical to understand how narrowly we think, how little we recognize, and how easily we're misled. Thoughts exist in a reality that is neither fixed nor free. For this reason, I've included more pieces addressing how we intellectualize.

Most of the essays in this section are about how we think, with some being reflective and others directive. In the effort to gain control of our thoughts, it's critical to understand how narrowly we think, how little we recognize, and how easily we're misled. Thoughts exist in a reality that is neither fixed nor free. They grow like vines on pre-existing structures we rarely think about.

I'm reminded of a presentation I made on the topic of how we think. I created it for and announced it to a professional group of fifty practicing psychotherapists, of which I was a member. Only one person attended: a 13-year-old boy who was brought by his mother.

This was no accident. Thinking is a creative act. The more you know, the less likely you are to think. Most of what we do is data retrieval, and data retrievers are not creative.

Two series of essays, Where the Thoughts Come From and To Be Confused, reach beyond what we know to how we know and the limits of what we can understand. You may find these essays difficult to read. They may seem irrelevant to readers more interested in filling in the potholes on the road to clarity.

I include these as encouragement to doubt everything; to recognize that your greater limitations are not what you know, but what you can know within your current framework. The best thing you can do to further your evolution is to discard most of what you know and start again. This will destabilize your personality and require emotional strength. Metamorphosis seems chaotic even when it isn't.

Much of what I've been taught in physics, brain training, and psychology is provisionally true at best. In physics, the boundaries of what's plausible are sometimes clear but rarely respected. In brain training, little is known for certain, and psychology amounts to a bunch of stories. I've concluded that I only know what I can do myself.

Introduction

Most of what we want lies beyond what we're able to understand. Being fixed on how we think creates an inflexible reality, but being flexible makes us vulnerable. So it is that some of the most capable thinkers are inflexible and frustrated. These people tend toward institutions, and institutions happily reward them. What such people need is a richer world of chaos that lies beyond what makes sense. This leads to mid-life crises, but any time is a good time for a crisis.

Creativity is the putting together of things that don't seem to fit. This can be funny or tragic; comedy and tragedy have always been connected. "Here there be dragons," and also there be gold. You can't get to a new understanding from the understanding you have. You will not see further standing on the shoulders of giants. You're looking for something others can't see.

New thinking always starts chaotically. It is not found along the well-ordered paths we've been advised to follow. We are taught to think without creativity because that makes us more docile and socially productive. We're taught to work on other people's projects. This insect-like trend toward mediocrity builds a stronger collective at the expense of individual growth.

There are two definitions of sanity: following consensus and gaining insight. Following consensus is medically, scientifically, and institutionally endorsed, but it will never satisfy you. Gaining insight is the path of personal and species evolution. Insight easily leads to things too big for us to contain. Consensus is collegial. Insights can destroy anything and everything.

If you're insightful, you'll be discouraged until you convince others that your ideas will benefit them. That's not a healthy aim because what most people crave is not good for anyone. You'll do better if you learn to live with discouragement.

To get beyond the hive mentality, you must embrace uncertainty, errors, chaos, and doubt. "You make it up as you go along," Jerry Lettvin, my psychiatrist and neurophysiologist mentor, said. The more correct you are for your own purposes, the more you'll deviate from the models taught to you, and the more people will contradict you.

The key to establishing a healthy reality is maintaining a healthy environment, and that particularly applies to the people around you. If you want to grow, don't fraternize with uncreative people.

Emotions

Emotions are an often ignored counterpoint to our decision-making process. When properly applied, emotions are the energy of wisdom. But emotions are huge, spanning the gamut from instinct to insight. Like gasoline, emotions are a fuel that comes from the earth. But more than that, emotions contain elements of wisdom. Emotions make us wise.

Your desire to punch someone in the face, and your desire to live a life in service to humanity, are both emotional. The first is narrow and immediate; the second is broad and forward-thinking. There is an emotion for every inclination, and they need to be handled differently. All are useful, and without them, you would be inactive and indifferent.

Emotions are feelings that arise from within us. We manage them with empathy and honesty, not with intellect. It's not intellectual truth that's important, as that's fabricated on whatever evidence we choose or with which we ply our trades.

Emotional honesty is less rooted in truth and more rooted in commitment. It's the truth you believe in and the things that are important to you. Small-T truths form the landscapes of the lives we build as children; the things we take for granted.

Big-T truths are the accomplishments of which we're proud; the monuments to which we bow. They are our emperor's new clothes. Beware of big truths.

It turns out that I'm empathic, which surprises me. I thought I was analytical. Being empathetic means that I get sucked into the lives of the people I work with. I'm not sure if this is something one can learn or unlearn.

I need to be careful to set boundaries because everyone seems to rock my boat, but I find each person to be a curious mystery. I'm tempted to lose myself in every maze—I love getting lost in the woods—and the most unpleasant people are often the most curious. Like emotions, empathy is a power that can be used for good or ill. I work to contain it.

Any situation that's meaningful to us, good or bad, must have some resonance in us, otherwise it would be foreign, unrecognizable, and irrelevant. I resonate with all of my clients, and sometimes I anti-resonate with them.

Introduction

Better understanding of our emotions is a necessary step forward in our evolution. As contradictory as it may sound, we need a better intellectual understanding of our emotions. At the least, we need greater integration. These essays are musings along these lines.

Sensations

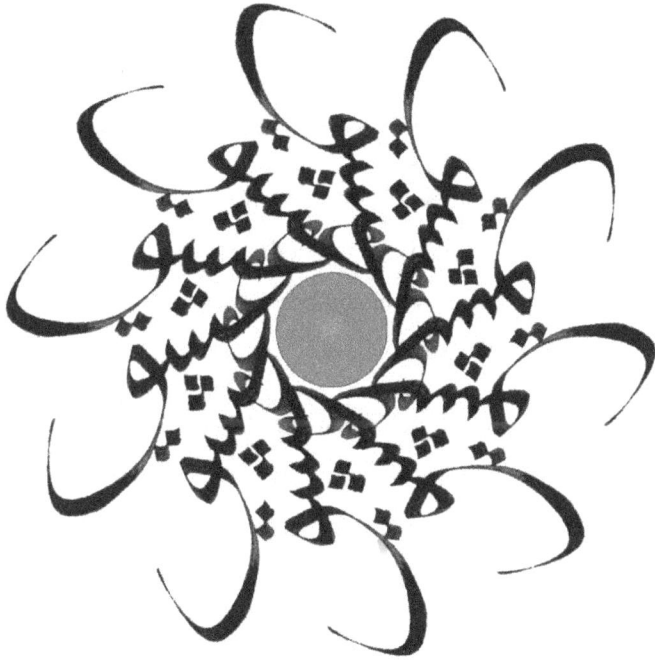

S1 – How Wise is the Body?

January 6, 2022

Trauma is a more common mind–body impediment than we realize.

"You need to believe in things that aren't true. How else can they become?"— **Terry Pratchett**, author, from *Hogfather*

Homeostasis

Because most of our body's operations are invisible to us, we presume the only effect we have on our body is through our intentional actions. We presume we do not have control of what we don't perceive, and that our thoughts and mental images don't affect our autonomic processes. This is the foundation of allopathic medicine. It is a reductive view of the body's processes, which claims our different systems regulate themselves independently.

This is partly supported for certain systems and weakly supported for most. The homeostasis of most of our body's systems depends on all the body's systems remaining in balance. When one of these systems is not in balance, we become more broadly out of balance. We attribute this to disease.

When I was discharged from my time in the hospital for Covid-19, my breathing was labored. I would not have been able to walk up my driveway without oxygen. I was given oxygen and a steroid inhaler, both of which help but neither heal. In fact, both work against regaining function and can be detrimental to long-term recovery.

> "Although encouraging patients to return to performing daily activities and to start low/moderate-intensity exercise at home is currently recommended for patients recovering from COVID-19, Humphreys et al. have described that patients experienced a lack of clear and consistent advice with regard to physical activity."

— **Jeannet Delbressine**, et al., (Delbressine et al. 2021)

Allopathic medicine, as it's now practiced, is normative. It aims to move you back into your body's expected operating range on the assumption that your body will regain control and reestablish balance, which we refer to as homeostasis.

The trouble is that when a system in your body has been pushed too far out of its normal range, it may not naturally return to its normal, healthy, operating state even though allopathic treatment says it has recovered. With too much stress, any of our systems become traumatized. Some aspect of ourselves has been distorted and will not return to normal by itself. This could be mental, muscular, or metabolic.

Returning to Normal

Allopathic medicine applies chemical and physical forces to push us back to a normal operating range based on a few parameters. There is little recognition of the interaction between systems—how one system affects another—and no recognition of the role of mind, intention, and emotion aside from taking one's meds and following the protocol.

My experience was that my lungs had forgotten how to breathe. It was not that I couldn't breathe normally, it was that some aspect of my breathing overreacted and interfered with my intention. If I took deep breaths, my diaphragm went into spasms, causing me to cough. I didn't feel the need to cough, but my diaphragm had forgotten how to operate normally.

This is very much like the condition of Post Traumatic Stress Disorder (PTSD). In PTSD, one's perceptions and reactions are hijacked by a past experience, and attempts to behave normally are short-circuited. Normal reactions, those that you do unconsciously and without thinking, are replaced by distorted reactions. Usually, these distortions reflect the traumatic threat or condition that affected you in the past. Your reflexive reaction has overwhelmed your recollection of how to react normally.

Recovering from PTSD requires an intentional redirection of your perception, attention, and reaction. In almost all healing modalities, someone other than you facilitates the healing. After all, if you could heal yourself, then you wouldn't seek help. But it is ultimately you who does the healing, because only you have the tools to maintain your balance.

I've since been involved with several doctors and, in each case, there is a reluctance to explore much of anything. Rather, doctors seem wedded to one protocol or another, not broadly informed about any, and reluctant to reveal their lack of knowledge. There is an unwillingness to reveal the lack of any well researched protocol and their professional requirement to follow the mandates set by their uninformed institutional managers.

This is for legal, financial, and administrative reasons. If you've been following the conflicts over the treatment of Covid-19, then you'll notice that it largely boils down to whether doctors have the right to apply their clinical experience to individual cases. Normally, they do, but in this case—to support what agencies want us to believe is an informed and unified front—they do not.

Few doctors are fighting for this right, and those who are fighting are the doctors who are establishing new protocols. Most other doctors, in my experience, are reluctant to entertain anything outside of the protocol their administrators tell them to follow. They do not use clinical experience and, as has been noted in medical education, they are increasingly encouraged not to.

Finding Guidance

I'm an advocate of learning. This means being aware of what's new and making accommodation for novelty. We seek outside help when we can't find the information we need. Regarding our health, we seek medical help when we can't heal ourselves.

Practitioners are increasingly less interested in providing us with knowledge. As standard medical care becomes increasingly formulaic, medical authorities become indifferent to their observations. Doctors become functionaries and as a result, learning stops. This approach is institutionally endorsed. Institutions, as you know, are not primarily concerned with your healing.

Some authorities are exploring new ideas. New ideas would not be critical if solutions were known, but here the solutions are not known. The institutions doctors look to for direction are slow, biased, morally compromised, and error-prone, and they always have been.

We're told that medicine is a science, but it is not. It fails nearly every test of science, as it lacks the freedom to explore the unknown. The only reason medicine makes progress is its connection to medical research and a "leakage" of creativity into an otherwise static field. This is heavily subject to hierarchical control. In the area of institutional control, your health is a political issue that's seen in terms of power, money, profit, and the advantage of others.

Teaching Myself

You can't presume healing is automatic. You have to learn how to heal, and each illness is different. One of the first lessons is being discerning about what advice to follow. In many cases, especially in the most dynamic of issues with the most conflicting of interests, the most obvious voices provide the worst information. Here, the whole of mainstream media should be avoided. There are no "fact checkers" because the facts are suppressed from public view.

There are facts that can be found in the original sources. Learning to read the research is difficult for people not trained in it. Learning the facts for yourself is the only way you'll become informed.

I've been following the science of Covid-19 for two years, since I contracted what I believed to be Covid-19 in March 2020. Some of the science has progressed from theory to experiment, but most conjectures that we hear are based on observation alone. Lacking a coherent story, the institutional narrative confuses, misleads, and causes harm in many more cases than is being recognized (Finley 2023).

It is statistically difficult to reach valid conclusions based solely on data, no matter how large the data sample is. It's for this reason that statistical techniques are used, such as randomizing and testing different groups within a population. It's essential that you know the size and independence of the populations used in any test. It's essential that you understand the basic statistics used in forming a conclusion. You must learn basic statistics if you are to rely on the conclusions that are extracted from statistics.

Using basic analysis and applying discretion will increase your trust in experimental answers, but these "conclusions" are entirely different from the theoretical explanations that are being tested. Explanations are theories. Observations can suggest theories, but you cannot reuse the observations that suggested an idea to substantiate it later. When someone tells you that such-and-such is the case because they saw it, this is nothing more than an idea.

S1 – How Wise is the Body?

I watched Stew Peters interview a doctor who claimed that the mRNA vaccine was causing visible deformations of red blood cells (https://www.bitchute.com/video/XLatr8YZkrYt/). The doctor presented a photo showing the claimed difference between healthy unvaccinated blood and unhealthy vaccinated blood. There was no experiment, no theory, no statistics, no control, and no data.

Both were aghast at the purported damage the vaccine was doing but, with no data, the photos mean nothing. These were supposedly intelligent people, though Stew Peters admitted he was a college dropout. The doctor—if she even was a doctor—had nothing to do with the research. She was not involved with creating the photographs and could not provide any verification of them.

Most doctors make poor scientists and, when outside of their clinical experience or scientific training, should be ignored. Lacking confirmation, most journalism should be ignored as a matter of course.

The public health directives have changed little since the beginning of the pandemic. They started out untested and uninformed and are still uninformed. Some theories are being tested, but the new knowledge is unreported, censored, or disparaged. As a result, public health recommendations have little relation to personal or public health. Some public health directives are dangerous.

Government-suggested protocols are not limited to scientifically tested, clinically consistent observations. Most doctors I've spoken to are reluctant to say what they know or what information they're using. This violates trust and undermines the medical system. Some organizations are following clinical protocols, such as those put forward by the FLCCC (2023).

Breathing

My problem appears to be one of poor pulmonary function. I was discharged from the hospital with an unlimited supply of supplementary oxygen, but without support or direction. Friends in healthcare have forwarded me useful directives on pulmonary recovery (Jin et al. 2021; Nici et al. 2006). The first is a professional paper published by the American Thoracic Association, and the second is from Johns Hopkins University and specifically addresses respiratory distress in recovering Covid-19 patients.

> "Anyone can benefit from deep breathing techniques, but they play an especially important role in the COVID-19 recovery process."
> — from *Coronavirus Recovery: Breathing Exercises*, (Lien 2021)

Both publications endorse the idea that one has to take some initiative in order to regain function. There are exercises and a routine one should follow. Breathing is under your voluntary control, so you need to exert voluntary effort to regain control after it's been lost.

Everything your body does affects your awareness, and anything you're aware of has some effect on your body. This is the basis for both sound judgment and medical hypnosis. Your mind and body collaborate to function at their best. This doesn't mean you have complete intentional control, but it does mean your mind plays an essential role.

Stomach and chest muscles are essential for proper breathing. My diaphragm plays an essential role, as does the movement of my viscera. My lung's tissues both absorb oxygen and release carbon dioxide. My heart should synchronize with my breath. This synchrony is almost under voluntary control.

The trauma of illness and treatment caused parts of my body to forget how to breathe. My chest muscles and my diaphragm lost coordination. My diaphragm behaved erratically, reacting to trauma by seizing.

We can feel some of these things, and those that we cannot feel we can imagine. Using imagination has a direct and immediate effect on muscles. You can relax, release, and engage muscles using your imagination even if you don't have voluntary control over those muscles. It's been found that imagining movement triggers the same areas in the brain as performing those movements.

You can test this for yourself, as you perhaps already have. By imagining the contractions of your large intestines, you can activate your large intestines and feel the urgent need to defecate. You do this using your imagination.

I need to retrain my diaphragm, my ribs, back, and stomach. Instead of taking short, raspy breaths—as I did when my lungs were in distress—I need to return to smooth breathing that is more forceful on the inhale and relaxed on the exhale. My lungs cannot perform correctly if my muscles do not support them.

Having this direct experience, the experience of needing to coordinate voluntary and involuntary processes, has provided me with greater insight into how hypnosis provides benefits to medical conditions. It suggests that by imagining what your body is not doing and imagining that you can do these things, you can regain coordination.

I suspect something similar to this plays a role in healing other systems in the body. I suspect all of one's systems, and all our diseases, are affected by our imagination.

Hypnosis

There are examples of pain being remediated through focused relaxation. There are many examples of our autonomic systems being dramatically affected by the use of hypnosis (Ewin and Eimer 2006). I suspect all chronic conditions can be improved through the use of focused attention and imagination.

Hypnosis takes this to another level. In hypnosis, you seem to be in a deeper connection with your autonomic functions. We've heard stories of people healing themselves with prayer or meditation. I know of one therapist who cured her advanced cancer using self-hypnosis, and another who did the same using variations of it.

Recovering from Covid confirms for me the role of focused intention in healing illness. Consider for yourself how you try to "feel better" when you're ill. You try not to imagine yourself getting sicker but getting better. How much more effective would you be if you had a deeper connection between your imagination and your disabled body?

References

Delbressine, J. M., Machado, F. V. C., Goërtz, Y. M. J., et al. (2021 Jun). "The Impact of Post-COVID-19 Syndrome on Self-Reported Physical Activity." *International Journal of Environmental Research and Public Health, 18* (11): 6017. https://doi.org/10.3390/ijerph18116017

Ewin, D. M. & Eimer, B. N. (2006). *Ideomotor Signals for Rapid Hypnoanalysis: A How-To*

Manual. Charles C. Thomas Publishing.

Finley, A. (2023 May 12). "Officials Neglect Covid Vaccines' Side Effects." *Wall Street Journal.*

FLCCC (2023). Prevention Protocols, *FLCCC Alliance*. https://covid19criticalcare.com/covid-19-protocols/

Jin, L., An, W., Li, Z., Jiang, L., & Chen, C. (2021). "Pulmonary rehabilitation training for improving pulmonary function and exercise tolerance in patients with stable chronic obstructive pulmonary disease." *American Journal of Translational Research, 2021, 13* (7): 8330-36.

Lien, P. (2021 May 11). "Coronavirus Recovery: Breathing Exercises." *Johns Hopkins Medicine*. https://www.hopkinsmedicine.org/health/conditions-and-diseases/coronavirus/coronavirus-recovery-breathing-exercises

Nici, L., Donner, C., Wouters, E., Zuwallack, R., Ambrosino, N., & Bourbeau, J. (2066). American Thoracic Society/European Respiratory Society Statement on Pulmonary Rehabilitation, *American Journal of Respiratory and Critical Care Medicine, 173*: 1390–413. https://doi.org/10.1164/rccm.200508-1211ST

S2 – Cultivating Mind–Body Health

May 12, 2019

Don't wish it were easier—let it make you stronger.

"Brute animals are the most healthy, and they are exposed to all weather, and of men, those are the healthiest who are the most exposed." — **Thomas Jefferson**

Compliance

In medicine, compliance refers to a client's willingness to follow the treatment program. For mind-body healing, "the program" is the connection between mind and body, and compliance refers to a person's willingness to build that connection. The word sounds authoritarian, like "law-abiding," but it means little more than a willingness to work toward progress despite difficulty. In hypnotherapy, everything rests on the force of mind, and here compliance is essential.

There are three programs: my program, your program, and the program—if one exists—that the mind-body needs. We'd like there to be a fourth program: the program that heals, but that is an abstraction that often cannot be "program-atized," and so remains a higher goal. We could imagine many more programs, but these are the big three. Great things can happen when these three are in alliance.

There is a certain skill of intuiting this alliance before any treatment begins, and I would say success depends on whether these three programs are aligned from the start. Let's talk about them.

My Program

Hypnotherapy falls into two broad categories: the "tell them what to think" approach and the "enable them to think for themselves" approach. Let's call these the prescriptive approach and the proactive approach. For the life of me, I can't understand why anyone would want to be told what to think, but, in most walks of life, that is exactly what people want: they want a prescribed solution. The way I understand this is to say that people try their best, and, when

16

that is not enough, they seek direction and advice.

Why do so many people feel that they have done their best, and their best is not enough? Why do people so often give up before they start? When this is bred into us, we are disabled; and it is bred into us, and it is the primary aspect of our disabilities. It is the lack of faith in ourselves—nature, God, or something that should be available to us—that is our most common obstacle.

Now, I'm sounding religious, and that takes me outside of most people's program, yet this is essential: we are not independent entities and our health is not something that resides alone in our separate selves. The faith that's lacking is a faith in one's ability to see beyond and to grow beyond appearances. It is the faith to exceed what we've been taught. This lack of faith turns the dynamos of modern civilization by keeping people within the institutions they depend on. It underlies our inability to maintain balance and heal ourselves from imbalance.

My program has two parts, and it is prescriptive at the start. Wherever we begin, we are at the start. I am telling you where I'm coming from, and that I work to open your power. If that resonates with you, then our programs may succeed. I aim to establish this compliance before we begin.

Once we agree that enhancing your power is our aim, I become proactive. I play the role of ears and eyes in the territory where your power has been misplaced, and this is a vast landscape. Two minds are better than one, but they are hardly enough. This is a psychosomatic world of history, ancestry, culture, memory, intuition, intellect, and emotion. Your power is anywhere and everywhere.

Our intellects travel in straight lines: from A to B, from cause to effect, from past to future. I'm perfectly happy using logic in physics and mathematics, but the psychosomatic world is not connected in this way. To find your power, you must get beyond your intellect. You can do this using expansive hypnotherapy or some version of it. All mind-expanding tools are some kind of hypnosis.

Your Program

Do you have a program? I can ask you flat out, and you'll answer by going off on some tangent, or so it might appear. In the realm of mind-body, nothing is just as it appears. To use a detective analogy, everything is a clue, and your "program" may not look like what you or I think a program should look like.

It would be nice if your program had simple steps that could be followed, but more likely your program is what you're already doing, full of twists and turns, certitudes and uncertainties, health and illness, jackpots and terrible investments. It's best if you are honest, but you don't have to be as long as you are authentic. Actually, it's better to see your dishonesty than it is to avoid it. The psychosomatic world is not linearly connected.

You could have a clear and focused program. We're taught to like clear programs because they "make sense" and, when they do, we can better assess the risks and rewards. This is why we have a plethora of practitioners selling programs which, like the commodities that they are, come with an assortment of features at a variety of prices. All of these programs depend on your body's ability to heal itself.

When you tell me about the steps in your program, I listen, but I don't entirely believe. There are levels to who we are, and our different levels have different programs. You might say our levels are our programs, though we prefer to hold ourselves separate from them.

I don't entirely believe what you claim is your program because your full program is the entire landscape of your power and disability. You can't describe this because it's not describable. Yet, I've asked you for a description, so, right there, we're positioned to take off into the realm of what can't be said.

People come to me who are stuck in life and confused about their future. They ask me to explain what counseling can do for them. I give them the big picture: settling the past, organizing the present, and thinking deeply about the future. I tell them that building a big picture helps people and that deeper issues inevitably come up. Most times, these people never call again.

I believe these people don't want to change or improve, though they will say that they do.

They're actually in the descending trajectory of chaos that feels natural to them. They will continue heading down until they connect with the motivation of their deeper issues. Until clarity emerges as a crisis. Think of your intellectual understanding of yourself not as a map of the territory, but as the door out of the first container of it. I listen to your program not to help you follow it, but to help you get beyond it. This is perfectly fine and normal; it's a good way to approach all intellectual boxes. Don't take yourself too seriously because no matter how big you think you are, it's not big enough.

The Mind-Body Program

Your mind-body's program is your fate, destiny, work, and potential. It's hard to tame or draw a line around it, but it underlies everything. We work to restore, enhance, realize, and expand these things. This is our plan, our best-laid plan, but you never know what surprises lay in store. Humility is needed in all stages of any program.

There is the expression, "The universe will provide." I understand this to mean that when you're on the right track, things fit together. For example, when you're on the right track with a cross-word puzzle, everything gets easier. It's not that you don't have to do anything, it's rather that the more clues you decipher, the more are revealed. That is not to say the universe will deliver that to which you are entitled. It won't. What it says is that only when you're in synchrony can you hear the full melody of what's happening inside and around you. This makes sense and sounds logical, but it is not simple.

Are we in synchrony with our mind-body program? We can't be sure, but this question is essential because your progress requires the coordination of our programs. A good deal of our work aims to answer this question, because your mind-body's program is the master program. It is the only program that can prevail. All others must comply with it.

It can be a sad truth that your mind-body program is bigger than either of us. The expression, "The Lord works in strange ways," is the admission that we may never understand what you're here to do, which is what your mind-body program defines. This can also be a great truth, and I prefer to think of it that way: it's the path to uncovering one's potential.

You come to me—or any healthcare practitioner—with an ailment. My initial inclination is

19

not to fully believe you. You shouldn't entirely believe your story either. The situation is likely different from what you presume. From this "clue," which consists of your initial guess, we try to figure out how to achieve the best result. This is not really a medical task, and it may not be a healing or curing task either.

Your path through life is not straight. You don't need to be certain where this path started or where it ends, because neither your heritage nor your legacy are fully known. Your mind illuminates a part of it, like a flashlight through a dark wood. If you look with other senses beyond your eyes, you will see farther. That's what my work is all about: seeing farther. I'm just as curious as you are. In this project, we are partners.

Getting Specific

This has all been very general, and I'd like to get specific. However, you are anonymous and each person's path is different. More than that, where ailments are concerned, there is disempowerment and fear, and it's unethical to lead you into this territory and leave you there. So, I cannot get specific in that way. Instead, I'll try another way.

Often, when we get outside the box of our intellect, we find ourselves in no box at all. This can be disconcerting, strain our patience, and make us feel powerless and vulnerable. This is why we don't want to leave this box—this box of certainties surrounding the core of what we perceive to be our disability. Yet when we get outside the box, when we leave our preconceptions behind, it is a breakthrough. Breakthrough to what? Well, you don't know, and I can't tell you, but I can take you there.

"Leaving The World" is an audio induction that aims to take you into a space that is outside what you know. It's a simple task, really. It involves dropping all that is familiar in what you see and think while remaining alert and aware. You might compare it to an emptiness meditation, except in this journey, you are not looking inward, but outward.

Leaving The World (An Induction)

Leaving The World is a hypnotic induction. **DO NOT** listen to this recording while you're driving a car, operating machinery, or doing anything that requires your attention.

I want this to be a very fantastic piece, and I want you to appreciate all that you can do with your mind and all that you can evoke through imagery.

Begin by relaxing, finding a comfortable position, letting your head rest against a pillow, the head of a bed, a recliner, having your arms by your side, your feet up or on the floor, grounded, your weight comfortable. Breath normally with a certain ease and regularity, rhythmically. Slowly inhaling, pausing, and gently exhaling with no expenditure of energy.

Imagine on the inhale that you're sucking light up, like a wave, up through your feet, leg, chest, and torso, shoulders and into your head. And when you exhale, the light just radiates away, and with the next exhale a wave of light strokes up your skin, through your knees, hips, stomach, chest, shoulders, neck and head, and as you exhale, it radiates away.

Do this once more, bringing the light up and feeling it move past your skin. The sensation is heightened in those areas as it moves up to your head, and as you exhale, everything just dissipates, like heat from your body. Now close your eyes and follow this exercise.

I'd like you to look up to the top of your vision and then rotate your eyes to the bottom. Rotate up to the top.... And then down to the bottom. Now this time when you rotate, rotate as high as you can an imagine that you're looking straight up, straight up out of the top of your head, and hold it up there, and then imagine that you're looking all the way back, out of the back of your head, over the top, looking back, just imagining that you've rotated your eyes to look out the back your head. And then look down, looking down your back, and you can imagine what it looks like looking down your neck, and then looking forward under your chin, back to the point of your lowest vision moving back up to the horizon to look straight forward again.

And then move your eyes all the way to the left, back to the center, all the way to the right, back to the center. And now when you move them all the way to the left, hold them there and imagine that you're looking right out past your left ear, and you're looking beyond your left ear and you're looking beyond and behind your left ear until you're looking all the way out the back or your head having rotated your eyeballs all the way around until you can imagine looking straight out the back of your head, and then moving still further to look out the right side, behind your right ear, having rotated perpendicular, looking straight out from your right ear, and moving forward to come back to the horizon, looking straight forward.

If you practice this, you'll find it's a kind of imaginary creation. And it feels funny because if you actually do practice it, it feels like you're rotating your eyeballs 360-degrees in their sockets.

Now I'd like you to use this kind of imagination, that kind of whimsical imagination to imagine that you're walking down a wooded slope to the beach, and we've all walked to the beach, sometimes over sand dunes, sometimes over wooded glades, and this time you're walking down a set of wooden stairs, through the beach dune, down to the sand. As you step down the stairs, 5, 4, 3, 2, 1, down onto the beach, you can imagine what it looks like, clouds scudding across the horizon, sea air, the smell of the beach, the smell of the salt, and you can walk straight forward, down the compressed sand to where the surf is, and then the sand becomes heavy and you can feel your impressions hold as you move your feet beyond until you reach the water, and you walk straight into the water, and we all remember the feeling of first touching the water as it burbles around our ankles.

But in this case, in this imagination, you walk out and you don't sink into the water, but you don't go any further than your ankles and you continue to walk out into the ocean, as if you were walking on something firm, but now you are walking out beyond the surf, and as you keep walking and the waves are gentle, and the horizon envelops you, until there's nothing in front of you or around you but the ocean, and you keep waking.

And you take a breath and you relax and you feel that there is a depression in front of you, something like a stairway, and it's a stairway in the ocean, and there's a hole in the ocean, and the stairway leads down into the dark blue, and you walk down it, 1, 2, 3, 4, until your eyes move down below the height of the ocean, and you're still walking down, 5, 6, 7, until you're surrounded by blue, and now you can't tell whether you're walking in water or air because the temperature on your skin is completely neutral, and you look around and everything is blue.

In front of you, you see a doorway, a doorway kind of hanging in the water or the air, and the doorway has a handle and you reach for it and you lower it like a lever and you pull the door open and it's not blue anymore, it's black, there is blackness through the door and it's a rich and velvety blackness, a sparkling blackness like night air.

And you walk through this door and you find yourself floating. You can move forward, but there's no sense of ground under you, and you're surrounded by a deep and endless blackness. Move forward through this. As you move, it's difficult to tell where you are and it's difficult to tell whether you're moving any more. Take a breath and relax and fill your imagination with emptiness. Boundless, infinite emptiness, and you feel yourself leaning into it, and moving through it.

I'd like you to imagine that this would be the world you would enter when you moved out of life. When you were in a space that was completely in another world, whether it was inside you or outside, it would at first seem empty and featureless. It would have nothing, and you would feel as if you were nothing. And I ask you to immerse yourself in that feeling, so that you don't have to not think because there's nothing of you to think. And be patient and be calm and imagine that you have transformed out of yourself and out of your world and into some intermediate place, foreign, empty, quiet, and boundless.

And I'll ask you only to orient yourself to up and down and front and back and to get a feeling through some internal sensation of passage, and in front of you conjure, or evoke, a sense of presences in the distance, presences that are spirits, senses of yourself, disconnected from history or obligation with no need to make appearances or have appearances, and there may be several or there may be one, and you feel them or you sense them, and you bring them closer to yourself through your own motion or your attraction of them, until you feel them around you.

And let this sensation have a kind of color, a kind of black-light luminescence which surrounds you like a membrane or a cloud, and although it doesn't speak, it doesn't think thoughts; it conveys its awareness through emotion. It has a mood, and it imbues you with a mood. And it's the mood of joy and the mood of friendship and health. And let that feeling completely define you, so that without thoughts, all you have is a happy, joyful mood.

Now let yourself rise up, out of that environment as if you were a bubble that formed on the bottom of the sea and now it's broken loose and begins to rise, and as you rise, you flatten and you break into little bulblets shaped like a jellyfish now rising moving silvery and as you get closer, a light dawns and it's the bluish-green of seawater, until it's thin enough for you to see the reflections on the underside of the waves, and you break through the surface and then you lift as if you were a cloud forming in the sky, and you float over the land.

And then you settle, and as you settle like cool air, and a body appears, and it has legs and arms and eyes, and it is you and you are walking, you are walking up the beach, and you are walking up the stairs, and you are walking back to the room, and you are walking to sit down, or lie down, or recline in whatever position you are in, and things come together like iron filings to a magnet until the world has reassembled, and you are whole again, and you are still, joyful, and contented.

Leaving The World is a hypnotic induction — **DO NOT** listen to it while driving a car, operating machinery, or doing anything that requires your attention.

Listen to a streaming MP3 audio reading of *Leaving The World*:
https://www.mindstrengthbalance.com/mindwp/wp-content/uploads/2019/05/Leaving-the-World.mp3

S3 – You Are the Echo of Memories You've Forgotten

March 29, 2023

Your memory is not about who you were, it's about who you can be now.

"You can't depend on your eyes when your imagination is out of focus."
— **Mark Twain**

Memories differ from associations. Memories are snapshots and associations are the connections between them. Most of our memories are combinations of both that trigger each other and extend in various directions to the limits of our shallow interests and abilities.

A continuous memory, something like a video, is a series of memories sequential in time. No memories are as continuous as a film or audio. Our memories are more like a quilt of patches connected in more than three dimensions.

If your memories were presented to you as you actually experienced them, it would drive you crazy. You wouldn't know what is real from what was real. We accept the twisted spaghetti of our memories in the same way that we accept the fantasies of our dreams.

We remember aspects of events, bits of pictures, elements of meaning, and implications. I remember few sounds and those that I can remember are more like words with feelings, not audible sentences. I remember feelings associated with circumstances.

My smartphone takes still pictures with half-second videos attached. This is how I remember most images, with a bit of motion, but only enough to orient my attention. I remember even the most emotional experiences as a series of short videos lasting only as long as the peak of my attention, which is less than a second.

These memories, taken by themselves, lack connections, and it's only the larger recollections—situations along with their associations—that trigger our thoughts and feelings. Associations bind the collage of thoughts and feelings into relevance. The lines of these collages craze outward like the fractures of a struck glass pane. Cameo tapestries and tree-like extensions—more like lightning than waves—fracture outward from a central event.

Memories are lightning storms, metaphorically and neurologically. Even the softer ideas that come during meditation are distant thunder. They are never like ocean waves, whose continuity, expanse, and even textures impress us. But beneath these memories are layers of textures, of which only the peaks and whirlpools catch our attention.

Without associations, memories are a random jumble. Lunatic collages; abstract mixtures of fear and longing disconnected from the tempo of waking life. Dreams are much more a reflection of our real selves than is our waking personality. Dreams follow pathways through emotional mountains that we're not willing to travel. You create the reality you imagine, and there are many things we won't dwell on because of what they trigger in us.

Your Personality Is Not In Motion, It's In Neutral

At this moment, your normal self is paying attention to me. This is not your full self, but you still act and react in ways that are typically you. You aren't aware of or remember anything outside the current moment until you're triggered by some direct or associated event. We gaze in our outward focus and graze on what's in front of us. We are illuminated when something catches our attention, and we are deer in the headlights. Thinking is largely an involuntary act.

Science offers useful exercises because its ideas purport to be logically connected. Like jigsaw puzzles, science offers a pallet of problems with missing pieces you can think about. Scientists are people who prefer well-phrased problems over the illogical problems of life. Scientists tend to have difficulty with life's normal problems, which is why you should be cautious when following their advice.

The attraction of logical puzzles is the illusion that we experience a logical world. That's a comfortable illusion, similar to what religion offers. "Spiritual bypassing" is the phrase used to describe the substitution of dogma for judgment, which results in a disabled-follower mentality.

Logical puzzles can offer intellectual bypassing, which results in a disabled-leader mentality. This happens when we accept other people's rules instead of crafting an understanding from our own experience.

People enjoy these exercises. Sometimes we indulge in them as games. At other times, we insist we have real insight, but these games are not constructed in the ways we construct ourselves. Logic often plays the wrong game.

Games allow us to evaluate our moves and find rewards at their conclusion. Life is not structured in this way. Our attraction to simple conflicts reflects our animal nature.

We chase contrived puzzles in the way that dogs chase cars, instinctively and with enthusiasm. In the 30,000 years we have been with dogs, we have become like them. We have learned to succumb to conditioning.

These recreations exercise our preconceptions and our inclination to put things in order, but otherwise serve no real purpose. I'm a firm believer in the fertility of chaos over predictability. Order is good when things stay the same, but repetition often teaches us to overlook what's new.

Your Potential Is Not Limited By Who You Are

Behind your wall of perceptions and presumed relationships lies a network of alternatives and revelations. Beneath the floor of your normal amnesia lies a labyrinth of unrecalled experiences and implications. It's what you don't remember that shapes your personality, like long-gone rivers that carved your disposition.

The little you remember comprises the small amount of leverage you have to recognize your feelings. Most of your emotional foundation is well below the waterline. When it comes to insight and inspiration, most of us are couch potatoes.

You may have heard the expression, "What fires together, wires together," which masquerades as an explanation of memory. When applied to human thought, this is little more than the tautology that habits are repeated behaviors.

What fires together is not what's wired together, it's simply what happens to be firing collectively or in sequence. Many things in the brain are happening as the result of other things, and the miracle of the brain is that they are not wiring together. The brain remains fluid and conditional. Patterns develop, but patterns are not mechanisms.

There are always alternatively wired pathways, they're just not used. Thought networks are not hard-wired; the mind is not defined by hardware, it's re-programmable. It's like the thruway exit that you always take. It's not hard-wired in your brain, it's just habit.

The learned neural structures seen in primitive animals are not causal. What appears because of conditioned learning are not "thoughts," they're reflexes. They are automatic, like the muscles that result from exercise.

Neural changes are not the cause of your memories, thoughts, and personality, they result from them. Changes in neural structure correspond to changes in behavior, but this is not thought. Classical conditioning is conjectured to explain memory, but it is only a small part of it. This is important: neural connections do not make thoughts they support thoughts. It's thoughts that make neural connections.

> "This analysis pertains to only relatively simple and short-term behavioral modifications, a similar approach may perhaps also be applied to more complex as well as longer lasting learning processes."
> — **Eric Kandel** (2000), neurophysiologist, referring to his observations of the nervous system of the sea slug Aplysia.

I see no evidence that thought patterns are rooted in slow-growing neural wiring. The emergence of new ideas and rapid changes in personality show memories and associations are not the result of neurons wiring together. You conceive of new ideas on a much larger scale and on much faster time-frames than neural structures grow.

You Are Not Aware of the Limits of Your Potential

To put it another way: all that you are aware of cannot describe the limits of your potential. As long as you limit yourself to what you're aware of—reactions, attitudes, preconceptions, reflexes, and reasonable certainties—you won't get beyond them.

If you think you can think your way to a greater understanding of yourself and others, using thought alone, you're fooling yourself. Thinking for greater understanding is great, but don't trust your conclusions.

All that is "in the box" is more of the box. There's a time and place for everything, and the time and place for reasonable thinking is understanding what you're limited to, not what you're capable of. The time and place for being a fool is when you're committed to change.

They say, "If you meet the Buddha on the road, kill him." This is a coded way of saying that you should eliminate all rational projections. And while you're at it, kill the projectionist as well. The projectionist is your view of yourself.

I don't mean kill your physical self; I mean kill your logical self. What's left is your emotional self. Your emotional self is both foundational, nonlinear, irrational, and the guiding force for who you can become.

When you meet your emotions on the road, embrace them. Intellect answers the question of how to continue without change. Emotion yields insights into questions that make little sense.

As a therapist, my clients struggle to learn and change. Their conflict is between what experience is telling them and how they understand it. If behavior was just a matter of firings and wirings, then people would not get so tangled up in conflict.

If you want to change, improve, or grow up at all, then thinking out of the box is somewhat of a deception. "The box" is all that can make sense, and as long as you resolve your situation sensibly, you are still in the box. To grow and change is to get out of the box, and the thought structures you find there will not make sense in that context.

New solutions require new people, which is why most existing people, along with the institutions they have created, generate nothing new. You can either wait for old thought forms to die—which usually requires the death of the people who support them—or you can create new ones. And the new ones will be unrelated to what you've learned and who you are.

Creativity, imagination, chaos, and reconnection; you don't need reason, but you do need emotion. Forget the goals, grasp the distinction between positive and negative.

Intuition is your guide at whatever level it has developed. Follow it and educate it. To gain control of your mind, pay attention to the silences between your thoughts.

References

Kandel, E. (2000). The Nobel Prize in physiology or medicine. Retrieved from: https://www.nobelprize.org/prizes/medicine/2000/kandel/biographical/

S4 – Origin of Chronic Illness and the Nonsense of Medical Hypnosis

December 25, 2018

The origin of chronic illness lies in the struggle with our emotions.

"Anger, hurt, emotional pain, and sadness generated in childhood will stay with you all your life because there is no such thing as time in the unconscious."
— **John Sarno**, MD

The conflict in ourselves is between the controlled person we have created ourselves to be and the emotional person who exists inside us. From this arises a disconnection with ourselves, a failure to sustain the health of disconnected parts, and the dysfunction of the organs, systems, and complexes related to them.

From this disconnection arises such somatic issues as immune, skeleton-muscular, gastric, circulatory, neurological, cardio, and pulmonary dysfunction. At the same time, there arise psychological issues of denial, depression, anxiety, anger, fear, violence, and mania. Left unresolved, these become chronic and develop into a rigid level of habit or addiction. An addiction is a coping strategy aimed at resolving underlying discomfort not otherwise addressed. Healing lies not in further denying our repressed feelings, but in embracing them.

> "Generally, people find it difficult to conceptualize the idea of unconscious rage. Some find it abhorrent, while others simply can't believe it can be there inside them without their knowledge. The idea that emotions—raw, heated, towering emotions—can exist outside of consciousness is hard to accept. Even when people intellectually acknowledge that these might exist, they find it hard to imagine them because they don't feel them. We live in the world of the conscious, and most of us think it is our only world. We acknowledge only what we are aware of, what we feel consciously."
> — **John Sarno**, MD (2007, 109)

Seeds of Illness

We unconsciously create the seeds of illness in our struggle to attain complete control over our past and orient ourselves to a socially fabricated future. Trends in illness move epidemically along social lines: heart disease, chronic fatigue, depression, cancer, and more recently, autism, attention deficit, obesity, and drug addiction. The prevalence of these disorders varies with class, culture, and community. These are not entirely physical and not entirely mental. They are both. They are psychosomatic.

Illnesses are not entirely individual in their cause. They are not aspects of a "germ theory," in which one's physical defenses have been breached. Not only do we have our weaknesses, but our health also exists at social, genetic, and historical levels. Many of our diseases are not just dysfunctions of the individual; they live at the interface between what we authentically feel and what we force ourselves to be. They are socio-somatic. Addressing them symptom by symptom, and person by person, is ignorant at both the biological and social levels.

> "I had removed one symptom only to have its place taken by another."
> — **Sigmund Freud**

What I have said may seem unconventional—you won't hear it from mainstream health practitioners—but it's not speculative. The emotional foundations of health are affirmed by those who engage in the psychological and somatic aspects of client health, personal relationships, and social movements.

Adding another layer makes this more understandable: there is a parallel between machines and humans in that both can be seen as having aspects of hardware and software. The body is the hardware; the body is a given. One cannot live without the body, and with small exceptions, one cannot replace it.

The mind is the software. The mind has some preassigned elements, namely those necessary to keep the body going, but much of what we consider to be "us" is re-programmable. One might say that our identity is "loaded in" after our bodies have booted up. And just as in software, not everything that's loaded into us is benign, authentic, or welcome.

The Fabrication

There are lots of parallels we could play with here, but I want to focus on just one. What "one" thing do you think is most important? For me, it is this: that our identities are a complete fabrication. There is no reality to who you think you are. It is entirely of your construction, and it is entirely unnecessary in its details. At the same time, it is both difficult and requires much effort to reprogram you. And for this reason, the method by which you are reprogrammed is largely that of illness.

Our minds organically develop as a kind of guidance system. We are self-correcting, but only if we are aware, and our ability to self-correct is relative to the cost of making adjustments. And because the process of life is expensive, the costs of readjusting our personalities are high. If you compare us as individuals to how we present ourselves in society, you could say we operate under the tyranny of our egos. Our egos direct our socially appropriate behavior and dictate, for most of us, that we take short-term profits and live short-term lives. And what happens when our body's long-term requirements conflict with our mind's short-term goals? We become vulnerable, and we get ill.

It has become increasingly clear to me that resolving physical disease lies in readjustments of the mind. Not that a change of mind alone can fix disease, but that failing to change one's mind can be the key factor in sustaining disease. It's not a question of cause. It's not a question of whether the disease or the attitude came first. That question is not important, and may not even make sense.

The hardware, the software, and the environment all work together, operating on different scales of time, distance, energy, and reality. What may appear as a cause from one perspective may appear as a correlation from another. Is physical stress caused by a poor relationship, or is it the other way around? Is your health determined by what you eat, the bacteria in your mouth, or the flora in your gut? For the purpose of regaining balance, it doesn't matter. All are interdependent, and all must change. Different forces are required to instigate and sustain different changes.

The Healer

Western doctors don't like to admit it publicly, but their success owes more to the patient than it does to them. This might seem to empower the patient, but it is rarely seen that way. We patients are more interested in deflecting blame than accepting responsibility.

Such is how the ego works: it exists to protect itself, and the less it's responsible for, the better. That is one of the defining aspects of Western-style medicine: it deflects blame. In Western medicine, the doctor and the disease are partners. Onto them, we project our dysfunctional selves, both the good and the bad. We let them fix us, even though they really can't. We insist they make it appear that the problem is external, and the fix requires no readjustment to ourselves.

When it comes to psychotherapy, the only people who change are those who decide to change. Western psychotherapy's false claim of authority is why it often cannot achieve a lasting effect. All external efforts at change fail until a person accepts responsibility, regains authority, and changes her or himself.

I bristle at analytical methods and prescriptions, which is what I find in most of psychology. The root of sustainable change is emotional, not analytical, and certainly not pharmaceutical. This is because the root of your identity is emotional. The analytical part of you, your self-obsessed ego, is the entirely fabricated, self-controlling aspect of your software.

I accept my identity as a hypnotherapist because hypnotherapists are undefined and unconstrained. Historically, I feel myself closer to a sage or a bush doctor, but those labels are misunderstood. Hypnotherapy, as I practice it, is almost entirely somato-emotional. It is not limited by what makes sense or can be sensed by anyone except my client.

When I develop rapport and elicit compliance, my work is tremendously effective. Without those two elements, it is not at all effective. That success lies in the compatibility of my mental software with that of my clients. I achieve this by presenting myself authentically and, in doing so, challenge my client to do the same. It is a challenge most prospects decline, and that is just as well.

We all have egos, we all talk and analyze, and all this a fiction. Or rather, you might say, it's just advertising. It is the self we have erected, which we protect, and which is giving someone grief. The path to healing, if there is a path to healing, lies beyond the ego, talk, and analysis. For me, that means going beyond data, diagnosis, evidence, and model. It means going to, and finally embracing, the emotion. I believe that is the shortest, cheapest, and only-est path to change.

References

Sarno, J. (2007). The *divided mind: The epidemic of mindbody disorders*, HarperColins.

S5 – How the Placebo Effect Implies Learning, and Learning is Hypnotic

August 17, 2022

Chronic illness involves forms of mental dysregulation to which we are attached.

"Our client's problem is that they have lost rapport with their unconscious mind. Our job is to help restore that relationship."
— **Milton Erickson**, psychiatrist and hypnotherapist

The Mind-Body

Besides thinking, your brain directs your awareness, collects information from your body, and synchronizes basic functions. Hormones produced in association with your brain manage your daily metabolic rhythms, attention, and arousal.

Even though your nervous system extends throughout your body, it's not clear how involved your brain is with your body's many functions. Many of your muscles operate autonomically, such as your heart, lungs, and circulatory system. Aspects of your intentional muscular control are handled by your cerebellum, a component of your lower brain, but there remain aspects of movement that are unconsciously linked to hearing, sight, balance, and orientation.

The mind and body affect each other at many levels. There is no single way to describe this structure. Control is a combination of hierarchical, serial, and parallel connections. To a large degree, organs of your body perform their regulation, communicate with your brain, and affect your mind on unconscious levels. Their operations rarely come to your conscious awareness, and when they do, their effects can be both direct, through pain or pleasure, or indirect, through moods and metabolic adjustments. This much we can agree on.

There are aspects of our body's functions that appear in our consciousness, and there are aspects of our consciousness that affect our body's function. No one should be surprised that this happens at a superficial level of concern, perception, and intention. We are all concerned about our health and take action to maintain and protect it.

Just as we have physical or mental dysfunctions, we also have psychosomatic dysfunctions. There are mind-body connections that can improve or degrade. These holistic mind-body connections—our mind's regulation of bodily function and the body's ability to direct our minds—lie outside of psychology and somatic medicine. These connections between mind and body are not cognitive or intentional but have connections to both. They can enhance or impede health and function.

Unconscious behaviors elude your awareness by being rooted in reflex and habit. Some of these behaviors you may have learned, and others may be intrinsic or instinctive, such as needing to sleep or eat. They may be good habits, bad habits, or simply familiar patterns.

Justifying What's Unhealthy

Unhealthy behaviors can be rooted in memories and associations. You are not conscious of many of these, at least not immediately conscious of them. They are thought patterns that developed under different circumstances which you no longer fully remember and may no longer make sense to you. Dreams reveal the kinds of associations our minds can make when unfettered, psychedelics can similarly unleash our minds, but the conscious mind is rarely creative to this degree.

Our conscious mind always justifies itself to itself. Our justifications, which only appear when we question ourselves, help us be accurate and consistent, but we do not require them to reflect high certainty. We don't make a federal case out of every decision, we usually shoot from the hip. When we are completely confused, we look to others for guidance.

Allopathic medicine offers to take over responsibility, redirect our environment, and re-pattern our behavior. We must surrender to it, and the doctor takes responsibility. Medicine prescribes new patterns for better health that include changes in our diet, environment, chemistry, and behavior. Prescriptive psychotherapy, following this model, suggests better ways to think and address situations. The goal is to enlist your full compliance in adopting healthy patterns of thought, behavior, and function.

But there are areas below consciousness that not only contribute to your behavior, but determine it, and sometimes these subconscious patterns conflict with your better psychosomatic judgment. You may want to eat less, but you may be unable to. It is these areas that we address with medical hypnosis.

Placebo

A common image of the placebo effect is an action that appears to work, but either doesn't work or only works superficially. The concept is mechanical. It presumes that a remedy works on you, not with you, and that it either repairs a mechanical error or does not.

This is a false, mechanical view of medicine. In reality, many paths connect cause and effect, and virtually none of the body's mechanisms are understood well enough to trace all causes to all their effects. Even saying something as simple as "an analgesic relieves pain" is full of caveats and presumptions.

To gain a better understanding of cause and effect in medicine, break the action into a cause, perception, and result: what's being done, what we feel is being done, and the result of what's been done. We would like to know if we can rely on these occurring together, even if we don't understand how one connects to the other.

An action can be considered a placebo when we do not see, or current theory does not predict, a connection between it and what results. In the mechanical view, we're only interested in the action and the result. The mechanical view considers perception to be irrelevant, and most medical theories exclude awareness as playing any role in connecting an action with its effect.

By considering the trio of cause, perception, and effect, we can better clarify placebo action. Consider these cases:

- The action has a plausible effect. There may or may not be any perception of the action, and a result is seen.
- The action has no plausible effect, but the action is felt, and a result is seen.

The first case is not considered to be a placebo effect because the effect exert a "real" influence. In the second case, the cause is considered a placebo because it's implausible that the effect caused the result.

With a placebo, we might dismiss the effect as an illusion, but we should be cautious. The effect we're looking for might be a skill that requires learning and practice. The beneficial result might become stronger if the actions are repeated and one's intentional role is learned.

We might call any skill a placebo since we don't know the mechanics of learning. For example, none of the initial actions of walking, swimming, or relaxing generate immediate or initially enduring results. They all take practice, require perception, and develop in ways we never fully understand. Once we learn to master and control these actions, their effects become obvious, and the results are enduring.

If we take an ineffectual pill, learn mindfulness, and cure our depression, we might say the pill was a placebo and mindfulness was the real thing that had the verified effect. However, clinical trials show that most antidepressants have no more effect than dummy pills with no chemical activity, yet antidepressants continue to be given credit for resolving depression. Many clients insist their pills are effective and depend on them.

Hypnosis

We can learn to control important aspects of our physiology by managing anxiety, fear, stress, and depression. In addition, our subconscious minds can control blood flow to selective tissues, the ratio of different antibodies in our immune system, our circulation, metabolism, hormone levels, and potentially much more.

We don't know how our subconscious mind accomplishes these feats, but we have found through hypnosis that the mind can enhance and enable these effects. What we don't know, and might never know, is how much conscious control we can learn in those subconscious areas where we can have an effect.

These should be considered skills since not everyone has them and, like skills, their development requires attention and practice. Not everyone is equally adept, open to this kind of learning, or the goals of it.

Would you want to learn to control your circulation if your life depended on it? Probably yes, if the effort recovered your health, but probably not if it wasn't necessary. Quoting

Voltaire or Spider-man, depending on who you read, "With great power comes great responsibility."

We're better at acquiring power than upholding responsibility. This is the source of many people's ambivalence to learning to control themselves; they would rather take a pill and be done with it.

Learning

A broad definition of hypnosis identifies it as anything that engages the subconscious or unconscious aspects of our minds. All learning is a hypnotic experience. This would include learning to ride a bicycle, paint a picture, learn a language, control your brain, or manage your emotions.

Hypnosis can be considered a placebo effect in the same way that learning any skill involves initially ineffective mechanisms that are made effective through perception, interaction, and application. Most times, and perhaps for most people, these skills come naturally without therapy, teaching, or distress. Some people lack the self-regulatory skills needed for learning, and these people are liable to suffer a range of distresses and diseases because of it. However, even those of us who can learn will not learn if we're discouraged from trying.

The biggest mystery of hypnosis is not that it works or what it can do, although learning through induction is mysterious. The biggest mystery is why those people who need these skills resist learning them. Is the prospect of creating a new reality so frightening that our clients don't want to try, or are they frightened that they might succeed?

I have found that chronically ill clients do not have the self-regulatory skills that hypnosis requires. They reject the suggestion that they could learn these skills, and they resist the learning opportunities offered to them. For these people whose illness involves a lack of self-regulation, allopathic medicine promises an escape from needing to self-regulate.

For certain chronic disabilities, this promise is an illusion. For most disabilities, improving one's skill at self-regulation is beneficial. It could easily be life-changing.

S6 – Attachment, Resistance, and Secondary Gain

August 2, 2022

Chronic illness can be improved by a program of mind–body learning.

"To a very large extent, men and women are a product of how they define themselves."
— **Jeremy W. Hayward**, senior teacher of Shambhala Buddhism

Awareness

We have both conscious and unconscious awareness. Conscious awareness works with our reasons and intentions. Our conscious perceptions are those we recognize and remember. We direct conscious awareness like a spotlight.

Our unconscious awareness moves on a separate track and has a form of intentionality that feels different in the rare instances when we're conscious of its effect, but we rarely are. Seen as "the silent observer" our unconscious awareness is said to monitor and express our deeply felt and less readily expressed identity.

It's our unconscious awareness that tells us we're being looked at from a direction in which we have not looked. We are only unconsciously aware of many things. We can become more consciously aware if we pay attention to small signals, and we will gain greater control of many things if we do.

Our unconscious awareness reflects our values, sense of place, and sense of self. Rooted in our memories and associations, it is not directed by and does not answer to our intellect. Unconscious awareness is not intellectual, not immediately perceptible, and not strongly emotional, but it taps into these under various conditions.

Ideas come into consciousness in the same way that you might think you're being watched, or be inclined to be curious, or perceive a strain in your neck. If you focus on, follow, and explore any of these indications, then you'll find more ideas waiting for you. One might say that the conscious emergence of unconscious awareness is pragmatically spiritual in the sense that it's more fundamental than perception and more substantial than a concept.

Most of our thoughts originate in our unconscious awareness. We can't see how they form, but it's likely a combination of stimulation, associations, and emotions. The product of these is an idea that emerges fully formed in our conscious awareness. Such an idea might express itself to us as a statement, such as, "This feels right," "I am reluctant," or "That makes sense."

Since our unconscious awareness cannot be isolated or analyzed, we cannot be sure of its extent. We don't know if it's tied to our bodily systems or if it's separate from them. It's possible that unconscious awareness is partly cognitive and partly somatic. That it's partly in our heads and partly in our bodies as extensions of our nervous, endocrine, cardiovascular, hepatic, lymphatic, and digestive systems.

Our latent fears, hungers, hesitance, and excitements arise from our unconscious awareness. The connection between our two forms of awareness can be loose. We may feel drawn to or repelled by some circumstances without being aware of the reason. It can take anywhere from minutes to months for clarity to emerge.

Behavioral Medicine

There is a vaguely defined field called Behavioral Medicine which roughly refers to anything having to do with the behavior of people giving, receiving, or experiencing medical situations. It can refer to social, technical, or personal elements pertinent to wellness. Behavioral medicine is a field that has no real boundary.

Behavioral medicine is mechanistic. Practitioners of behavioral medicine have an allopathic, linear view of medicine as being mechanical rather than regulatory. It is always simpler to ignore what is not obvious, and this seems to be a general philosophy in medicine, but it's surprising to find this attitude in the psychosomatic realm, where the situation is not mechanical.

Mechanical conditions involve no thought or intention; regulatory conditions stem from both conscious and unconscious actions. Regulatory problems do not admit mechanical solutions.

Even mechanical issues, such as a broken bone, are rarely resolved by mechanical remediation alone.

Half of those practicing behavioral medicine are trained as psychotherapists. Current psychotherapy espouses a rational approach that does not recognize unconscious awareness. This is because of the failure of mistaking relationships for causes. Greater insight is apparent in neurology, where one is more able to see the absence of the links between the state of the body and the state of the mind.

Self-deception

> "The first principle is that you must not fool yourself, and you are the easiest person to fool."
> — **Richard P. Feynman**, physicist

When one's conscious and unconscious awarenesses are in conflict, conscious awareness becomes superficial and unconscious awareness goes into hiding. This is like a family conflict in which the family members cannot communicate, both because they don't speak and don't listen.

If aspects of oneself are repressed, one becomes neurotic, but if aspects of one's conflict manifest physically, one becomes ill. The psychological conflict is real, and the physiological consequences of it are also real. The result is a somatic illness with psychological elements.

These elements are not causes in the sense of coming before, they are factors in your self-regulation. The psychological dysregulation contributes to and sustains the illness, and together these create the symptoms.

The influence of your unconscious easily escapes your awareness. Your body's dysfunction cannot recognize the role of your mind, and your mind won't take responsibility for your body. To recover this awareness, you must overcome the obstacles of fear and self-deception and become more conscious of your body.

Think of this in the family metaphor. The failure of family communication results in a collapse of family integrity and the ill health of its members. Communication restores health, not because it results in an agreement, which would rarely come about, but because it results in an engagement. With engagement comes synchrony, and with synchrony comes balance.

In my role as a therapist, I insist my clients take an increasing role in solving their problems. This separates my clientele into two groups: those who accept a larger role and make progress, and those who refuse and fail. Those who succeed recognize the role of their psyche in framing their distress, while those who fail reject responsibility. It's these people, those who cannot resolve their psychological conflicts, who can manifest their psychological conflict as a physical sickness in their bodies.

Fear

> "When one is frightened of the truth, then it is never the whole truth that one has an inkling of."
> — **Ludwig Wittgenstein**, philosopher

I've had clients who presented chronic illness and who denied that their psyche played any part in it. In some cases, I agreed, and I worked to help them focus on finding strength, comfort, and healing. In other cases—most cases—I disagreed and felt their illnesses had psychological components.

These clients were frightened by the suggestion that their state of mind might be a cause of their condition. Our work to effect healing was quickly subverted by their rejection of responsibility. They could not admit they were doing this, as that would require them to recognize the role they were playing. Instead, they found trivial faults in our process, such as schedule conflicts, bungled billing protocol, or conflicting social attitudes.

To be clear, when these clients made progress and their psychological issues emerged or their physical problems were at risk of being healed, they fled from treatment. Their bodies needed healing, but their minds refused to allow it.

I cannot be certain of this, and it was rarely obvious, but I see the pattern. It occurs when I can both see healing begin on the physical level and witness rejection on the psychological level.

These clients were not trying to be offensive or contentious, but they were not honest either.

They justified their reasons to stop treatment on grounds that seemed marginally rational to them, but I could see their reasons were contrived. Evading responsibility is a recognized trait of psychosomatic clients.

Courage

> "Courage is not the absence of fear, but the mastery of it."
> — **Mark Twain**

You cannot argue courage into existence. If it's not there, then there is little you can do about it. Courage can be brought forward through a threat, enticement, or deception. In a functional sense, courage is commitment. Without commitment, whether you call it courage, you can't achieve anything. Healing always involves a measure of courage. Courage to address a negative life situation for which you're unprepared and without assured success.

To approach one's illness using mind control takes courage. It feels like you're going into battle naked. While your mind has more control over your body than we're led to believe, most people would rather not believe it. Most people would rather agree to the ministrations of those who are endorsed as competent in offering safety, then rely on themselves. We're taught to think this way. Making use of medical hypnosis requires us to think otherwise.

The stern approach to medical hypnosis insists clients make some commitment. An easy commitment is financial, and a simple means to ensure it is to ask clients to commit to multiple sessions of hypnotherapy soon after starting. If medical hypnosis were more widely understood and endorsed, people would be more comfortable with it. But both the goals and the means of the approach are poorly understood.

To counter the likelihood of a client abandoning therapy, the therapist can request payment for multiple sessions before starting a medical hypnosis program. Treatment is not piecemeal, and abandoning a program of treatment halfway through defeats the client's stated intention, achieves little, and furthers the misimpression that there is no mind-body connection.

I have not yet taken this hard-line approach, as my preference is to follow my client's direction. But medical conditions are different, and they represent a mind-body conflict in which it is the client's direction that is contributing to their condition and derailing their progress. A person may heal themselves, but it's not an intellectual process, and their intellectual decisions both to engage and continue in hypnotherapy cannot be relied upon. Medical hypnotherapy must present itself with more authority than hypnosis used in psychotherapy. Medical hypnotherapy focuses on an actual condition with the goal of an objective resolution. It does not lend itself to moving the goalposts.

To instill greater responsibility, the authoritative hypnotherapist gives his or her clients homework. This amounts to a program of action of the sort a person would naturally develop. However, it is just such a lack of natural inclinations that are typical of chronic conditions. Most likely, a person with a chronic medical condition is not taking care of themselves as best they could.

A hypnotherapist assigns homework to break the process of habit change into traceable steps. Homework could be regular relaxation, exercise, or disengagement from stress, listening to recorded audio material, journaling, dreaming, or reporting on certain issues. If clients don't complete these assignments, the program either halts at that point, focuses on the source of the resistance, or develops a new strategy.

This is the disciplinarian's approach: the client makes a financial commitment before their fear of healing arises. When and if this fear arises, choosing to flee from further sessions carries the prospect of a financial loss.

Ian Wickramasekera is both a therapist and researcher in behavioral medicine. He describes what he calls the Trojan Horse procedure for securing the compliance of a client experiencing a psychosomatic condition. He presents the client with authoritative evidence of the success of the treatment that does not raise the specter of their fears.

Being assured of a non-psychological program—falsely, as it turns out—the client has little reason not to comply. It is only after the client commits to a lesser goal, something less than a release of their attachment to their physical illness, that Wickramasekera approaches the psychological issues that play a role in maintaining their condition.

Support

The origin of the somatic illness is partly one of dysregulation based on conflict and fear. Addressing the dysregulation requires addressing the fear that's hidden in the body. This is what the client does not want to encounter. The somatic condition plays a collaborative role in keeping the fear hidden.

> "They are patients whose somatic complaints have been unresponsive to multiple, conventional chemical and/or surgical interventions. Often, the referrals are poorly made. Without rapid and effective patient reorientation by the behavioral medicine practitioner, these patients are unlikely to make or keep an appointment, or if they come in, to return after the first visit."
> — **Ian Wickramasekera** (1988, 135), psychologist

Wickramasekera works to shape "the patient's cognitions into an educational model of illness, as opposed to a biomedical model in which the patient is the passive recipient of treatments… Shifting to an educational model (requires the client to) disable secondary gain or the rewards of the 'sick role' and physical symptoms."

In most cases of somatic illness, we assume the client wants to recover. The client is quick to say they do. But with many psychosomatic conditions, this is not the whole story. The client may declare their desire to heal, but their symptoms run a mysteriously unresponsive course. There is no obvious benefit to being ill because the benefit lies in the absence of what can't be seen, and which the client is loath to consider.

Resolve

For most conditions, we aim for progressive improvement. Even with purely psychological problems, we expect symptoms to reduce to issues that can be addressed. This is not the case with some psychosomatic conditions because the symptoms are not caused by the problems, they are barriers that obscure them. When these barriers come down, the genuine problems come up.

> "The course of learning real control of symptoms is not a short, positively accelerating course for which there is a 'quick fix.' Rather, it is an uneven course, with gradual elevation interrupted by regression as physiological self-regulatory

competencies develop."
— **Ian Wickramasekera** (1988)

Conflicted clients who abandon treatment are not ready to face their disability. I don't know the reason, and it is unlikely my guesses would be welcome or helpful. This doesn't apply to all clients and all treatments, but is particular to treatments that require the client to take responsibility for their unconscious conflicts.

People must take responsibility, and I prefer they take it honestly. For a person to act without honesty sets them in opposition to the practitioner and themselves. If I hide behind a mask of authority—which many practitioners do—the scheme is a fraud.

> "The fourth and final component in the psycho-physiological role induction is directly and openly to investigate the psychosocial antecedents and consequences of the patient's symptoms. Now that the patient is no longer an imposter, he or she is out of the closet and is a psychotherapy candidate… At this fourth step, the patient's symptoms have typically shifted from predominantly somatic (pain, dizziness, etc.) to predominantly psychological complaints (e.g. phobias, anxiety, depression, etc.)."
> — **Ian Wickramasekera** (1988)

Caste in this light, psychosomatic illness sounds like a combination of Post Traumatic Stress and Dissociative Identity Disorder. Forcing a person into a realm of terror where their problems are clear may sound logical, but if they have already damaged their body to bury the issues, exposing their issues will only cause further damage. Their emergence must be organic and voluntary.

I suspect all illness has a psychosomatic component, and being at odds with oneself plays a role in all dysregulation. To resolve psychosomatic illness, the client must build a bridge across a chasm that only they can see.

There is good news and bad news. The bad news is that your doctors cannot cure your chronic illness and prolong your life. The good news is that you can. I suspect many cases of chronic illness can be improved or resolved entirely by a program of psychosomatic learning.

> "Unexpressed feelings come forth later in uglier ways. Psychosomatic illnesses often are the reincarnation of cumulative resentment, deep disappointment, and

disillusionment repressed by the Lose/Win mentality. Disproportionate rage or anger, overreaction to minor provocation, and cynicism are other embodiments of suppressed emotion. People who are constantly repressing, not transcending feelings toward a higher meaning, find that it affects the quality of their relationships."
— **Stephen Covey**, author of *The 7 Habits of Highly Effective People*

References

Wickramasekera, I. S. (1988). "Psychophysiological role induction or the Trojan Horse procedure, chapter 7." In *Clinical behavioral medicine, Some concepts and procedures*,143-54. Plenum Press.

S7 – Trauma and Healing

December 23, 2021

You cannot fully heal if you're in a disempowered state of mind.

"Healing involves discomfort, but so does refusing to heal. Over time, refusing to heal is always more painful." — **Resmaa Menakem,** psychotherapist

Trauma is a conscious component of injury and is an obstacle to healing. My days in Intensive Care, being unable to breathe effectively because of Covid-19, taught me something about trauma.

Healing is something you do yourself. When it happens naturally, we suffer, struggle, and prevail, and this becomes the foundation of our experience. Our bodies and our minds learn this is the healing process. The suffering motivates our struggle, and our struggle appears to us to be a definitive part of healing. We take credit for our recovery, even if we normally take little credit for anything else in our lives.

Struggle creates focus, and the struggle and the focus may be necessary components of healing. But the actual healing process, or the details of the process, may not depend on any of your willful actions. You don't heal because you are rested and warm. Healing forces you to rest and seek warmth. You are following your body's directions.

Your immune system, organ functions, and blood chemistry are self-correcting systems. Your struggle and focus may direct you in working with your body, but it's likely that your healing would proceed regardless, and force you to comply with it. What we think of as our choice, such as how to take care of ourselves, is really our mind responding to our body's command.

Resting, keeping warm, doing what seems to help are voluntary actions, but anyone who tries to ignore these signals and "get creative," such as attempting freezing therapy, will quickly be reminded of what their body wants them to do. But what happens when you follow your body's directions and it doesn't work?

Something different happens in your mind when your healing fails. When this happens, you are left feeling that you are not capable, powerful, or good enough to prevail. It's not enough to rest and sleep; it's not enough to focus, act, or know; ultimately, your being is insufficient and there is nothing you can do with any of your resources. You are insufficient. You do not have the power to prevail. Your inner self can be deeply injured by this. It is a deeply confusing experience that can cause you to panic or become numb.

Action

There is something about being able to act that creates faith in oneself. It is less important that you're successful or effective. What's important is that you have something to do and some way to do it.

At higher levels, we find support in family, community, and nature. Yet when this all seems to fail, we risk coming to the belief that either we are not good enough, or we have been abandoned. Our options are to freak out, fight, or collapse. It is at this point that we may become deeply frightened: we are slipping away and there is nothing we can do about it. We make choices all the time along these lines and, to some extent, we suffer small traumas.

We might put our faith in the healer. Until this point, the healer was a secondary, supporting character, but when everything you do fails, the healer becomes a transcendent figure, the person who will determine your survival. Here is where the prayers to God become fervent, or the appeals to the healer become desperate.

At this point you enter a mentally malleable state, your mind becomes neuroplastic and who you are may change. This is a critical, unstable point. If having faith in oneself is critical to healing, then being supported in one's faith in oneself is necessary.

The action that one needs to take need not be physical, although physical progress would be most welcome. One is looking to merge one's energy to a more unified sense of purpose. In this, support can be as important as progress.

Inaction

When I was in Intensive Care, I was isolated and alone. Without my cell phone and charger, I would have been traumatized much more. The hospital had no sense of me as a person, spirit, mind, or being. I was just numbers on a machine being managed by nurses and doctors who had brief contact with me, and who seemed to have no idea what to do with me. Under these conditions, most people die from lack of mental support.

I was having trouble breathing, but that's not what I remember. I remember holding on to survival. People were giving oxygen to my damaged lungs in order to see numbers read out on their machines. Numbers were the goal, not healing or supporting my ability to heal myself.

Is this the limit of allopathic medicine? Is this how most people are treated? Put into an antiseptic bubble and dosed with pharmaceuticals until they either prevail or succumb? I have a new disrespect for medicine!

> "We need to pay special attention to the breath because it is a very powerful and centrally important system. Somewhat like the flywheel in a car engine, the breath regulates all the other autonomic systems, including brain function."
> — **Peter Levine** (1997), psychotherapist, from *Waking The Tiger*

Recognition

We are told that the body heals itself when healing occurs. How does this happen?

We are led to believe that few of our executive decisions affect our physiology. I don't accept this, and I don't know how anyone could. I think there is a physiological consequence to almost everything we think, whether or not we take action.

When I was young, nothing happened unless I made it happen. Public education was a warehouse in which students and teachers spent their days empty of insight and useful experience. With every passing year, students' personalities became thinner and their output less interesting. The only valuable things were those things that people did themselves.

My teachers were flatulent personalities, repetitively expelling inert, digested material onto the food trays of imprisoned students who were expected to eat it. With few exceptions, teaching was just like any other job, and the result of it was as poorly formed and indigestible as any other cheap plastic product.

I believed what my parents believed, which is what other parents believed, which is what everyone seemed to believe. I grew up in an affluent neighborhood, but I knew a few less affluent kids and their parents seemed to believe the same things. In a fit of dissatisfaction, I spent a few months exploring private schools, but they all seemed to follow the same program.

It was at this point that my father woke to the recognition that I had a problem, and there was something he could do. My mother could not wake up, but my father took me under his wing and made me his photo assistant. On the shorter jobs, where the equipment was lighter, I flew with him to cities around the US to photograph colossal, empty office buildings either set amid tens of acres of magazine-perfect gardens, or monument-like intrusions into busy cityscapes.

This was a breath of fresh air. The environments may have been contrived and yet to be occupied—he was sent to photograph them before they were put into operation—but at least they were real investments in the future. And while these architectural subjects were not yet occupied or alive, I could explore new towns, cities, and forests, flying to places I'd never heard of and would never remember.

When I was 12, a 15-year-old friend returned from Outward Bound wilderness school and introduced me to the idea of exploration. Until that point, all I'd explored was shoplifting and vandalism. The shoplifting was mildly empowering, but the vandalism was pathetic. The problem was that I had no emotional support and I was angry.

I was taking steps beyond climbing trees. I was looking at my hands and wondering what they could accomplish. I was developing a sense of creativity. I distinctly remember returning to my high school after my first summer in the big western mountains. I put photos in the library. People looked at them unknowingly in the same way that the Indians in Florida looked at Columbus's boats as things not of their world.

Mallory answered the question of why he wanted to climb Mt. Everest by saying, "Because it's there." The real reason is because extreme experiences force us to realize ourselves.

Mountains become personal when we risk our lives in getting to know them.

Nature tests us in complex ways and rewards us with experiences we do not expect. It punishes us fairly and rewards us by simply by allowing us to pass into places that few, if anyone, ever see. This offer is made everywhere, in faraway mountains you've never heard of, or nearby ravines, swamps, and cliffs that only plants have explored.

Reaction

You must attend to your mind. Notice the speed of your thoughts and the rhythm of your attention. As my hospital stay progressed, I was aware of the gears of my mind disconnecting. I felt like an engine whose governor was malfunctioning. I had to engineer operations that would otherwise have been natural: eating trays of hospital food; navigating to the bathroom while connected to machines by tubes and wires. Attempting to stay warm.

I listened to Spotify music for the duration of the long nights. I tried Audible's spoken books, but they seemed so trite. When you're considering your mortality, who cares about some author's creative self-indulgence?

I listened to Robert Kiyosaki's *Rich Dad Poor Dad* until I could no longer stand the repetition of its one-sentence plot. I listened to Brené Brown's *The Gifts of Imperfection*, as she extolled inaction and indecision as virtuous vulnerability until it made me sick.

I listened to Merlin Sheldrake's *Entangled Life*, about the ecological and evolutionary role of fungi. I listened mostly because he is Rupert Sheldrake's son and a friend of mushroom evangelist Paul Stamets. Sheldrake's entire book was a description—not an explication or analysis—of how networks discover solutions without using reason. This is something worth considering, but Sheldrake stood before it, perplexed.

Recovery

One has to create a recovery frame of mind. This is a state of mind that capably manages your executive functions and even, if you're lucky, achieves greater insight. The hospital experience seems designed to undermine your awareness. You're told only to eat the food, shit in the potty, and generate the numbers. I would not be surprised if, in the future, they put everyone in an artificial coma. Once human nurses are replaced by robots, they probably will. Once they do that, most people will probably die. They'll blame it on some new disease.

Luckily, an induced coma was not my fate, though they threatened it under some perverted belief that the more fear and power they could take from me, the better off they would be. They presented the option plainly: let us intubate you if we feel it's necessary or we'll let you die. The Grim Reaper could not have said it better.

Where does the trauma occur? It occurs where your spirit weakens. It was the threat of intubation, the experience of being unable to breathe, and the sense that whatever was going to happen to me might be a corporate decision or a medical experiment.

Not only were the nurses and doctors unaware of what they were doing, but they didn't care. You are an animatronic entity that will either go out the front door in a wheelchair or the back door in a bag. In either case, they will remain doctors and nurses, manage the ward, report the numbers, and develop their careers.

Throughout my first night in the hospital, I could hear an angry person shouting. I felt their energies were counterproductive. But after spending more time in the hospital, I think anger may be the right response.

Untraumatizing

I was happy to take part in a survey of my experience conducted by hospital services after I was discharged. I told them that no one paid any attention to my becoming healed, and there was no recognition that I might need to play some role in it.

Trauma is your inability to put yourself right. If you can't do it, then no amount of well-behaving physiology is going to do it for you. There is a body-mind, and a well-body will support a well-mind. But there is also a defeated and disconnected mind, and an unwell mind will undermine your physical state. In fact, an unwell mind might kill you.

The survey questions rated the hospital's performance on a scale of one to five. They did not ask the right questions. There was no interest in healing because no one was responsible for it.

I put my comments as succinctly as possible at the end.

I was first referred to Mental Health Services, and then to the Office of Patient Quality Services. What I was looking for was the Office for Human Beings, but there was no such office. I considered contacting Patient Quality Services, but I felt I'd be wasting my time.

The fifth step in Peter Levine's nine-step prescription for remediating Post Traumatic Stress is replacing the mental construct of defeat and helplessness with one of balance and engagement. If you cannot do this, you're screwed. This is something you must do Post Trauma but also Pre-healing. You cannot heal if your mind remains in terror, powerless, and disengaged from your body.

It's clear to me that the allopathic model will kill you, and it will do that because there is no "you" in it. You must take an active role in your existence or you will not exist. This is the ultimate "use it or lose it" proposition.

People who are spirit channels may entertain the notion of ghosts as people whose minds are so disconnected from their dead bodies that they are not aware that they've died. How such a person might communicate is not explained, but from a first-person perspective, this describes what I was feeling.

> "We are left highly activated, with an incomplete motor plan still going round and round in our brain."
> — **Peter Levine**, psychotherapist

When I climbed with other mountaineers, we occasionally did death-defying things because we wanted to, but most of the time because we had to. We didn't climb "because it was there," we climbed because it felt great to be there, or because it felt great to get out of there.

Rarely was I traumatized in mountaineering because I handled everything I did. Scarcely anything happened for which I didn't take blame or credit. This is the state of mind you need to overcome adversity. That's not to say you can overcome anything, but if you don't believe you can, you won't. To become untraumatized is to reject the notion that you have been overpowered. It doesn't matter whether or not it's true, it's a state of mind.

References

Levine, P., Frederick, A. (1997). *Waking the Tiger, Healing Trauma*, North Atlantic Books.

Sheldrake, M. (2021). *Entangled life: How fungi make our worlds, change our minds & shape our futures.* Random House.

S8 – Memory, Amnesia, and Your Self

June 1, 2022

Perception is full of holes, and memory is mostly empty.

"The true art of memory is the art of attention." — **Samuel Johnson,** author

Memory is not a record of the past, it's a resource for acting in the present. You remember in order to know what to do. Your memory does not exist for nostalgic purposes.

Every experience we have is far richer than we can perceive or remember. Take a moment to observe yourself watching and listening. After you're gone through the motions, go back and repeat them, but this time look beyond what you were looking at before and listen to what you didn't notice.

For the smartest beings in the universe, we certainly don't see, hear, or remember much. There have been savants who remember everything, and their brains appear no different from ours. We could remember so much more, but we don't. And the reason we don't is that it would be a waste of resources. The question we might ask is, given the incredible things our brains are capable of, why aren't we doing more with it?

Kim Peek, the real person on whom the character in the movie *Rain Man* was based, liked to memorize things: street maps, phone books, and books of zip codes. He knew the phone numbers of tens of thousands of people, as well as their street addresses, zip codes, and the precise street directions to get between one address and another… across continents. Besides eidetic memory, meaning that he didn't forget things, he had a photographic memory, meaning he could see things once for a second and remember them exactly. He could read two pages at once, one page with his left eye and the other with his right eye.

To be fair, Kim had abnormal neurology, but most savants are otherwise normal. We know so little of how the mind works that perhaps these savants have exceptional structures we don't perceive. Since we don't see this, let's assume it's not true. Let's just say that we're tuned to a more modest level.

Amnesia

You cannot function without a recollection of the past and a vision of the future. People who have lost their memory don't know who they are. People who can't form new memories can't function. There appears to be an equivalence between the ability to remember and the ability to foresee, as some amnesias prevent you from conceiving of the future (Tulving 2005). Without memory, we have no control.

Memory is not identity. A person can have a deep, balanced, and stable self-awareness and full cognitive abilities and yet have no episodic memory. They can have absolutely no recollection of any episodes of their lives and still converse, think, run, act, perform, contemplate, and calculate. From this, it's clear that memory is stored in different parts of our brains.

We're not conscious of much of what we remember. At this moment, somewhere in your mind, you possess countless memories from your childhood. You're not thinking of them and don't even know what they are. Yet with effort, concentration, and some reminders, you can recall a biography of details you don't currently remember.

Without such efforts, all we have is a pseudo-memory of what we remember. We think we remember and that we could remember, but we don't have access now, and there is no index. We can't say much about our memories in the current moment except that we think they're there.

We might assume there is a kind of pyramid structure to memories in which a few narrow peaks offer paths down into wide forests of detail. We think these forests of detail exist to support whatever isolated peak we can recall, but until we explore these memories, we can't say much about what details they contain.

Memories are not single things stored in isolation. If they were, then when they were recalled—given how full of errors our memories are—they wouldn't fit together. What we remember is a broad complex such that when we recall the wrong person in an old scene, we will recall the same wrong person in all the old scene's memories.

Recall

We remember more than we're conscious of. There are reports of hypnosis drawing out memories of facts or feelings that we thought we forgot or were unaware we knew. Attention and focus training can improve recall and doesn't require hypnosis. We confirm this with neurofeedback training. We have more recall than we presume, and we have memories we didn't know we had (Kihlstrom 1995).

It's also found that this sort of evocation leads to the recall of more false than true memories, on an objective and factual basis. However, just as past life memories can be labeled as false, that does not mean factually untrue memories are of low value.

The erroneous memory you have might be well suited to aid in solutions to your present problems. As I said, memory is not there to record the past but to guide the future, and the false memories that are recalled—at least in the therapeutic context—often provide valuable guidance. Memories may be factually false and functionally useful.

A person induced into a state of dissociative trance, in which they are unaware of the outside world but are aware of what's being said to them, can memorize a list of words perfectly and be asked not to remember them unless they are given a command. When taken out of trance, these subjects can't remember learning anything but, upon the proper command, they can fully remember the list of words.

There are two prominent kinds of recollection: direct recall, otherwise known as explicit memory, and indirect recall, known as implicit memory. Direct recall happens when you need to think of something and it spontaneously appears: a word, name, or location. Indirect or implicit memory relies on association, takes longer, is strengthened by establishing conceptual relationships, but it is nonetheless mysterious.

With direct memory, we feel helpless when we draw a blank. It's like a magic trick that didn't work. With indirect memory, we are more patient, though hardly more involved. With indirect memory, we say a few magic words, such as describing a person's appearance or personality, and then their name appears: the rabbit jumps out of the hat.

The hypnotized learner cannot consciously remember the list of words they memorized until commanded to do so. These unremembered words are still in their memory but can't be retrieved directly. Direct recall seems to involve some executive function that can be halted when a person agrees not to use it.

The hypnotically amnesiac person can be tricked to locate by association the words they can't remember. The words can be drawn out of them. They'll speak the words, but they won't know that they learned them!

The forgotten words will appear with much greater frequency than similar words that were not memorized and forgotten. The forgotten words will just "appear," as if from nowhere. The forgotten, memorized words will be the first words they'll pick in a test of word associations, although they have no explanation of why these words are so prominent, as they have no recollection of memorizing them.

Even when the hypnotized person has unconsciously agreed not to remember, their associative memory "leaks in." This shows that our associative and our direct memory functions are distinct, there are different paths to the same recollections. Just as we don't know how we remember, we also don't know how we forget.

Trauma and Significance

Nothing is remembered accurately, and the most consequential things are remembered the most inaccurately. That's right: what we remember most clearly, we remember most poorly. That's because what's consequential is not what's factual. While we judge accuracy based on fact, we judge memory based on impact. To clarify, we might say that what has the greatest impact on us is remembered with the greatest distortion: a kind of tunnel vision effect.

If you've had an upsetting experience, then what you'll remember is what's upsetting, not the facts of the experience. This is obviously much more useful. For example, the fear of a stranger pointing a gun at you may be easy to substantiate, but the fear of walking in the dark through a bad part of town is much more useful.

I have a distinct memory of a spanking I received from my father as the result of my many efforts to piss my parents off. I remember flying in the air, a sense of the darkness in the room.

My father pointlessly carrying out his obligation, indifferent to my mother, who fussed and fretted on the sidelines. I have no traumatic memory of the event, and no recollection of what it was about.

I doubt this memory is accurate. My parents were probably present and may have behaved as I remember, but what's important is how I remember it, not what actually happened. The memory is a flash recording of ineffectual parenting that was easily recalled and needed no explanation. The memory isn't really about the spanking at all, it's about my relationship with my parents.

I have clients who semi-remember traumatic events. I don't know if their memories are accurate, whether they would benefit from remembering more or remembering more accurately. The memory could be a condensation of many events, or it could be a feeling that provides a summary and sense of direction. Alternatively, the importance of these memories could lie more deeply in the details that have been forgotten and may never be remembered.

Regression

> "Regression is first and foremost a product of the imagination, and any accurate memory produced is likely to be blended with a great deal of false recall."
> — **John F. Kihlstrom** (1995), psychologist

Regression is a hypnotherapeutic technique in which a client is asked to go back in time, step by step, to important scenes in their past. It's a contrived backward walk that follows seemingly historical events in order to gain greater insight into important past situations.

It is a process of better understanding circumstances connected with the present. It's presented as a path to better recall, but it's really a path to better conclusions. Regression appears quite rational, but there is no evidence that it is. Like all memories, regression is woven from thin cloth.

Hypnosis empowers regression by freeing us from our rational minds, which are ineffective on two fronts. First, we don't remember enough details, if we ever knew them. And second, human behavior isn't reasonable, it never makes total sense. We need to use our imagination.

I don't presume that you need to enter a dissociated state in order to find new ideas. Each person is comfortable with their level of creativity and may or may not need outside permission to go there.

If you're deeply attached to your story, you will be averse to regressing to disturbing memories. Such memories may cause deep confusion and probably won't be helpful. Using psychedelics to expand your memory and associations might break open your closet of secrets, but this might be a bad idea.

Everyone has the right to choose for themselves what sorts of demons they unleash from their past, and for that reason, I do not endorse the use of psychedelics as medicines. Using psychedelics should be based on the process they trigger, which is different for each individual, and not as a prescription for a preconceived goal.

Creativity in memory is helpful; your best ideas are probably out of reach. This is the entire purpose of counseling and coaching. It's what I feel is lacking in approaching problems too rationally. You need a space to think crazy thoughts without the need to explain yourself. I help people build this space. Calling this therapy, counseling, or coaching seems misleading. There is no formula; it's your reality.

> "Hypnosis may in the future provide a means to restructure personal identity by reshaping memories… to create a network of pseudo-memories to shape a positive and functional self-identity… [that exists] between mood and autobiographical memory."
> — **Mazzoni, Laurence, & Heap** (2014)

References

Kihlstrom, J. F. (1995 Dec 1). "Hypnosis, Memory, and Amnesia." *Journal of the Neurological Sciences, 134* (1–2): 6. https://www.ocf.berkeley.edu/~jfkihlstrom/hypnosis_memory.htm

Mazzoni, G., Laurence, J., & Heap, M. (2014 Jan). "Hypnosis and Memory: Two Hundred Years of Adventures and Still Going!" *Psychology Of Consciousness: Theory, Research, And Practice, 1* (2): 153-167. http://dx.doi.org/10.1037/cns0000016153

Tulving, E. (2005) "Episodic Memory and Autonoesis: Uniquely Human?" In *The Missing Link in Cognition: Self-knowing Consciousness in Man and Animals*, edited by Terrace, H.S. and Metcalfe, J., 3-56. Oxford University Press.

S9 – Imagination

March 24, 2021

Imagination is the key to growth, learning, invention, childhood, and healing.

"I sense the need for a new kind of mind of individuals who are integrators, as distinct from the reductionists… in the human dimension, as distinct from the molecular/cellular, trying to understand the whole which is far greater than the sum of the parts." — **Jonas Salk**, **MD** (1991), inventor of the polio vaccine

We're so often called to think more broadly that our eyes glaze over. But, as Salk also noted, you cannot develop what's needed at the time it's needed because by then it's too late.

We must develop some prescient guidance before new ways of thinking are needed. This will not happen in a mechanical world that only responds at the moment. This is the old argument against evolution by random mutation and natural selection: random changes cannot build a coordinated foundation. This is not a rebuttal of evolution, it is not even an argument, it simply makes the point that random mutation plus natural selection is necessary but insufficient. Evolution in unlikely directions must involve more than an immediate reward.

Consider a blind organism. If greater light offers a reward, then photosensitivity may develop, but an eye would be far more than what's necessary. Single-celled organisms have photo sensors that allow them to change their behavior in the presence of light, but they don't have eyes.

Beyond photosensitivity, visual discrimination could offer an additional advantage, and a lens would be beneficial. But a biological lens is far more than a discriminator—it's not a static object. The benefits of a lens in the eye only accrue when there are other parallel perceptual and cognitive structures in place to make use of the image. They will not all randomly occur at the same time, and without their simultaneous presence, there is no sight that can be rewarded.

If a simple shutter would suffice, then a lens would not develop as, lacking additional structures, there would be no reward for it. And once a shutter evolves, there would be little reward to extend it to include a lens, which is an entirely different structure.

Consider a house. To let light in, we create openings. To keep the weather out, we create shutters. A window and a shutter satisfy both needs. There is no need to develop a glass window pane that will do both at once. The feedback that would lead us to develop a glass pane differs from what leads to a window with a shutter. And if we already have a window with a shutter, then the need for light and weather protection doesn't give the feedback that would lead to a window. For that, you'd need additional needs and concepts.

To make the connection between the technology of glass and the benefit of windows requires our minds to connect the two ideas. We do this easily, and we understand the development of glass panes as a new solution. Nature does this all the time in the evolution of forms. Nature is constantly developing forms that are more capable than they need to be, yet we don't ascribe a mind to nature.

Hands

Consider our hands. They have changed little in form since we developed fingers. Something far less flexible than ten, 3-jointed fingers would certainly have sufficed for simple grasping and locomotion. A three-toed sloth uses three curved claws, and that's all. Yet we developed a complex hand and then, when our brains gained the ability to manipulate concepts beyond sticks, our versatile hands were ready for use.

Consider an octopus, a relative of the clam that no longer grows a shell. Clams don't have brains, but the octopus has nine brains, one that's central and an additional one in each arm. It has suckers with the tactile discrimination of a fingertip, photo sensors in each arm, and arms with the ability to wholly regenerate if amputated, brain and all. These features are unnecessary for the development of the individual and they are not incremental improvements to the clam.

Consider physical illness as it can arise from habitual states of mind. Physical conditions are often—some would say always—expressions of physical pressures extruded by the pressure of mental resistance into the shape of a physical ailment.

People come to me for relief from a physical ailment through a change of mind. These people show me they have latent mental abilities to affect their physical health. They can make progress in gaining awareness and control, and they can do this one step at a time. In almost every case, they resist. They vigorously refuse to develop these skills and they make up reasons to explain why they can or will not. These reasons draw on their emotions of fear, blame, or guilt.

Stress

It is almost a tautology that a person who has confounded their stresses into a somatic expression will resist attempts at relief. It is as if the body-mind has said, "Look at this! Attend to this and do not try to think me away from it!"

My clients come insisting that I help them do exactly that: to think away their discomfort, fear, guilt, and shame. Their emotional structure carries this burden or impediment. Their intellect wants to resolve it, and their emotions refuse their intellectual manipulations.

Our efforts start cautiously and clear-headedly, they are sane and organized. We have some clarity, resolve, certainty, and commitment. We believe we can, but we have doubts. It is not too long before less sane thoughts emerge. Clarity and certainty recede like failing memories. Resolve and commitment are pushed aside as stronger emotions rise: fear and chaos. My clients will blame me or themselves. They become overly sensitive, almost neurotic, and they may flee under some implausible pretense. This is what you'd expect if you tried to help an injured animal with whom you couldn't communicate. People seem to be no different.

Psychosomatic illness is a dysfunction that bridges the separation between the mind and body. It's a lack of sanity expressed in the body but, if you try to think it away, delusion inflames the mind.

I can almost predict my client's success at regaining elements of their physical health. Just at the point where their path is clear, they start acting pathologically. It is the nature of their dysfunction that, in the realm of the critical issue, they become frightened, horrified, petrified, or aggressive. They'll do anything to avoid the issue that, almost by definition, they could not confront in their minds alone.

Here's an example from my life. I've become increasingly successful in my private practice and then, yesterday, my back went out. I did nothing to injure my back, it just went out, and now I have difficulty standing. Just when my career gains strength and resilience, my back loses both. I have the sneaking suspicion something psycho-somatic has occurred, but I cannot see it.

If I had a counselor that told me my back pain was mental, I might object that it is quite real. But I am a counselor, so I know this is a real possibility. My back reflects what my mind does not see and directs me to confront it. The enlightened view sees this as an opportunity, but an opportunity to do what? It's an opportunity to be more attentive.

Solving a mind-body problem requires a mind-body change, not a change in just one or the other. If you want a change in your somatic situation, you must work toward psychological change as well. This is not just a change in patterns, but a change in spirit: a fundamental change of character. But the ego will not agree to this. It is not sufficiently well connected to the body to coordinate the change that's needed.

It is in this sense that the ego—your sense of self-reference and the confluence of your intellect and emotion—gets in your way. The problem is not that you have an ego, as some believe, but that your ego cannot do its job of adapting yourself to or releasing yourself from your body. You must get beyond the ego, and few are ready to do this. Few have the clarity and resolve. As a result, I see most of my clients make a few steps into this unfamiliar territory and stop. Maybe they'll gather further strength and make further progress, or maybe they'll succumb to their somatic illness.

Time

Often the quickest solution is a dead end, and greater, long-term potential comes from the less expeditious solution. If left to themselves, molecules would have to explore and reject a multitude of dead ends before being rewarded for the "mistake" of a less immediate but more flexible solution. We don't see that happening in the evolution of either our bodies or our minds.

Using the lens in our eye and the muscles that control it, our receptors and nerves integrate perception into a 3-dimensional image. To develop an eye from a photo receptor requires foresight that's greater than the what's in the photoreceptor. There is some force that conceives what might be useful, uses a process of induction, and develops an imagination of the future. There are forward-thinking forces in quantum physics, but they have not entered the classical thinking with which we understand evolution and biology.

It is dawning on physicists (Castro-Ruiz, Giacomini, & Brukner 2018) and philosophers that causality may not be deterministic. Other relationships may exist between events beyond a simple ordering in time, a linear chain of causes and their effects. This is contrary to our worldly experience and it may contradict our notions of reality. It may be structurally inconceivable to us and, if it is true, it will generate experientially inconceivable predictions. Predictions which involve experiments that lie outside the envelope of what humans can experience. This is exactly what already exists in the quantum realm, but we don't know how to understand these phenomena outside of that realm.

How can people gain the courage and conviction to enter realms that lie outside their present experience? How can your ego be convinced to dissolve itself and reform differently? Perhaps we can use the metaphor of time to say that there is a way to a future different from what our ego is sure will befall us, and which our ego will do anything to avoid. Anything, including beating your kids, warring with your neighbors, or drinking yourself to death.

The path to a different future starts with imagination. The realm of alternate reality starts in your mind. It need not be a literal image. It could be a feeling or a lack of feeling. It could be embodied in a new connection or a new disconnection. I'm not saying that imagination is reality, but that you must imagine a new reality first. Imagination welcomes chaos and fosters new ideas.

Play

Children have good imaginations: they grow into forms that fit their physical world. It's not enough to have an imagination, you must use it. You must apply it to your life. It's not enough to paint on canvas, play music, or dance. You must paint, play, and dance your life.

Therapy is about leading you out of the corner of your mind and back onto the playground of imagination. I object to most psychotherapy as it amounts to further negotiations with a hostile ego, something akin to convincing your parents that you're grown up. This is neither spontaneous nor imaginative.

Altered state work is the alternative: hypnosis, dreamwork, psychedelics, and somatic experience. Each of these takes you out of your container and offers you a chance to reorganize and to open your frame of mind. Psychedelics, extreme somatic experience, and naturally altered states of creative immersion are authentic paths to change.

References

Salk, J. (1991, May) *Academy of Achievement Interview*, San Diego, California. Retrieved from https://achievement.org/achiever/jonas-salk-m-d/#interview

Castro-Ruiz, E., Giacomini, F. and Brukner, C. (2018). Dynamics of Quantum Causal Structures, *Physical Review, X8*, 011047. Retrieved from https://journals.aps.org/prx/abstract/10.1103/PhysRevX.8.011047

S10 – Interoception

January 7, 2020

The ability to imagine, sense, explore, and control events within your body.

"Finer and finer performance is possible only if the sensitivity, that is, the ability to feel the difference is improved."
— **Moshe Feldenkrais,** physicist and physiotherapist

The Mechanical View

Interoception refers to a perception of what's interior. It's a simple word whose use has been stimulated by techniques that enable us to see what's going on inside living systems. The term is evolving and has split into alternative definitions that reflect what people are looking at or looking for.

Reductionists look for the smallest units of things: the unit of memory, feeling, or emotion. Mechanists explore the connection between what we sense and how we act. At a higher level, we want to understand what feelings and perceptions are, whether these are real things, and if they're related.

The general feeling among reductionists is that physiology generates events in the brain. These build into forces that eventually come to awareness. There's a seemingly endless amount published on the results of searching through the haystack of images, structures, and signals looking for thoughts. These approaches lack insight, and this stuff feels empty. This will always be the case when you're using lifeless tools to look for lifeless things.

The Vital View

"Learning how to 'see' into the body, to perceive subtle movements, and to feel energy surrounding the body are all nuanced skills essential to psychedelic guides, shamans, and somatic therapists."
— **Rachel Harris** (2023), psychotherapist

Explorations that begin with the seed of what you're looking for are disparaged as unscientific. This is the fundamental reason that reductionist science—which is essentially all of current science—segregates itself from questions of essence. All explorations that contact actual feeling begin with some element of it. None reduce to the inanimate. Here are some examples.

Eastern Medicine, including Traditional Chinese Medicine, acupuncture, and Ayurveda, all include fundamental life force. Spiritual healing, whether Western or Indigenous, depends on a link to power or direction. These cosmologies don't work to explain these forces, they focus on how these forces develop.

Applied kinesiology, or AK, is muscle testing. It involves asking verbal questions to a patient and expecting their musculature to answer. AK posits a connection between vital forces and mechanical actions and exists in the zone between the spiritual and the mechanical. AK asserts you can ask questions to the self, the "wholly other," and get answers from the body.

Applied kinesiology gets to the heart of the vital view, and this view is full of uncertainty. I've seen it used by practitioners I trust to help direct them, and I've seen it used by charlatans I don't trust, who use it for their own benefit. The inability to discern who's competent from who isn't excludes vitalist approaches from scientific exploration.

Applied kinesiology is a psychosomatic technique with an interesting mechanical component. Other mind-matter approaches go much further. Rudolf Steiner's biodynamics took permaculture into the mystical, while Wilhelm Reich took psychology into crazy realms. Both broke ground from which new ideas are still emerging nearly one hundred years later.

I would like to do the same with hypnosis. Aside from simple manipulations, no one really knows what hypnosis is. Of the many effects of hypnosis, one is an enhanced ability to recover from surgery. Besides decreasing pain and doubling the rate of post-operative healing, there are reports of significantly reduced blood loss through the clients' apparent ability to control bleeding while under anesthesia.

It's well established that there is what's called "a hidden observer" when a person is in hypnosis. This observer is an aspect of awareness present even when the conscious self has been disabled. This hidden observer is a rationally self-aware self during deep hypnotic states.

The hidden observer may not be able to speak using one's voice, but they can use hand signals.

Contact with the hidden observer is only possible during hypnosis, when the conscious mind is disabled and has been moved out of the way. While under deep hypnosis, a person's hidden observer can express itself,. This "person" is not the same as their conscious self. It sees, hears, feels, and remembers things of which the conscious self is unaware. Who the hidden observer is, and how different its thoughts, feelings, and plans can be, remains unknown.

The Emerging View

In 2016, psychologists Norman Farb and Wolf Mehling (2016) wrote:

> "Interoception, the representation of the body's internal state, is a growing target of scientific research, buoyed by a growing respect for contemplative traditions relating interoceptive awareness to the cultivation of well-being. An emerging interoception literature cuts across studies of neurophysiology, somatic anthropology, contemplative practice, and mind-body medicine.

> "Key questions include: How is body awareness cultivated? What role does interoception play for emotion and cognition across the lifespan and in different psycho-pathologies? What are the neurophysiological effects of interoceptive training in Yoga, mindfulness meditation, Tai Chi, and other embodied contemplative practices? What categories from other traditions might be useful in this investigation? How might the cultivation of interoceptive awareness improve resilience in chronic health conditions?

> "Such questions have historically been ill-addressed by Western science, which is still influenced by a 400-year Cartesian tradition that treats cognition as something distinct from sense-perception."

The reductive neural, electrical, and mechanical approaches are scientific, but they are not insightful. Their taxonomy of perception establishes correlations with no understanding of what perception is or what's perceived. They are like botany before genetics, where everything was about categorizing, without the slightest idea of what might lie behind it.

Granted, the hypothesis of "vital force" doesn't say much about what underlies it, but it suggests a dynamic approach. It suggests perception exists to achieve a balance. Assigning sensations to brain centers will no more explain perception than assigning emotions to brain centers explains what's felt.

One of the more pernicious and unreported drawbacks of the scientific approach is that it does not question itself. It does not question the authority of its practitioners, and it does not question their preconceptions. After all, the goal of science is to discover answers, but the deepest inspiration comes from toppling old answers and building new questions.

You'll find scarce few scientists who will plow under the gardens of their thoughts. Your average nonscientist has a healthier skepticism about what they believe. This lies at the root of scientific arrogance, which I presume we have all encountered. It feeds into the celebration of authority and a disdain for the creative.

The Pragmatic View

We should not pay so much attention to the brain. It's an intermediate organ that stands between perception and apperception. Most of the brain's function is to disable sensation, as there is far too much going on for us to handle. All this brain imaging is tantamount to a study of the gears of a clock in the search to understand time. We should improve our perception by perceiving more and more subtlety. Let's see what arises in the higher plane of consciousness. Event potentials, ion concentrations, or enlarged grey matter tell us nothing about consciousness.

Consider the meme from *The Wizard of Oz* in which we're told to "pay no attention to the little man behind the curtain." He's the one who makes things happen, but, as that fable tells us, he knows nothing. Consciousness, which is what we're after, lies beyond the reach of our thoughts. It seems grand and mysterious, as embodied by our perception of a Great Oz. But it is beyond that, the smoke and mirrors that produce it. Consciousness is not the mysterious nerves and their signals, and it is not the perceptions and recollections, it is an organized structure that arises from these things.

You can learn to walk barefoot across burning embers without getting blisters. You can learn to push a sharpened knitting needle through your forearm and suffer neither pain nor bleeding. The reason you don't learn to do these things is because they serve no purpose, but you could learn them.

There are things you can learn that are of less risk and greater benefit, but they may take you outside the zone of normal thought and perception. The reason you don't go there, don't learn those skills, and don't gain those benefits are discussed in Malcolm Gladwell's book *Talking to Strangers: What We Should Know About the People We Don't Know*.

Gladwell argues trust has developed as the basis of collaboration. Trust lies on top of perception, and in its support, we adhere to consensus notions of communication and behavior. Rooted in this is the distrust of novelty, and the dis-attraction to nonconformity. We have so internalized this that to engage the different is, for many of us, a distraction.

The Historical View

Being sensitive involves overlooking convention. Introspection—looking at yourself—is a questioning and creative act. Most people are thoughtful—their heads are full of thoughts—but not questioning. Questioning involves being self-critical and prevailing against outside criticism. If you are injured by criticism, your creativity will orbit what's popular, like a captured planet.

Intellect has a bad rap. It's poorly employed and poorly understood. As children, we experienced the adult world around us in its use of logic, knowledge, and language. Adults used these things as tools and weapons. If you want an easy lesson in hypnotherapy, listen to adults talking to children, and notice children's dazed responses.

When it comes to children, most adults are intellectual bullies, not skilled thinkers. It is our experiences from childhood that make us wince when someone starts "explaining" things to us. We've learned what condescending means in our experiences with parents and teachers. Once you learn that sensitivity and self-expression bring pain, you will numb yourself to criticism. If you've been traumatized, you may shut down entirely and feel nothing. Becoming sensitive again is to become expressive and requires adjusting your old patterns of avoidance.

Our aversion to intellectualism also has cultural roots, as beautifully explained in Richard Hofstadter's 1963 book *Anti-intellectualism in American Life*. Intellectuals have historically been linked to the ruling class, and the early US colonials were attempting to escape the ruling class. This led to the odd combination of a need for invention and a rejection of expertise. This took root in the independence of Baptist churches, and the regionalism of the cultures in Western states that are manifest in Idaho, Wyoming, Texas, and others.

We see this still today, in the appeal of individualism and novelty associated with the West Coast, compared to the tradition and institutionalism of the East Coast. The West Coast is North America's creative and injured child; the East Coast is its abusive, colonial parent.

Novelty triggers our innate sense of risk aversion. We celebrate creativity only after its benefits have been demonstrated. As authors Scott Barry Kaufman and Carolyn Gregoire write (2016) in *Wired to Create, Unraveling the Mysteries of the Creative Mind*:

> "Why are paradigm-shifting ideas throughout history consistently, and predictably, ridiculed and rejected? It's because, as a culture and as individuals, we're deeply biased against creativity…
>
> "Unconventional ideas that break from tradition or challenge our existing ways of thinking, which nearly any important creative achievements do, often push us out of our psychological comfort zone. As a general rule, we don't like things that challenge our habitual ways of thinking, which makes creative work a dangerous endeavor."

Our aversion to novelty is amplified in school. The primary purpose of compulsory schooling is not training but conformity, as this sort of schooling offers no opportunity for creativity: you cannot create within a context; real creativity happens outside of a context.

This lies at the root of the diagnosis of ADD/ADHD, as I explained in my 2014 article "ADHD as Emergent Institutional Exploitation," in *The Journal of Mind and Behavior*. It's not that most students labeled ADD/ADHD can't pay attention, it's that they don't want to. They are languishing canaries in a poisoned atmosphere.

Cars are a good barometer of the social nature of identity and individuality. As I drove my son to school one morning, I considered what a nineteenth-century person would think of cars today. Shapes have changed, but society's adherence to conformity hasn't. Today's cars all look the same. They all have the same not-really-aerodynamic aerodynamic look, and they're still priced according to their sex or authority appeal. Cars epitomize what society considers futuristic and creative, and really isn't.

A Body of Work

I will write a book called Interoception. It will encourage readers to explore new perceptions within their bodies. The insight for this comes from what we know can be accomplished using focused attention through hypnosis, and from the expanded awareness we get from controlling our mental frequencies.

I have developed a sensitive stomach, and this seems to derive from my stomach's reluctance to secrete juices and mix its contents. I have found I can communicate with, exercise, visualize, and imagine myself doing these things, and then they happen. My digestion improves.

We all have had the experience of sitting on the toilet and waiting to move our bowels. We succeed when our colon executes peristalsis and our anal sphincters relax. I have found that when I imagine, sense, and encourage these things happening beyond the limits of my direct perception, they happen. I rarely squeeze or strain. Of course, I am in collaboration with my body, and my requests are appropriate. This, too, is based on perception.

The HeartMath Institute (https://www.heartmath.org) has a patented way to facilitate your heart's optimal function. This occurs when your heartbeat and breath are properly coordinated. It's achieved by amplifying these signals to a level you are conscious of, at which point your natural inclinations take control. With these heightened perceptions, most people's bodies naturally move into greater coherence, and they do so fairly quickly. Those with the most trouble coordinating their pulse and breath are people with cardiopulmonary dysfunction. The HeartMath Institute provides data supporting the health benefits of improved heart-lung synchrony.

Interactive Metronome (https://www.interactivemetronome.com) is another biofeedback approach that amplifies perception. Through the use of electronically assisted feedback, you can learn to improve your visual, muscular, and cognitive timing, and by that means, your coordination and perception. Everything in your body works through a process of coordination, and this depends on timing and sensitivity.

Each system, be they muscles or organs, must be ready and responsive. Each of these systems maintain their own internal rhythms as this is how they synchronize. The simplest task is to clap or tap with accurate timing. Beyond that, precise timing can be measured in microseconds. This level of precision is beyond what's sufficient for everyday responses, but discerning these small differences is critical for improved synchrony.

How do you learn to hit a fastball? How do you even see a fastball? Speed isn't everything. Precision, synchrony, and poly-rhythmic complexity go well beyond the speed of one's reflexes and into the realm of expanded awareness. It takes practice, and to succeed, you must develop enhanced perception. How do you learn to perceive what you cannot perceive? You begin by imagining it!

I recorded a guided visualization to improve your perception of your liver and another that is an exploration of your small intestines. These are exercises in enhanced internal awareness, and they are not that different from developing your awareness as part of the general process of personal growth.

It is likely that many of the things we internally perceive are, in fact, interactions with our external world. As amplifiers, we don't discern what's internal from what's external. The external world generates signals we perceive internally, and a deeper part of ourselves tells us what it sees. It's often unclear if these messages are inferences or perceptions. For that reason, I work to heighten external perception, which I prefer to call subtle perception.

We Hold Ourselves Back

There are many external perceptions we're unaware of because they're too subtle or too quick. In fact, we are unaware of almost everything that occurs in the world. This includes our communication, most of which occurs without our intent.

Paul Ekman (2009) has made a profession of teaching people how to understand others. See his book *Telling Lies* for an exploration of our ubiquitous, facial micro-expressions— expressions that reveal our feelings and intentions which we are both unaware that we're generating, and are not consciously aware of having witnessed. With exercise, we could do much better in a range of perceptual abilities.

However, there is a problem: we don't want to. Interoception, and perceptions generally, require our initiative and effort. Unlike medicine, school, and work, perception does not happen to you. Stimulus happens, but perception requires your compliance. You do this for yourself and until you learn how to alter your perception, you won't.

I had a client who was plagued with anxiety and discomfort. He was in such a state of alarm that everything was a threat or was seen as a threat. After some time, I made it clear we could focus solely on establishing comfort. The offer was rejected because they preferred not to take the risk of doing anything. Instead, they said they preferred to give all authority to specialists. As they were not willing to collaborate in change, I expect they won't change either in their attitude or their discomfort.

If you think you might gain greater comfort and control by becoming more sensitive, look on my website for guided visualizations that could help you.

References

Farb, N, Mehling, W. (2016). "Editorial: Interoception, Contemplative Practice, and Health." *Frontiers in Psychology, 7.*

Ekman, P. (2009). *Telling Lies: Clues to Deceit in the Marketplace, Politics, and Marriage.* W.W. Norton.

Gladwell, M. (2021). *Talking to Strangers: What We Should Know About the People We Don't Know.* Back Bay Books.

Harris, R. (2023). *Swimming in the Sacred.* New World Library.

Kaufman, S. B. & Gregoire C. (2016). *Wired to Create, Unraveling the Mysteries of the Creative Mind.* TarcherPerigee.

Hofstadter, R. (1963). *Anti-intellectualism in American Life.* Knopf.

S11 – Interoception, The Colon

August 20, 2021

You are no better than what you disdain.

"Nothing living should ever be treated with contempt."
— **Elizabeth Goudge**, author

Warts

As an intellectual person, I have difficulty believing one can affect a virus through the power of the mind alone. Despite my disbelief, there are repeated claims that hypnosis can cure warts. Unlike a bug bite, which heals more quickly if you stop scratching it, warts are caused by the human papilloma virus living in your skin. Healing only comes from the action of your immune system.

You can cure a wart by surgically removing the tissue that supports the virus. Alternatively, your immune system can kill the virus. If your immune system is your body's only internal power against a wart, then how can hypnosis cure warts?

I recently returned to the work of Dr. Dabney Ewin, a surgeon and medical hypnotist. His book *Ideomotor Signals for Rapid Hypnoanalysis*, written with Bruce Eimer (2006), presents photographs and case histories of medical ailments they cured by hypnosis alone. An extensive papilloma virus infection presented in one case was entirely resolved by a single session of hypnosis.

The gist of Ewin's approach is to uncover ideas fixed in the subconscious. These are not "your" ideas, or ideas that you profess. They are a secondary form of reasoning in conflict with your conscious thoughts. Because of this contradiction, the subconscious idea is rejected, overlooked, suppressed, or forgotten, but it is not removed.

Not everyone's minds are in possession of clear and contrary opinions. Yet, it's increasingly recognized in trauma psychology that problematic subconscious thought patterns exist. These thought patterns are hard to access, and their resolution can have a great positive effect.

Autonomic Control

According to Ewin and Eimer, hypnosis speaks to the subconscious mind, and it is the subconscious mind that has the power to direct the immune system. In cases of medical hypnosis, the client presents a medical condition that is not clearly of mechanical or exogenous origin. The origin of the difficulty cannot be found, or previous treatments have failed without explanation. It is to these cases—sometimes judged as psychosomatic, hypochondriac, or malingering—that Ewin and Eimer applied hypnosis hoping to engage the immune system.

The immune system is complex. It involves dozens of types of immune cells of different functions, a separate vascular system, as well as a kind of learning and memory for which there are no known theories. Yet, judging from the success of Ewin, Eimer, and many others, there is a powerful connection between the subconscious and the autonomic processes of the muscular, vascular, and immune systems.

From the outcome of hypnotic treatment, we can infer that the subconscious mind works in alliance with the immune system even though there is little understanding of how. There is no concept of "thinking" in the immune system, although emotion powerfully affects our endocrine system and our thoughts.

We don't understand the subconscious as an integral, rational system operating beneath our awareness. We don't really understand it at all. Our subconscious seems to have access to different memories from those we're aware of. We can only conjecture that these things exist: the immune system "thinks," the subconscious maintains a separate existence, and our conscious mind remains oblivious to both.

If ideas carried by the subconscious create illness, and the immune system can be directed by the subconscious, then the subconscious can cause healing. If the mind and the immune system are talking to, aware of, and responding to each other, then aren't they really two sides of the same system? Our preconception of the body and mind as being separate is an obstacle to their working together.

What I find most surprising about Ewin and Eimer's work is the simplicity of their treatments. It's possible that they're cherry-picking the results: that they're reporting only the successful cases. Skeptical readers would like to apply a scientific analysis to more carefully curated data. The trouble is that the scientific protocols for collecting physiological data and psychological data are different.

Issues, outcomes, measurements, and even notions of repeatability, falsifiability, and objectivity are different in these realms. To pursue psychosomatic medicine will require methodological changes. For now, we rely on clinical records and case histories. It would not be difficult to build a more compelling mind-body science, but, so far, we don't have it.

Interoception

If it's true that the subconscious can cure illness, then we want to know how it works and how to apply it. Why wait until the psyche and the soma are out of balance before one intervenes? Why not foster greater balance to begin with? The focus on disease is dysfunctional; working with the subconscious is fundamental to health.

On August 15th, 2021 an article by David Robson (2021) appeared in *The Guardian* titled, "Interoception: the hidden sense that shapes well-being." Robson says, "There's growing evidence that signals sent from our internal organs to the brain play a major role in regulating emotions and fending off anxiety and depression."

The word "interoception" refers to both conscious and non-conscious perceptions of the internal state of the body. "Non-conscious" can mean both unconscious, as in reflexive, and subconscious, an alternative awareness.

The article quotes psychologist Manos Tsakiris who says, "We are seeing an exponential growth in interoceptive research," with academic conferences devoted to the subject and a wealth of new papers. Research on interoception is now one of the fastest-growing areas in neuroscience and psychology.

I would like to make a modest proposal that we all have greater control over our autonomic systems than we are aware of. I suggest we can improve this awareness with little difficulty if we are subconsciously encouraged to do so.

Following this suggestion, I have been creating a series of self-hypnosis audio files anyone can listen to in order to improve their self-awareness. To become more interoceptive.

The Large Intestines

I have a growing set of self-hypnosis audio files that address various systems in the body. One of these concerns the gut. I divided the gastrointestinal tract into the stomach, small intestines, and large intestines. Each recording is about 20 minutes long. You can find these interoception audios on my website at: https://www.mindstrengthbalance.com/product-category/mind-body/.

These self-hypnosis explorations are informative, perceptual, and interoceptive. In addition, they are positive and empowering. Some were difficult to create. In particular, the exploration of the large intestines presented me with a problem.

People are averse to the subject of defecation, yet no treatment of the large intestines would be complete without it. The subject of feces is taboo. We can employ the topic for invective, and engage it for humor, but in normal conversation it seems out of bounds.

I didn't find the right perspective until I had a client whose problems related to the large intestines. There was no avoiding it: I needed to fully address interoceptive issues of the colon, including evacuation.

By connecting what I know about the enteric nervous system, the immune system, and the gastrointestinal tract, I have completed the third and last self-hypnosis audio in the gastrointestinal series. You'll find the link to this audio file below.

Listen to this audio when you're in a contemplative state. That could be before meditation, relaxation, or sleep. I suggest listening before sleep because sleep is a time when your subconscious and autonomic processes take control.

You don't need to do anything. Let your conscious mind relax and drift into a light sleep. In this state, your thoughts are more plastic and your concepts are fluid. You're more likely to experience moods and associations that you would not have during daily life. New connections are made in these situations. Try it, it's free.

The Gut Part III: Large Intestines (An Induction)

The Gut Part III: Large Intestines is a hypnotic induction. **DO NOT** listen to this recording while you're driving a car, operating machinery, or doing anything that requires your attention.

We think of our stomach and intestines as organs in our bodies, but they are actually the lining of a hole that goes through us like the hole in a donut. And because they are extensions of the outside of our bodies, they can be infected by what we eat and breathe. I'll guide you on a descent into this elongated hole, down your throat, into your stomach, through your intestines, and out the other end of the alimentary canal.

We've visited the upper gastrointestinal tract in other guided visualizations. In this journey, we'll explore the great large intestines, and you'll see why it's so great when we get there.

Begin by relaxing into your body and leaving your external sensations behind you. Place your right hand at the right edge of your belly with the right edge of your hand against your right pelvis. Place your left hand at the left edge of your belly with the left edge of your hand against your left pelvis. Your fingertips should be touching. Between these hands runs your colon, starting on the right, rising up to cross behind your navel, and descending down to your left.

Imagine preparing to turn yourself inside out, leaving your sensations of the outer world and turning your attention to what's happening inside you. You are powering down sight and senses of the external world. You are powering up your insight and insenses of what's inside you.

Open awareness and refine your ability to communicate. Recognize that awareness is both sensual and visual and that you start to see what you start to sense, even though this vision does not come through your eyes. You see what your brain senses and sight is a form of knowing that goes far beyond your eyes.

Close your eyes, focus on your breathing, and locate some place in your body where you can feel your pulse. You are taking a trip on a boat that will be cruising down your alimentary canal. Your breathing will be your sails and your pulse will be your propeller. You control both and they work together, never fighting, moving in the current of your body's rhythm, even when your insight is fogged and unknown. You trust them and they carry you forward.

We are visiting a part of your body that does the most mysterious chemistry, deals with the most toxic substances, and creates the most valuable resources. Your colon performs inhuman chemistry that our body does not understand or control but only manages to the mutual benefit of the organisms that live in your gut.

This is a safari, and you move quietly and without disturbance. We are visiting processes that create toxins, collect and expel toxins, and you'll keep those areas quiet even though they'll recognize your presence. They will remain calm and they will keep to their quiet rhythms, contained and patient, gentle, and relaxed.

Your heart beats slowly in the center of your chest. A true organ that's all muscle and always in motion. A slow motor. Feel your pulse as a slow idle of the motor of a riverboat. And we're on that boat, passing down a river that is inside you.

Take a slow breath first to fill your chest and then exhale...

For your next breath, fill less in the front of your chest and more on the sides... and then exhale.

For your third breath, hardly move your chest at all, but lift the top of your belly just below your rib cage.

And for your fourth breath, breathe still deeper, bypassing your chest and stomach, and moving all the way down into your pelvis, your gut, to the base of your spine.

As you move down into your body, as you move down through this channel that is really flowing outside the inner surface of your body, the hole that goes through your body. Settle into this deepest breath as the way you'll breathe for now. This is the breath that accompanies your heart in this passage through your system. Inhaling down into your lower belly... and imagine the exhale passing right through you.

Sink down into the chair or bed, through the floor, and into the earth, and let your pulse tap the energies below you. Your breath turns from the movement of the air, and the two together are a kind of synthesis that combines air and water, by the chemistry of your lungs and gut, into the energy that sustains you.

You are the rhythms inside you. Release yourself to these rhythms.

Take a breath, relax your face, let your jaw drop. Move past your teeth, across your tongue to the back of your throat, and slide down your throat past your vocal cords into your upper chest, past the bronchial tubes leading to your lungs, and down toward your stomach.

This environment is preliminary. Food chewed and enzymes added, pulverized, and hydrated to a kind of slurry. What once had a taste is mixed and broken and you accompany it to the first chamber of preparation and transformation, which is your stomach.

Your stomach is the immigration center to a new world, a vast hall where what once was whole begins a journey into its parts. Move through it as a cathedral, the heart of a mountain, funneling into a small gateway, leading off through a sphincter into the small intestines.

Through this sphincter, your stomach slowly and carefully, selectively, passes the food you've eaten with cycles of pressure; your stomach's fingers squeezing a pastry bag, passing a few tablespoons each minute.

The small intestines act chemically through the action of enzymes, acids, and bases. The small intestines are a test tube, a chemistry set in which only a small part of your food reacts. Only a small amount of what you eat is digestible. Here, your food is washed with chemicals that search for small nutrient particles to bind or cleave: proteins to peptides, fats to acids, starches to sugars.

In a voyage of 36 hours, food only spends 6 to reach the end of the small intestines, spiraling through at the rate of an inch each minute. Most of the liquid and nutrients are removed from what you've eaten and its further passage is blocked by another sphincter, this one leading into the cecum, the start of the large intestine. And your riverboat passes through it, and now we're here, in the cecum, at the start of the large intestine.

The cecum is a kind of stomach that adds liquids and churns its contents. It can be small because it's not filled by your sudden appetite and can push the food it receives upward into the ascending colon. Into the cecum flows a well-mixed, chemically reduced chyme the consistency of soft oatmeal. The cecum's size relates to the small amount of plant material we eat, larger in herbivores and smaller in carnivores.

In the cecum you add cellulose digesting enzymes, mixing them in. But more dramatically, here is the chaos of your gut biota, one of the densest populations of bacteria on earth. An unfathomable collection of 40 trillion micro-organisms. 5,000 different species, each with their own life cycle, their own life's rhythm, and their own DNA.

More numerous than all the cells in our body combined, amounting to a volume half of our brain, which doubles every four days. Their lives are short, and we expel one-quarter of them—half of our stool—each day just to keep their population from growing. Only half of our stool is what we've eaten; the other half is what's been born inside us.

Our large intestine is a still that ferments the food we've eaten. Six feet long and thickly mucus lined, home to trillions of bacteria, fungus, and viruses. Some of these live in the soil, water, and vegetation around us. Some we know as serious diseases: shigella, salmonella, and others similar to cholera and the plague. We kept them in check and they serve our digestion.

Most can't live outside our bodies. We can't even raise them in a laboratory because they're killed by air. We are their home, their universe, and their source of life. We can live a short while without them, but not well and not for long. We feed them, they feed us, and of course, there is communication. One-tenth of our brain's tissue surrounds our large intestines. Here, our immune system learns of the bacterial world around us. We manufacture many of our brain's neurotransmitters in the colon.

The colon manages kinds of chemistry we don't understand. We've only started studying our gut biome, where it comes from, and what it does for us. Of course, those organisms are aware of each other. They communicate with chemicals in the lining, the liquid, the stool, even the gas. We are aware of them through our immune system and the nervous system in our gut. And they are aware of us, maybe like we're aware of whatever runs our universe. They're surely aware of what we eat and sensitive to it.

Focus on your right hand over your right pelvis. Your cecum is below your palm. Here, countless bacteria, yeasts, and viruses are being mixed into the food you've eaten. The whole affair begins to decompose, the cellulose breaking down into fats, sugars, and acids. These liquids from our slowly fermenting stool are absorbed into the walls of our colon, allowing nutrients to enter our bloodstream. For nearly 30 hours, this ferment travels the six feet up and across our abdomen and then down the left side.

Focus on your left hand over your left pelvis. Below this is the base of your descending colon. Following that is an S-shaped extension that brings the large intestine to your centerline, in front of your sacrum, above your anus. Here is the location of your rectum, the final reservoir of your stool, a cone-shaped repository that funnels down to the sphincters of your anus.

Your rectum has its own rhythm, purpose, and musculature. It's your rectum that signals to you when you need to evacuate your bowel, and when it contracts, which it does in coordination with your anus, it is to empty itself. In doing this, you are relieved, and when done fully, you are fully relieved.

We have such taboos around defecating. Modern cultures seem to have particular trouble with evacuating, but even traditional cultures keep bathroom issues private. Because of this, we don't learn. We don't learn the most basic things about what our shit should look or smell like, what its consistency should be, and what it means when its form is not normal. No one knows, and no one tells.

It's as if sex was so taboo that it was never spoken of, and no one knew anything about it, how it was done, or what its results were. It's as if we engaged blindly and ignorantly and never spoke about, coordinated, recognized, or understood it.

How do we transform the food we set our lives around and talk about almost incessantly into something unmentionable, unthinkable, and forbidden? Yes, we are finished with it, but what's left behind tells us the final grade we've earned after each course of digestion. How do we know if we've done everything right, if we aren't aware of what's going on inside us?

Follow the work of your large intestine from its start to its finish. It's true that there is little to nothing human in your feces, but even as feces, while it's still in your body, you are extracting nutrients from it. Think of your colon like an assembly line in reverse, not one in which things are built, but where things are taken apart. At each step, your stool is adding to you through the essential elements you take up into your bloodstream.

In your mind, imagine the organ that is your colon and the very slow palpations that take nearly a day to move your food that remaining six feet. It's an organ full of muscles, surrounded by billions of nerves, irrigated by major blood flow, host to the center of your immune system. The least you can do is to be there and pay attention, watch, listen, sense, and maybe you can learn.

And why is it so unpleasant to think of your rectum? Do you disparage the garbage truck? Can you imagine where you would be without it? Accept that you are your body's garbage man. Pay attention to the success or failure of your digestion.

Imagine you have navigated through your colon. Imagine you have been fasting and your colon is empty, slick, and thickly carpeted. A pink-skinned tube like your throat but at the other end.

Now you've navigated the S-shaped curve and settled into the lagoon that is your rectum, like the gentle shallows below a waterfall held back by a dam. Relax your perineum and imagine a sense of calm in your anus. Merely relax it. You can do this by releasing nothing because your anus is more relaxed when it's closed than when it's open. Like your lips, it prefers to keep closed.

Passing downriver, past the dam, imagine allowing yourself out of your anus. There is nothing negative here. You are no longer averse to one of the most complex and involved processes of your body.

You cannot explain it to others. They're not ready to understand, but you can understand yourself. You not only accept your colon, but realize that you are it and it is you, and so are the trillions of foreign organisms that live there.

Not unlike living in a real ecology, you are a shepherd and you are what you protect and you must know it in every way with humor, sensitivity, awareness, and compassion. Accepting your colon may be one of the most important steps in accepting yourself. You have passed; you are out.

Continue traveling along the surface of your body. Travel up your sides, across your back and belly, up to your shoulders, and back into your head. Back into your eyes and nose and mouth.

Open your eyes and remember. The language you use is not the only language of your body. The being that you are is just one of forty trillion for whom you're the host. You're just here to keep the others safe. Keep them safe by listening to them. Make it a habit. Listen to your body.

> *The Gut Part III: Large Intestines* is a hypnotic induction — **DO NOT** listen to it while driving a car, operating machinery, or doing anything that requires your attention.
>
> Listen to a streaming MP3 audio reading of *The Gut Part III: Large Intestines*:
>
> https://www.mindstrengthbalance.com/mindwp/wp-content/uploads/2021/08/Large-Intestines.mp3

References

Ewin, D. & Eimer, B. (2006). *Ideomotor Signals for Rapid Hypnoanalysis.* Thomas Books.

Robson R. (2021 Aug 15). "Interoception: the Hidden Sense That Shapes Well Being." *The Guardian*. https://www.theguardian.com/science/2021/aug/15/the-hidden-sense-shaping-your-wellbeing-interoception

S12 – Conversations With My Anus

November 30, 2018

Hearing a separate, audible speaking voice that was a part of my body.

"Through organ dialect, the body's organs speak a language which is usually more expressive and discloses the individual's opinions more clearly than words are able to do."— **Alfred Adler, MD** (1956, 223), psychotherapist

Dissociation

To move from the superficiality to the seriousness of this title requires some background. First, consider the notion of dissociation, or the splitting of parts of one's personality into separate personalities of their own. While this is normally seen as a sign of illness, it isn't. It's common but subtle. Psychedelic drugs can amplify it.

Imagine parts of your body having their own personalities. These personalities can split from what you consider yourself, and they can speak. The question is, when this happens, are we hearing something new or are we just "making it up"?

We all experience our nervous system "speaking" to announce pain or trouble. We have a headache, bruise, or indigestion and we "get the message" without dialog. The head, tissue, or gut have authority in their domains and they speak somatically. Like the frowning mother who needs only to point to our messy room, we understand without further instruction.

Indeed, were we to feign ignorance, the frowning mother, like the bruise, would make their point through demonstration. The bruise or gut need not engage in rhetoric or polemics. Yet under the influence of psychedelics, this can happen. To me, it has.

Ayahuasca

Ayahuasca is a natural, psychedelic "tea" that has the unusual property of creating a dissociated world while leaving your "I-ness" intact. Under its influence, you can journey to other worlds while remaining cogent, verbal, and aware. The notes you take make sense when you return. They make sense, more than your average dream.

Ayahuasca irritates one's alimentary canal. Your gut is not just irritated, it's infuriated. It responds with projectile vomiting and explosive diarrhea. It's not enjoyable, but one copes. How many times does one take ayahuasca for fun? Once.

In the Sci-Fi comedy *Dark Star,* hapless astronauts argue with the artificial intelligence of a malfunctioning thermonuclear bomb preparing to detonate while still attached to the ship. Unable to release, the astronauts attempt to use existentialist philosophy to convince the bomb it does not exist, and so should not explode.

I found myself in the same position, somewhere in the jungles of Ecuador, when the bolus of my ayahuasca reached the terminus of my intestines. I could not detach, and I did not want to explode. My only choice was to talk to my anus and convince it, somehow, that it could deviate from its natural inclinations.

It was an odd situation because—ayahuasca being what it is—my anus talked back. But I tell you this: unlike a bomb with artificial intelligence, the anus is not endowed with much. Its world is simple and its task straightforward. Thinking is not its strong point. The crew of the *Dark Star* perished because of their poor undergraduate education, but my arguments succeeded, and I lived to see another day. Let it not be said that philosophy isn't worth shit.

After the Flood

This was the end of it, but far from the beginning. At the beginning, after the wretched nausea of swallowing this concoction, my stomach had quite a bit to say about this adventure. Once the beta-carbolines and tryptamines perfused my system, these gastric complaints were communicated to my mind in plain English.

Your stomach is far from stupid. Your enteric nervous system, a wholly separate nervous network, is one-tenth the size of your brain. I have a renewed respect for the intelligence of my gut because of these conversations. And whereas I rarely get an answer outside of a dissociated state, I now always announce my intentions, and my stomach knows I'm listening.

These conversations took place over a decade ago. Since then, I've developed benign hemorrhoids and acid reflux. It recently dawned on me that these two conditions, at the entry and exit of my alimentary canal, are controlled by the same characters I once engaged in conversation.

I am wondering if the dissociation that began in the jungle has developed into a situation where the characters I brought to consciousness cannot reconnect to the subconscious world from which they arose. Or maybe now that I'm conscious of their affairs, I'm expected to take an active role, whereas I used to be exempt.

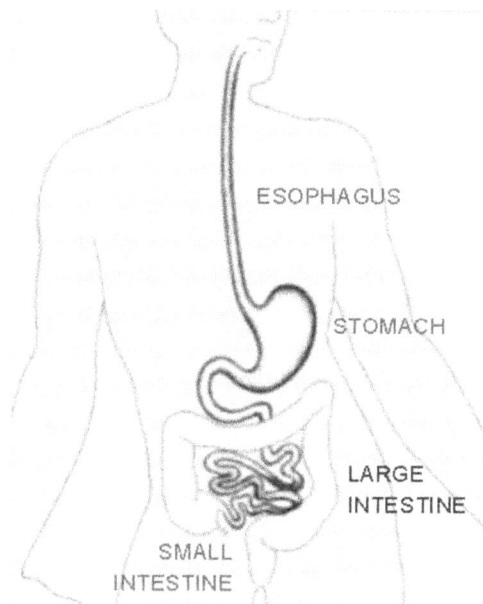

Figure 1: The alimentary canal is a continuous tube with separated stations, functions, chemistries, and kinds of awareness.

Home to Roost

There is something of merit here. I'm not sure if damage was done by the trauma of the ayahuasca, or by my conjuring into existence entities from inside myself that would have been better left undisturbed. Shamans say that disempowerment is a sign of loss of soul connection, and ayahuasca is about as shamanic a thing as one can get.

Yet, the idea is not so different from the idea of "organ dialect," put forward 100 years ago by Alfred Adler. Today Adler is called "the father of humanistic psychology," but most of his work has been forgotten.

Adler's idea was that the body harbors an understanding of systems of which the mind is only faintly aware. From this follows the idea that trauma can root in the body and that dysfunctions of the body can migrate to conflicts of the mind.

His idea of "organ jargon" was not meant literally, but he was serious in saying that our "fiction" of reality becomes our blueprint for development and behavior. This is pretty close to saying that one's dialog with others, oneself, and one's organs become your operating manual.

The implication is that changing the text—the fiction—creates an actual change. If this is the case, the "fiction" is not entirely fictitious. After all, we never perceive reality, only our fanciful version of it.

My conditions have improved since I made a personal investment, "rolled up my sleeves and got to work," you might say. It cannot be denied that directing conscious energy—simply attending to the flow of energy—through a troubled organ creates a higher level of engagement and attunement than remaining powerless and disengaged. But what is the prognosis?

How far can we take this? I do not know, but I've met some characters who might.

References

Adler, A. (1956). *The Individual Psychology of Alfred Adler*. Edited by H. L. Ansbacher and R. R. Ansbacher. Harper Torchbooks.

S13 – Liver and the Lack of Sleep

February 10, 2019

In Traditional Chinese Medicine, the liver is the body's most important organ.

"One of the liver's main functions is spreading and regulating the flow of Qi (energy) in the body and in the mind. It is similar to springtime when there is a burst of motion and life, as compared to winter when the energy is still and low."— **Michael Perfetto**, MSOM, LAc, acupuncturist & Chinese herbalist

TCM and Gut Function

"According to Traditional Chinese medicine (TCM)… the liver holds 'the soul'; it is associated with the fire element and it is considered more important than the heart, an organ full of energy and powers, making it extremely important to cleanse the liver regularly. The liver manages everything, including moderating mental activity. In TCM, it is thought that if qi (chi, our vital energy) is unable to flow along the liver meridian, it ends up concentrating in the organ and showing up as irritability, insomnia, depression, anguish, melancholy, and doubt…"
— **Dr. Irina Matveikova** (2014)

TCM provides a unique description of physiology during sleep, and the psychology related to it. It divides up the period between 11 PM and 7 AM into four sections, with a distinct energy dominating each. You'll find summaries of this on many websites. TCM ascribes insomnia to imbalances of these energy systems.

A comprehensive 2016 article by Leslie Korn reviews gut function from a Western perspective, focusing on digestive chemistry and recent insights into the Enteric Nervous System. Chapter 7 of Roger Jahnke's (1997) *The Healer Within, Using Traditional Chinese Techniques to Release Your Body's Own Medicine*, deals specifically with meditation and deep relaxation.

The Body Clock

According to Traditional Chinese Medicine, the periods between 11 PM-1 AM, 1 AM-3 AM, and 3 AM-5 AM have the following associations.

11 PM - 1 AM: Gallbladder

According to TCM, the gallbladder "is responsible for what is exact and just." Waking during this time could involve the processing of indecisiveness and resentment. It is also associated with insufficiency—specifically, being fearful about choices or outcomes; a lack of courage, initiative, and assertiveness. The gallbladder is a pivot between courage and fear.

1 AM - 3 AM: Liver

During this time, toxins are released from the body, and new blood is made. Waking during this time could involve problems with detoxification. Waking between 1AM - 3 AM may result from repressed anger, resentment, frustration, irritability, or bitterness. The eyes are the sensory organ related to the liver.

3 AM - 5 AM: Lungs

If woken, consider nerve-soothing exercises involving breathing and body relaxation. Your body is heating up, so you will be more comfortable if you keep yourself warm. The lungs are associated with feelings of grief and sadness, either the expression or the repression of them.

5 AM - 7 AM: Large Intestine

The large intestine is all about "letting go" physically and emotionally. Emotions like depression, irritability, discouragement, distress, separation, compulsiveness, confusion, guilt, and regret. Physical issues of elimination pertain to the colon, rectum, skin, bloating, or dehydration.

I don't hold to a rigid interpretation of the TCM clock or its times. The quoted segments of the clock are flexible, as the methods by which we understand the clock are flexible. And the "organs" referred to by TCM are not the organs we know in Western medicine. TCM organs are analogs of those in Western medicine, but do not perform the same functions. TCM is concerned with energies and coordination, not objects operating separately from each other.

The TCM clock offers useful suggestions for insomnia, but your clock may differ slightly depending on your constitution, habit, schedule, genetics, health, life situation, and the season. I invite you to consider the idea of a sequence of physically different cycles and emotional states throughout the night.

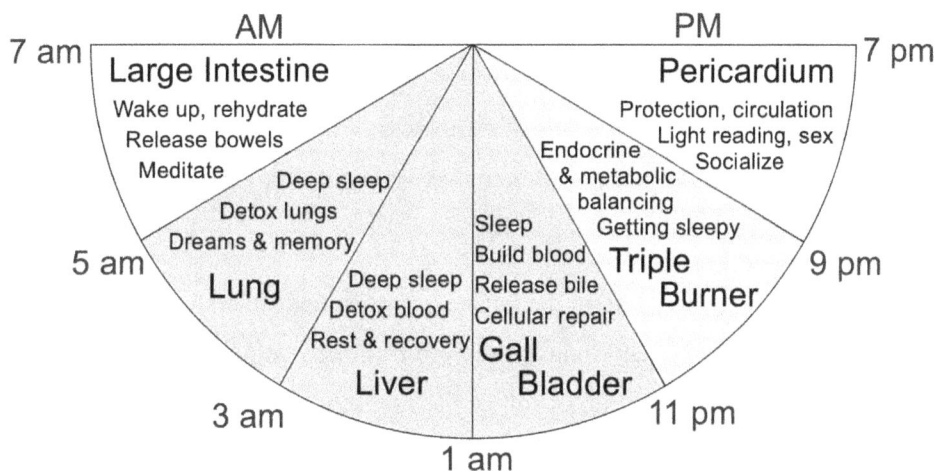

Figure 2: Traditional Chinese Medicine ascribes times of day to metabolic processes.

Trance and Guided Visualization

I work with these issues using guided visualizations, trance, and hypnosis. I use these tools to help my clients isolate their feelings, amplify their sensitivity to those feelings, and better coordinate their connections, resources, and needs.

Our physical body, daily schedule, and emotional pathways are dynamically interconnected and relatively invisible to us. We see the surface of our body, but cannot see and rarely envision what's inside it. Trying to focus one's attention, follow the body's clues, and reconfigure one's energies feels like chasing a flock of birds, or a school of fish: they seem to go every which way.

It is relatively easy to attend to the breath, pulse, or digestion, and so to focus on the lungs, heart, and large intestine. It is hard to imagine sensations of the liver and gallbladder, as their musculature and operations are beyond our conscious control. For these, we must use our imagination by recalling whatever sensations and emotions are familiar. By creating a picture and feeling, we can reconnect to these otherwise overlooked parts of ourselves.

We can do this by relaxing and focusing on selected perceptions. Then, we move into a state that invites the emergence of feelings, ideas, and emotions. Finally, we attune to inclination, intuition, and subtle perceptions that we otherwise obscure with agitation, cogitation, irritation, tension, and our nearly incessant mental chatter.

We want to experience multiple levels of awareness and recognize ourselves as composed of multiple personalities with different levels of awareness. We want to recognize our obsession with certain issues and how we react in compulsive ways, to relax these reflex behaviors, and to regain the ability to regulate ourselves.

I have created a guided visualization to connect you with your liver. The purpose is to gain a perception of yourself and your environment viewed from a place where clarity and purity are paramount. This might be a new sense of self or the strengthening of an existing self.

This is the personality that you want to evoke and adopt when you awake between 1 AM and 3 AM, when the Chinese medicine clock says your body is working with these energies. Also, it is an awareness of self based on purity and cleansing, such as would serve you if you're dealing with chronic liver issues. This will benefit all of us by supporting our liver's function at all times of day.

After completing this visualization, I can place my awareness in my liver. I hear bodily signals. From this state of mind, I believe I can better pay attention to my liver and its signals, much as you can suddenly hear each word of a muffled conversation once you know what words are being said. And it cannot be denied that you have liver sensations. They say the liver itself has no sensation, but its membranes and ducts do.

Listen to this audio file daily, for seven consecutive days. As with all hypnotic audios, only listen when you can give it your full and undivided attention, and when there will be no danger should the tape put you to sleep. In fact, expect to fall into a light sleep. As always, do only what feels right. Be consistent, educate yourself, and be flexible.

Liver Connection (An Induction)

Liver Connection is a hypnotic induction. **DO NOT** listen to this recording while you're driving a car, operating machinery, or doing anything that requires your attention.

Let's distinguish two types of emotions in our thoughts: emotional reactions and emotional inclinations. Emotional reactions are reflexes of peace or threat that originate in our lower brain. Inclinations are feelings of synchrony or conflict seated in our second brain, our enteric nervous system, our gut. This may not be clear to you, it may not seem right to you, so let's ask your gut to help explain it.

I want to talk to your organs as if they were parts of your mind. If not parts, then personalities with particular voices and attitudes. Let's start a dialog with those parts of your body with whom you rarely speak. I would like to give voice to your sense of clarity, the sense that things are cleansed and flowing smoothly. I would like to build a dialog and give voice to your liver.

Find a relaxed position, settle into it, and let awareness sink into your body. Take a slow breath, fill your lungs, pull air into your belly and close your eyes. We'll count down from ten as a way of sinking into your body.

Begin at ten; slowly exhale and feel your awareness moving down from your head into your neck. Then count nine and feel yourself seated in your throat, in the place of your voice. With eight, exhale to a place between your shoulders, feeling the weight of your shoulders. Exhale to seven, to a place high in your chest, behind your collar bone. Six, exhale, and relax into your heart, getting a sense of your pulse. Five, going down into the center of your chest, behind your solar plexus, a place of sensitivity and power.

Now we're at four, and I want you to relax into the sensation of being inside yourself, leaving your external sensations far away. Feeling the space in your lungs, shielded by your ribs. Three, moving lower, feeling yourself centered in your stomach, muscular, enclosed, and contained. Relax your stomach. Exhaling to two, finding a place beyond or beside your stomach, at the edge of awareness, beyond your sensation. This is your intestines, your upper gut. A second skin, fully contained but external and alien in every way. Inhale... exhale, to finally arrive at one, behind the gut, to the mediator of what's outside you and what's inside you. If your gut is a machine, then this is who controls it, a very natural intelligence. This is the domain of your liver.

It's paradoxical we feel little connection to our liver. It is our largest internal organ, holding much of our blood, having a greater chemical effect on the rest of our system than any other organ. If the brain is the center of our electrical awareness, the liver is the center of our chemical awareness, yet we think nothing of it. Let me suggest that this is not so. That we think so much from our body's chemical point of view that we are totally at its service. That it has a hand in all our aspects.

You may need to go back and forth a few times. Move back to your stomach, then down to your intestines, and then down farther still to what lies beneath it. Imagine thoughts are chemicals. Maybe not the whole thought, but aspects of it. And it's true: each thought has many colors and meanings, many directions, memories, and consequences. If thoughts were faces, then consider their many features. If your awareness is a stage, then your brain sets the characters, and your liver sets the lighting, and how little we are aware of the lighting of the scene.

Look for the visceral, look for the chemistry that, like weather, blows in from overhead. Our fear of blood and our sense of life are rooted inside us, not in the lungs, the heart, or the bowels, but in the liver. That very large and central place between our heart and our bowels where chemicals are made and molecules assembled. It is our financial district, where it's all business mixed with nuance and implication.

Take this moment to place yourself very small in that central space inside yourself. Be silent, ask for permission to be present, ask for an audience. Commit to keeping your brain and mouth closed, and your ears and eyes open. Create a picture of this place in your mind. Maybe it's a garden, an armchair, or a view out a window over a distant landscape. See or hear what may seem like static at first, as if you are reading a ticker tape of your own internal chemistry. A sound like wind, crickets, or pebbles in a stream. Listen to the fleeting feelings, nuances, and subtle suggestions. What comes to you?

Imagine you're in a space with the odd shape of your liver, pushed into the corner of a cube. Pushed flat between the balloons of your gut and lungs. Such a squeezed shape for such a soft and sensitive organ. An organ as delicate as your brain but flexible, protected by the muscles and ribs around it, located at your center. Imagine its feelings are central, too. Feelings and associations are central to you, the first flickers of insight and inclinations that lead to insights. Ask yourself what do you feel about your own ability to make thoughts pure, clean, and vital. To make your body pure, clean, and vital.

If thoughts were voices, these voices would come from elders with calmer, quieter tones. Take a calm breath, slow your breath down, and settle into your elderhood, a kind of undercurrent of your own personality, a space inside yourself. Focus on awareness, focus on subtle feelings. What sort of clarity do you need? What kind of cleaning out would benefit you? If you were clearer, what would you see? What would you feel? Feel that now: clear, light-hearted, unburdened, connected. Clear, light-hearted, unburdened, connected... Are you able to hear the origin of your own voice, sense the quiet between your thoughts? Are those spaces clear? What does clarity feel like? What feelings come to you?

Settle into those feelings now, rafting down a gentle river, flowing under a crescent moon. Imagine that your body has tides, and the tides rise to sweep away old thoughts and the debris that settles around you like dust and broken twigs. Like a sudden cloudburst whose flood waters course through your ventricles and arteries, and your liver, more than just a filter, metabolizes everything from fats and carbohydrates to proteins and hormones.

Imagine if you had to know what your liver had to do. You would not know where to start. We make decisions, we shop for groceries, we do the laundry, but can you imagine an organ that handles all the biochemistry for your body? We talk about higher intelligence and wonder about life on other planets. How would they think, how would they act, what would they want?

There is an intelligence in your liver that was born knowing, that is constantly adapting, dealing with new things, and maintaining balance despite what you do and how you live. Where are all these instructions? Do you think this organ is just some kind of vending machine? Is it anything less than a supercomputer? Is its intelligence "artificial"? Do you think that you're aware of much? Doesn't your liver speak to you? Doesn't it stand to reason that it would? Can you hear it? Can you hear it if you try?

Take another breath and try, or imagine, that you are breathing for your liver, that you are breathing for the chemistry of your body, and that the gases your lungs exchange, that you can feel in the difference of your inhale and your exhale, mix, exchange, release, and distill in well-ordered sequences handled deep inside you. Take a breath, hold it for a calm instant, then let it out.

At the count of ten, you are at the center of your body, in your liver's foreign and blood infused world. Counting down to nine, let yourself out, to grow larger, to move out to some perspective. Eight brings you back to your stomach, outside your inner body, passing the world you eat. Seven takes you to your lungs, back into the air and light. Six, and you're passing your heart, mixing the blood and air which never touch. Five and you're up beneath your collar bone, holding up a shoulder on either side. Four to your esophagus that channels air and liquid, but always in different directions. Three into your throat that sometimes speaks the thoughts you think. Two, rising through your face, into your head, into your mind and the small thoughts that have nothing to do with the infinite complexity of how your body works in every second. And one, to be back watching the world outside, like a sentry on eternal guard duty whose shift ends once each day, when you sleep. And zero, the empty mind: this world, this day, this room. Eyes open, clear, remembering the journey, sensitive to your body.

Liver Connection is a hypnotic induction — **DO NOT** listen to it while driving a car, operating machinery, or doing anything that requires your attention.

Listen to a streaming MP3 audio reading of *Liver Connection*:
https://www.mindstrengthbalance.com/mindwp/wp-content/uploads/2020/02/Liver-Connection.mp3

References

Jahnke, R. (1997). *The Healer Within, Using Traditional Chinese Techniques to Release Your Body's Own Medicine.* HarperCollins

Korn, L. E. (2016 Dec). "The Second Brain: Trust Your Gut." *The Neuropsychotherapist, 4* (12). https://drlesliekorn.com/wp-content/uploads/2022/11/2_SP_The-Second-Brain_Trust-your-Gut_2016.pdf

Matveikova, I. (2014). *Digestive Intelligence: A Holistic View of Your Second Brain.* Findhorn Press.

S14 – Sex Addiction

September 15, 2021

In the chakra system, sex addiction relates to a blockage of energy at the second level.

"Once we open up to the flow of energy within our body, we can also open up to the flow of energy in the universe." — **Wilhelm Reich, MD,** psychoanalyst

Context

Sex addiction is a compulsion to sexual thoughts and actions that blocks emotional awareness. It creates an unconscious separation between healthy and unhealthy behaviors.

The first three chakras are survival, reproduction, and power, which all focus on the forces of life. Sexuality follows survival and precedes power. Sexual addiction is a retarded growth of sexual energy that both compensates for and prevents the development of power, love, communication, intuition, and spirituality.

A sexually addicted person cannot manage their sexual behavior. It does not mean more or less sexual activity. It means sexual injury blocks a person's development. The situation is an addiction because one's behavior cannot be controlled. One acts compulsively.

Sexual perversion is common in our society because we emphasize power but deny our access to it. This is power in all forms, in particular the power to be independent. Lacking autonomy and burdened with a sense of scarcity, many people's consciousness festers in the sexual energy that is the limit of what they have access to and control over.

Compulsivity is defined by actions taken in public and private, and social norms operate in both realms. The notion of obsessive thoughts requires a measure of how often and how strong normal thoughts are expected to be. Social metrics are an inaccurate measure of what is healthy for any individual. They are only a rough gauge of what is compulsive.

Sexual thoughts are triggered by our environment and our hormonal levels. In order to define sexual thoughts as excessive, it's necessary to establish what's normal. The notion of sex

104

addiction is contentious among academics, as most academics have a limited understanding of the intellectual, emotional, and spiritual breadth of the issue. Sex addiction is as much an issue of hypo-sexuality, or sexual anemia, as it is of hyper-sexuality.

Vaguely defined as a sexually centered maladjustment in the 1987 third edition of the Diagnostic and Statistical Manual® (DSM), mention of it has been removed from subsequent editions. The objection to its inclusion in the latest version of the DSM, the DSM V published in 2013, was that the idea lacked both research and definition as an addiction.

In 2016, the American Association of Sexuality Educators, Counselors and Therapists, the official body for sex and relationship therapy in the United States, stated that the notion of sexual addiction lacks "empirical evidence to support the classification... as a mental health disorder" (AASECT, 2017). Those who apply the term today apply it based on the social norms of a sexually distorted society.

Sexuality

A person's sexuality is affected by age, family, culture, social role, self-image, metabolism, and history (Hall 2011). Any of these could amplify or reduce desires or fixations otherwise considered normal. Disruptive developmental events include exposure to pornography, sexual abuse, religious training, a mentally disturbed environment, limited maturity, social or family expectations, and drugs.

Since one's personality is created in childhood, child abuse is life-changing. Childhood sexual abuse can both amplify or reduce the future role of sexuality. It can distort sexuality into abnormal, unhealthy, self-destructive, and anti-social forms. It is interesting that sexual addiction is singled out as an excessive fixation on sexual behavior when unhealthy sexuality can manifest as either excessive or insufficient thoughts or actions.

What our society considers healthy sexuality is not healthy; our society is sexually perverted. Sexuality, a canary in the coal mine, has been sick for thousands of years. Civilization's lack of spiritual balance has its roots in its unbalanced attitudes toward sexuality. We are fixated on sex because we cannot achieve healthy relationships that include sexuality.

Like all things spiritual, sexuality cannot be defined by thoughts and behaviors alone. Normal acts and ideas do not define sexuality just as they do not define psychology; one needs to understand emotions and awareness. A person can talk and behave normally and still be compromised. Without a full description of sexuality—such as what might be present in the chakra or some other body-mind system—it's not possible to describe the normal or recognize the abnormal.

Maladjustment

Family conditions that predispose a person to sexual maladjustment include child abuse and compulsive or addictive family behaviors. Families that are emotionally or morally impaired pass this on to their children, who manifest these imbalances in adulthood. If a child cannot repair their damaged patterns, they'll display them as adults, and likely pass them to their progeny.

There are arguments in the literature regarding the genetic factors of sexual behavior, and while behavior is not associated with one's chromosomes, it is shaped by one's epigenetic predispositions. A person predisposed to being sensitive and frightened will be damaged by an insensitive and exploitative family environment and likely carry childhood traumas into adulthood.

Social forces mix character and family issues to amplify or degrade a person's sexual behaviors. Sexual degradation of women, which has prevailed in Western culture for millennia, has created sexual dysfunction at all levels. Sexual attitudes that prevail in social castes confuse sexuality, gender, morality, power, authority, and spirit. The gender dimorphism and related ambiguities we see today have more to do with systemic sexual perversion than they do with gender.

Sexual addiction is typically associated with impulsive desire, excessive engagement, and being unable to control behavior that negatively affects one's life. Not recognized is what could be called sexual aversion, anxiety, phobia, or frigidity. These are widespread, almost to the point of being taken as normal. A lack of sexuality also leads to compulsive, distorted, and dysregulated behaviors.

Sexual addicts are recognized by their extreme character, but the notion of extreme is relative. Some symptoms may be obviously excessive, but there are many in-obvious symptoms of sexual maladjustment that may never be noticed or recognized for the dysfunction they really represent.

Maladjusted behaviors might include an obsession with intercourse, but may also be an obsession with an aversion to intercourse. Sexual maladjustment can throw any aspect of the psyche out of balance. Ultimately, it isn't sexuality that is the problem; it is the management of the sexual energy that underpins the psyche.

Lust is a dominant theme associated with negative traits, such as exploitation, anger, dominance, frustration, power, or self-worth. One's erogenous zones can become overly sensitive, active, or responsive. They can also become deprived of sense, activity, and response so that sexual satisfaction is impossible (Mayo Clinic).

Religious traditions that eschew sexuality are dysfunctional. Sexuality is a necessary component of survival. Sex-denying traditions reveal their role as exploitative institutions. Not that they cannot serve a positive social role, just as the military can serve a positive social role, but they cannot foster full human potential.

I recall an extreme cult I encountered years ago in New York City based on a combination of Gnosticism, asceticism, and Catholicism. The leader insisted adherents reject all sexual thoughts, become celibate, divest all material attachments, and give money to him.

My partner at the time was being sucked in by this cult. I thought the malicious intent was obvious, but I did not understand the nature of my partner's illness. I pulled her out of that orbit, but other manifestations of the dysfunction ultimately prevailed because the problem was in her.

> "What is hell? I maintain that it is the suffering of being unable to love."
> — **Fyodor Dostoevsky**

Therapy

Sexual addiction emerges from a chronic lack of satisfaction rather than an addiction to what's satisfying. If the behavior is excessive, it's excessive because its attraction fails to reward. Sexual addiction is related to psychotic and neurotic behaviors and cannot be understood based on actions alone. For those who are addicted to porn, porn is not the problem, it's their coping mechanism. The problem is their inability to fully express themselves and be recognized for themselves.

Typical addictive behaviors are compulsive stimulation, multiple affairs and hook-ups (one-night stands), uncontrollable pornography, unsafe practice, exhibitionism, voyeurism, pedophilia, and exploitative sex (sadistic or masochistic). Uncontrollable urges are closely related to how one views the world and one's place in it (Francoeur 1994, 25). A person who excessively fixates on sex lacks adequate reflection rather than reflects on sex excessively. They are sexually starving even if they don't recognize it.

Typical underlying beliefs include worthlessness, seeing oneself as unlovable, inability to access deeper meaning or find it in others, an inability to reconcile with one's abuser, who is typically a parent, and a lack of spirit in oneself. The neurochemical high of orgasm temporarily compensates for pervasive emptiness, which is all a person has ever known.

One's addiction can be rooted in anger, frustration, and traumatizing experiences that cannot be accessed through any other means. Frustrated deprivation—indulgence in sex or aversion to it—is an attempt at gratification in the same way that taking more of a drug is an attempt at getting what you need. It's a kind of fixation on one's disabled self that takes you more deeply into what you don't have. As a method of compensating, it's like narcissism.

The sexual addict who seeks therapy is admitting their dissatisfaction. However, people differ on what makes them feel satisfied and in control. The distinction between one's vision of healthy and unhealthy sexual behavior is left largely up to the individual who seeks treatment. A personal balance cannot be based on today's social norms.

Goals

To see sexual addiction as engaging in too much sex misses the underlying dysfunction. To think of sex only as intercourse misses the energy orgasm can carry.

Sexuality has dramatic and distinct aspects. We can hardly manage the physical, emotional, and spiritual energies separately. Behaving as if sex is only intercourse reflects the shallowness of our discourse.

Given how ineffective it is to talk about things we don't understand, it makes sense we cannot see the many parts of sexuality. It makes sense that we have created spirit, emotion, and physical nature as separate and that we project these separate aspects onto others and manifest them as separate presentations.

When you separate things that have a complex relation to each other, it's hard to put them back together. It's like taking apart a jigsaw puzzle. It's hard to speak of them as a unified concept using a language that castes them as different.

One way to regain unity is to invite all the voices back to the table, to engage in a comprehensive conversation. This is the aim of group encounters and group therapy. When insightful voices combine, a greater whole can emerge. The risk is that a voice is missing. If the group lacks a necessary voice, that voice won't be generated through compromise.

I can envision a helpful group around alcohol addiction, but alcohol is simple compared to sex. I cannot envision the same progress from a discussion of sexual dysfunction.

Means

The literature on sex addiction endorses 12-step programs (Griffin-Shelley 1991). Standard addiction protocols focus on abstinence, while protocols for sexual addiction focus on redefining positive sexual activity (Gold 1998). It would be a mistake to aim for sexual abstinence, as one does with drugs and alcohol, since sex is necessary. Sexual addiction is the misuse of a necessary function.

12-step programs engage emotion and spirit, two things missing from clinical therapies of the last 50 years. Emotion and spirit are critical to one's self-image and a balanced relationship with others. They are critical elements of balanced sexuality. There is good reason to believe such programs can help broaden a person's awareness and help them build deeper sexuality.

The standard presentation of 12-step programs is formulaic. This is both a strength and a weakness. Whether one needs more of what these programs offer, or one needs more of what they cannot offer, depends on the person and the program. Joan Zweben (White 2014) shows that 12-step programs have a much greater variety than is supposed, and because of their variety, they should not be dismissed.

Experts, evidence, and standard protocols don't make a theory credible. What is needed is efficacious understanding. In order to draw a line separating normal from obsessive behavior, consider human sexuality in both its social and personal senses. There is no physiologically obvious line in diagnosing sexual addiction (Goodman 1993).

In applying the label of addiction to sexuality, there is the danger of making sexual abstinence a goal. To accept abstinence from sex as a path to recovery is ludicrous. The 2015 film *The Lobster* and the 1990 film *The Handmaid's Tale* are dark explorations of social control of sexual behavior. In both, normality is a nightmare, and medicine "normalizes" people to a degraded level.

Freud put forward a theory of psychological imbalance due to sexual repression. His star pupil, Wilhelm Reich, said psychological balance was based on sexual expression. Both are out of favor these days, but I find insight in both of them.

Reich was ahead of his time in recognizing sexuality as psychologically fundamental (Reich 1974). This is developed further in Tantric yoga, which has a variant in Western Tantra (Hyatt 2012).

It is not surprising that Western culture has smeared Western Tantra as anti-Christ occultism, and Reich as being insane. Academic sexology has avoided this modern witch-burning by casting itself as an eviscerated, objective science, returning sex to a mechanical act. Reich recognized this as dead sexuality, and his insights continue to be condemned.

> "The goal of sexual suppression is that of producing an individual who is adjusted to the authoritarian order and who will submit to it in spite of all misery and degradation."
> — **Wilhelm Reich**, MD, psychiatrist

Ends

Abstinence-based and redirection-based programs have different ends. These programs conceive of "sexual sobriety" as a form of control (Griffin-Shelley 1991) but sexual sobriety is actually a lack of control, it is a frigidity. I am reminded of the 1952 chemical castration of Alan Turing, which was an attempt by the British state to stop the crime of homosexuality. Until sexual addiction is seen for the sexual dysfunction it is, there is little hope of balance.

We live in a society that celebrates sexual sobriety, indulges in sexual excess, and endorses sexual perversion. Reich's endorsement of spiritual sexuality has always made good sense to me. Combining Reich's theory of psychopathy's origin in sexual perversion with Alice Miller's view of psychopathy's origins in childhood abuse (Miller 1998) creates an accurate picture of our perverted society.

References

AASECT (2017 Dec). "AASECT Position on Sex Addiction, American Association of Sexuality Educators, Counselors and Therapists." *Aasect.org*. https://www.aasect.org/position-sex-addiction

Bramwell, D. (2018 Oct)."The Godfather of the Sexual Revolution?" *The Psychologist, 32:* 84-87. https://thepsychologist.bps.org.uk/volume-31/october/godfather-sexual-revolution

Gold, S. N., Heffner, C. (1998). "Sexual Addiction: Many Conceptions, Minimal Data." *Clinical Psychology Review, 18*: 367-381.

Goodman, A. (1993). "Diagnosis and Treatment of Sex Addiction." *Journal of Sex & Marital Therapy, 3*: 225-51.

Griffin-Shelley, E. (1991). *Sex and Love: Addiction, Treatment, and Recovery*. Praeger Publishers.

Francoeur, R. T., Traverner, W. J. (1994). *Taking Sides: Clashing Views on Controversial Issues in Human Sexuality*. Mcgraw-Hill College.

Hall, P (2010 Aug). "A Biopsychosocial View of Sex Addiction." *Sexual and Relationship Therapy, 26* (3): 217-28. https://www.researchgate.net/publication/233377619_A_biopsychosocial_view_of_sex_addiction

Hyatt, C. S. (2012). *Secrets of Western Tantra: The Sexuality of the Middle Path*. The Original Falcon Press.

Mayo Clinic (undated). *Compulsive sexual behavior*. Mayo Clinic.

https://www.mayoclinic.org/diseases-conditions/compulsive-sexual-behavior/symptoms-causes/syc-20360434

Miller, A. (1998). *Thou Shalt Not Be Aware: Society's Betrayal of the Child.* Farrar, Straus and Giroux.

Reich, W. (1974). *The Sexual Revolution: Toward a Self-regulating Character Structure.* Farrar, Straus and Giroux.

White, W. (2014). "Clinical Leadership in Addiction Treatment: An Interview with Dr. Joan Zweben." Chestnut Health Systems. https://www.chestnut.org/resources/eb026800-5f96-4e7f-918b-b6daa3616f9e/2014-percent-20Dr.-percent-20Joan-percent-20Zweben.pdf

S15 – The Worlds Inside You

October 13, 2021

Chi is the sum of the energetic frequencies that run through your body.

"Your family will appreciate that the more Chi-full you are, the more cheerful you are."— **Kenneth S. Cohen**, Qigong Grandmaster

There are things we can think about and there are things we can't. Awareness is an outpost at the boundary, something like a monastery in which we study our reflection. Life seems to drift toward greater awareness, but the force behind this is unclear.

Studying one's reflection is fairly safe. It doesn't compel you to see or act and it has few repercussions. It might lead to insight and action, but that becomes a choice. Self-study is vague and intangible. It offers no guarantee that you'll learn anything.

There are other ways to encounter yourself that are more compelling, that require more of you and have greater returns. Some of these are sex, addiction, illness, depression, mania, service, sacrifice, and exploration. There are others I have pondered but have not tried, and which may also offer paths to some kind of enlightenment, such as war, violence, and insanity.

The obstacle to learning is usually your notion of self. That is why, in shamanic training, one always reaches a point where it is necessary to disintegrate oneself. Anything that takes things apart gets some credit for the subsequent putting of things back together, but neither redemption nor reassembly is guaranteed.

There is no single path to full awareness. But more than that, no one path is sufficient. One needs to follow several paths and gain overall views from several vantage points. There is more to become aware of than any one personality can express.

To stretch the idea to its limit, there is no one personality from which the full scope of one's awareness can be seen. At least, not within what we view as the scope of personality. This is why past life regression therapy can be so liberating; I prefer to call it Alternative Live Exploration, as I believe that makes its value clear.

You either live to pursue many paths, or your path traverses many lives. In this respect, the Buddhist notion of reincarnation makes sense, as full awareness requires seeing the world from the perspectives of many people. Whether these "past lives" were real is a perfect example of how we cannot accept something for what it is, and instead attempt to control it intellectually. The human psyche is not "a reality," it's a construction.

Integrating opposites creates advancement. This is not compromise or reduction, it's expansion and epiphany. Advancement is a process of inclusion, growth, and greater control that differs from progress. Advancement is a state of greater balance, which brings together more cycles, more energy, and larger rhythms. In contrast, progress is simply the reductive process of moving to the next step up, down, or sideways.

Personal Awareness

Few people can stretch themselves enough to see their own reflection. Most people seem averse to recognizing their ignorance. I can't deny it is a painful process, and one for which one is usually punished. You are both reprimanded for failing to join the consensus, and isolated once you achieve new insight.

Punishment comes from within the project, employment, or society that is averse to growth. Anyone who reveals the fallacy of what others believe to be true will probably be struck by the double-edged sword of rejection and dislocation. This is why few people are aware and most strenuously resist any effort to make them so. It is tragic—though it is natural—that the more knowledge you have, the more unaware you are encouraged to become. Creative people are seen as unstable. We keep them away from children. Those who we allow to teach our children are inevitably safe and boring. Teachers are traditionally matronly and nondescript. Prophets inhabit the unstable frontier.

"When I turned six or so... after a shopping trip to a nearby village, (my mother) stopped the car about three miles from home and let me out. She told me that I'd have to find my own way home by talking to people to ask for directions. By the time I arrived, many hours later, she was very apoplectic—she had not accounted for time to stop to look at bugs and inspect rocks. But it worked. I started to become more comfortable interacting with adults and expressing myself."

— **Richard Branson** (2016), business magnate and entrepreneur

Readers of my book *Becoming Lucid, Self-awareness in Sleeping & Waking Life*, explore the reality of our projections. These are the fundamental images we construct of what exists, and on top of which we build our ideas. Disassembling this reality is a good place to start if you hope to find new understanding, but your mind is not your only source of reality. Your body is another.

Tai Chi and Chi Kung (Qigong)

These two traditions are seen as movement arts, and they are that, but they are also arts of awareness. Tai Chi is mostly known as a set of movements that follow a strict order. That order is both a physical series, a series of stories, and a set of spiritual precepts. Most people who practice Tai Chi focus on it as a physical discipline and let its spiritual aspects arise as they will.

Chi Kung places a greater emphasis on energy in the body. It advances the idea that energy governs form. Where Tai Chi teaches that energy follows the form, Chi Kung insists that energy gives life to movement. I have always felt the two traditions are paths to the same destination. Tai Chi for the morning when movement emerges, and Chi Kung for the evening when movement goes inward.

Both traditions require you to release your mind and move into a larger awareness. It is hard to describe this awareness because descriptions are in the mind and of the world, while awareness is of the mind and in the world. Awareness is what descriptions represent. We can talk about greater awareness, but the talk does not make it real. Awareness is an experience, like sight or emotion.

I am working on a book on interoception, the ability to sense your internal functions. At the moment, the book is in pieces. It exists on my website as blog posts and hypnotic audios. The book will be an exploration of what you can sense by focusing on your internal physical self.

Energy and Mechanism

Most Western medical specialists today believe that your mind cannot communicate with the organs and processes of your body. They believe your body is autonomic, that it governs itself, and that your mind exists in a separate world of thoughts. They believe the only connection from the body to the mind is through sensations of pain or pleasure, from your organs to your mind. For these people, the body is a machine, and the mind plays no role in its operation.

This is not the case. The mind and body affect each other through the endocrine, neurological, immune systems and the gut, but these connections are neither obvious nor straightforward. The connections go beyond these mechanical avenues to a level where aspects of the mind actually inhabit our tissues.

I have little interest in arguing the point. It rests largely on levels of awareness that some of us don't have, rather than a deductive conclusion. Eastern healing traditions, which include Tai Chi and Chi Kung, strive to integrate mind and body. They accept the fundamental concept of Chi, or body energy, which is dismissed in the Western tradition.

The Eastern approach to the Western rejection of Chi and the disconnection of our parts is simply to ignore what is ignorant. I am inclined to do the same. This fails to achieve the kind of integration we need, but sometimes there is more to gain by moving forward than by argument.

The Body's Awareness

A chapter of my book on interoception will foster awareness of one's Chi. Perhaps this should be the first chapter, but you could say that learning to sense, follow, and direct your internal life force is the ultimate goal. I will consider it here.

Controlling Chi is part sensation and part imagination. We take sensations as real and what we imagine as fantasy, but this is a mistake. Sensations are as much a creation of our mind as any other image, and the images that we create in our mind can play as fundamental a role in our reality as any sensation (Seth 2019). Let's just say that all sensations are a product of our imagination, and every sensation must be imagined in order for it to become real.

The goal is to focus on any and every part of your body, whether or not you know what sensations are produced by it. We must start by recognizing that most of us have little awareness of any parts of our body other than what's connected to our external sensory nerves. In fact, unless they're athletic, most people in the West don't even know what it means to have a full body awareness.

Between the Hands

If you're standing up, sit down. And if you're sitting down, then drop whatever you're holding and relax. Focus on one part of your body. You could choose anything, and, after we're finished here, I hope you will choose different parts of your body. For now, focus on your hands. We'll do two exercises.

First, with your hands resting palms down, place your focus on the backs of your hands. Let your sensations guide you. Maybe you have sensations in your wrists or your fingertips. Don't stress or flex your hands, but you can look at them. Telescope into the backs of your hands with a tunnel vision that shuts out everything else.

The backs of your hands are aware of temperature. There are tissues and veins and there are many tendons that run over your knuckles and attach to your finger bones. These tendons gather as they pass through your wrists and attach to muscles in your forearms. Simply attend to the feeling in the back of your hands.

Imagine there is an energy that flows through the backs of your hands. It has a sensation that you are not accustomed to, but which is always there. Imagine it as a dark violet color, as if it radiates a black light that's partly heat but more than heat because it flows.

Imagine a pool in an otherwise dry riverbed fed by the stream that flows beneath the gravel. This energy, in the backs of your hands, is like the underground water that flows up from your wrists, across the surface of your hands, and back into your knuckles.

Feel the energy at the surface of your hands partly carried by the blood, but it's not a liquid and cannot not bleed. It's a coordination between all the cells in your hands, a kind of communication that has a rhythm. A frequency you can imagine as something pulsing gently, but also with fast ripples. Like the ripples on a stream that twists over and around large boulders. A flow of white noise, like the noise in your ears that first you hear and then goes away.

Now take a slow breath and feel your chest lift… and your shoulders lift… and feel the breath in your arms, down into your hands like a wave that rides up the beach and then sinks into the sand as the sea rolls back.

Turn your palms facing each other and bring them toward each other just to where each hand senses the other, or separate them so they're just where you feel something between them. Your palms are two to six inches apart and you feel a warmth, a tingle, or a field; something that you can pass your hands through.

Focus on the space between your palms and sense it as a gas or a vapor. It has a form and a boundary. It's something created by your hands that forms more strongly when your hands come closer and begin to dissipate as you move your hands apart. Take a breath… and as you inhale, imagine this ball of energy between your hands growing in form and substance, and as you exhale, feel it losing its color and becoming transparent.

With small motions of your hands, slight and almost imperceptible, sense the size and substance of this energy between your palms. Let the energy swell with the inhale and ebb with the exhale. Feel the energy within your hands, between your hands, created by your hands, and surrounding your hands.

Settle your hands back down, down onto your thighs, the arms of your chair, or by your sides. Let the energy that is lingering in front of you be soaked up by your eyes. It gives you the impression that you can see farther, more clearly, deeper, and into things. Your mind's eye can now see with greater detail, as if images have more meaning, and you can understand symbols and associations.

Let yourself follow this energy to float into a landscape of indistinct vistas and unrecognized characters. Let your images be populated by pleasant memories taken from welcoming opportunities from the past. And when you daydream, imagine this energy filling your mind to give you super-sight.

Think back to what we're talking about now, the awareness of sensation, imagination, and your mind. States of focus and concern, or states of reverie, dreams, relaxation, and emptiness. These are the mental aspects of physical awareness. You can use your body to explore the limits of your mind. Any body state that captures your attention is a vehicle to greater awareness.

If you're interested in going further with this exploration of sensation and awareness, then read my book, *Becoming Lucid, Self-Awareness in Sleeping & Waking Life*. You can get it from my website as a set of printable PDF files and downloadable audio MP3 files. Use this link:

https://www.mindstrengthbalance.com/product/becoming-lucid-access-to-book-and-audio-files/

Printed, audiobook, and digital formats are available through most major online booksellers.

References

Branson, R. (2016 July 28). My mother's unconventional parenting lessons. Richard Branson's Blog. Retrieved from: https://www.virgin.com/branson-family/richard-branson-blog/my-mothers-unconventional-parenting-lessons

Seth, A. K. (2019 Sep 1). The neuroscience of reality, *Scientific American, 321* (3). Retrieved from: https://www.scientificamerican.com/article/the-neuroscience-of-reality/

Thoughts

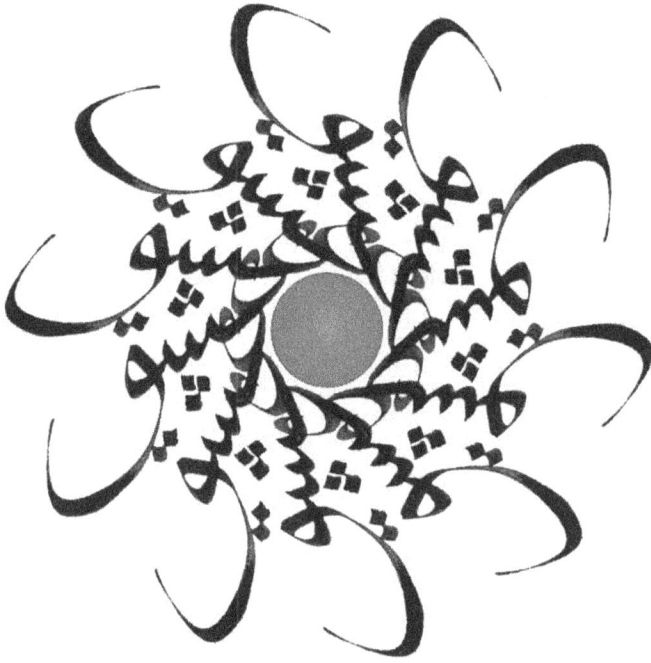

T1 – How Smart Are You, and How Would You Know?

April 27, 2023

No one is average, and no one's problems are the same.
Being unsure of yourself is a healthy attitude.

"I know that I am intelligent because I know nothing." — **Socrates**

Does Intellect Make You Smart?

This has to be one of the more useless statements ascribed to Socrates. But then, Socrates wrote nothing, so whatever "Socrates said," is being said by someone who isn't secure enough to say it themselves.

We're told that Plato spoke for Socrates and that Plato is no slouch, but who knows? Yesterday's Plato may have been today's Tucker Carlson. According to Peter Kingsley (1999), there was a lot of horse trading going on in Greece in the age before Christ, and Plato was a salesman.

Regardless of how arrogant or humble we might appear, each of us acts on what we strongly feel. This brings us back to the question: how smart are you? Most of us answer that question by deferring to authority to judge our success. But success is more of a reflection of the environment in which you operate than an indication of the depth or breadth of your skill.

We look to certification, education, or success to substantiate a person's authority. This may be the wrong thing to do because authority represents enforcement or consensus, not knowledge or insight. My answer is that a person's experience is the best indicator of their skills and intelligence. Having a good intellect does not make you smart.

At present, my greatest insights are ideas I'm still working to develop. They may never be published for others to see and they may never be recognized, but they won't be less insightful for that reason. I know something, and I don't care what that makes me.

The Dunning Kruger Effect

Ignorant

Confidence

Average

Informed

Knowledge

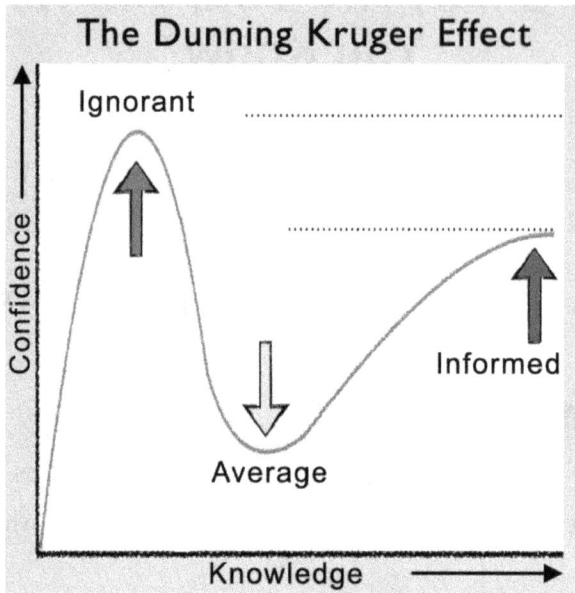

Figure 3: Knowing less fosters more confidence than knowing more.

The Dunning-Kruger Effect

The Dunning-Kruger effect refers to the tendency of poorly informed people to overestimate their insight, and well-informed people to underestimate theirs. The result is that most people who speak out are the poorly informed. Those with limited knowledge are more likely to form a consensus.

In addition, those who know best are reluctant to speak out. They do not make a majority and rarely establish a consensus.

Dunning-Kruger reminds us that the more you know, the more uncertain you are likely to be. This is not a simple contradiction. It does not mean that the more you learn, the less you know. It means the more complexity you appreciate, the less simplicity attracts you.

You can know the value of your ability without being certain of your conclusions. The real question is not "smart or not smart," it's one's ability to make progress. A trivia expert can sound smart, but a good memory doesn't make a person capable. It depends on the problem. The solution to an unusual problem won't depend on a good memory.

Some people are good problem solvers. It's a skill, but it doesn't mean you're smart. Problems are like puzzles. If you know the tricks of that trade, then you'll be a better problem solver. Some tricks can be learned by rote, but fully solving problems in context takes experience. The best solutions are simple from some perspectives, but not obvious.

I like complex problems, and the problems people bring to me are not simple. The most common elements in the problems brought to me are repetition and inflexibility. There are good reasons for these patterns, but they play an obvious role in causing and perpetuating the problem.

People say, "It's this way because…" or "I do this because…" and right there is the obstacle, staring everyone in the face. It's obvious to everyone, and pointing it out doesn't solve the problem, but it provides a path to the problem's root. Aversion to solutions grows out of the problem itself.

The path of flexibility is the path that people don't want to take. People suffer emotional problems because they won't change what they consider to be their reasonable attitude. The more reasons you have, the more difficult it is to reconcile them.

There is another type of problem: the disguised problem. Disguised problems are unusually reasonable. They make us feel certain that another party is at fault. The conflict is clearly in the spotlight, and you are separate from it. But if you want a solution, you must step into the spotlight.

What is hidden are the underlying interests and motivations. Like a proxy war, there is conflict, combatants, and a battlefront, but these represent conflicts over deeper issues. People who bring these sorts of issues to me are dealing with two problems. The first is for them to see beyond the problem they're presenting—and they don't want to. The second is to confront the real problem that underlies it. They want to do that even less!

Here is where "being smart" becomes ambiguous. The smart person finds a new solution by recognizing a different problem, but this will not win the proxy war being fought on the surface. This surface war might be their crumbling relationship or their lack of success in some endeavor.

The real problem is a deeper conflict, it's a conflict that a person is having with themselves. They cannot grasp this until they reformulate their conflict. Their problem is with themselves, and the solution is not a compromise, it's a reconstruction of the situation toward different goals.

I often see quite a different picture when I look behind the curtains, but those in struggle rarely want me to see differently, and will not consider an alternative. We are defined by the story we tell ourselves, and we cling to those stories for many reasons. Addictive behavior is typical.

The reason usually comes down to fear and pain: "Better the devil that you know than the devil you don't," as the saying goes. This means people would rather continue to fight the endless war they're familiar with. They conceive this as something outside themselves, and from which they have built protective battlements. They cling to their self-esteem and the illusion of control. They don't want to consider a new self-image that lacks protection and has an uncertain outcome.

Common Versus Average

Most of us deal with common problems. Most of these are not as common as they appear, and they'll have uncommon solutions. Our uncommon solutions will be particular to us. They won't be well known or understood, and we won't find much help with them. People come to counselors like me with their uncommon problems. My skill is discerning truth and recognizing need.

Dealing with common problems and living a common life is not the same as average. Average is a concept that can be measured. Common is a judgment that people agree on. We confuse the two. Many people live common lives with common problems; no one is average, and I have yet to see an average problem.

Average is a mathematical construct that I find to be largely useless. Allopathic medicine uses averages to diagnose and prescribe, which is why allopathic medicine rarely works for non-average people. It is also why allopathic medicine doesn't work for mental health.

Imposter Syndrome Can Be a Good Thing

"Talent hits a target no one else can hit; genius hits a target no one else can see."
— **Arthur Schopenhauer**

We confuse talent with intelligence, and genius with talent, and Arthur Schopenhauer is not helping. To hit a target is to show success on a pre-established measure. A measure that's clear and accepted.

The target of a problem that's intelligently approached is often different from what is presumed. And the target of insightful genius is rarely seen as a target at all, and may not even be a target in any game-like sense.

Imposter Syndrome describes the situation where a person presents themselves as capable, and is accepted as capable, in a role for which they feel incapable. In short, they feel themselves a fraud or a phony.

But return to the insights of Dunning-Kruger: the most capable people question their conclusions. The least capable people can be the most confident. The implication is that feeling unqualified is a sign of greater understanding of one's problems and oneself, while being firmly confident reflects an inflated self-opinion.

It's a given that no one is average, but many problems are common, and the more capable you are, the more circumspect you will be. Imposter syndrome should not only be expected, it should be required!

"The test of a first-rate intelligence is the ability to hold two opposed ideas in mind at the same time and still retain the ability to function."
— **F. Scott Fitzgerald**

And so it is that the most capable people are the first to recognize and reveal their limitations. Those who defer or deflect their limitations—the expert or the blameless—are the least trustworthy.

True Imposters Are Something Else

There are true imposters, and they present a difficult problem. These people do not doubt themselves; they are quite confident. They are also disconnected from the truth of the situation and from themselves. This is not mental illness or emotional imbalance, it's psychopathy, and it's much more common than is supposed.

A true imposter knows what to think and how to act, and they do these things, but they don't know how to feel. This would be acceptable under normal circumstances, but the true imposter maintains abnormal circumstances.

The problem with true imposters is they, like everyone, are guided by their feelings and not by their thoughts. We have criteria for evaluating thoughts, but few for evaluating feelings. The psychopath lives in a world of feelings you would not recognize, and so they keep their feelings hidden, if they have any at all. They contrive reasons and invent feelings.

Our thoughts are adaptable to any situation. We can justify any actions and our commitment to reason can always be revised. This is a good thing because reason can justify anything. You can't rely on reason for altruism, empathy, or good behavior. A civil society depends on people being in resonance with each other, and a true imposter has no resonance.

True imposters are the reason I reject religion. Religion is a fine container for the spirituality of feeling people, but it is a common hiding place for true imposters. Imposters hide in places where people's thoughts and behaviors are prescribed. We also find them in institutions, corporations, schools, churches, and the military.

The Special Danger of Religion

In most institutions, there remains a need for empathy, feeling, and resonance. That need may only appear within the level of your colleagues, but people still expect you to be human sometimes. Religion, in its attempt to provide a structure for spirit and morality, provides a complete map of virtue. If you follow all the precepts of your religion, then all of your virtues are accounted for. If you follow religious dogma to the letter, then you never need to reveal yourself to yourself or others.

> "Spiritual bypassing simply means that you use spiritual concepts, platitudes, or
> activities to 'bypass' or avoid dealing with your true feelings, especially the hard
> ones like anger, grief, fear, loneliness, envy, and shame. It doesn't work."

126

— **Alison Cook** (2023), faith-based psychotherapist

This presents a danger for all religious people. How do you know your piety is real? Do prayers absolve you of your sins? Who calls you to account? If you showed your true feelings, would you still be a good person?

One is not called to ask such questions of oneself in a corporation or the military, but you are asked to absolve yourself of sin in the church. And because you cannot, the church provides absolution for you. Absolution for anything amounts to absolution for nothing.

I believe these are questions we should ask ourselves. Outside of religion, where we take responsibility for our own moral choices, we can ask these questions of ourselves. As healthy people, we can see our failures, cope with them, understand their origins, and become better for them. We do not need to seek the forgiveness of a higher power. Flaws, like failures, are a normal consequence of learning. We redeem ourselves by questioning, trying, failing, learning, and improving.

We all need to know what we're hiding from ourselves. If you feel guilty of imposter syndrome, then you're wise. You're being realistic. If you feel immune from questioning yourself, or if you have no true feelings and are not bothered by this, then I urge you to call me before you do more damage. A person detached from their feelings is a danger to everyone, including themselves.

References

Cook, A. (2023 Jan 8). "The Danger of Bypassing Your Emotions." *ChurchLeaders.com*. https://churchleaders.com/outreach-missions/outreach-missions-articles/371050-the-danger-of-bypassing-your-emotions.html

Kingsley, P. (1999). *In the Dark Places of Wisdom.* The Golden Sufi Center.

T2 – Why It's Dangerous to Believe What You Think

Jan 6, 2023

People who believe what they think don't learn otherwise.

"Memories of emotional events are stamped on running water." — **Aristotle**

James lives in the house next to mine. He was born with Klinefelter syndrome, a relatively common genetic condition that can go unnoticed. George Washington is purported to have had the condition. In James's case, Klinefelter has seriously impaired his development. While chronologically 57, James is an adolescent. He looks like an adult but has the mind of a young teenager.

We make many assumptions about people's thoughts and behaviors. This is the reason age groups segregate. By limiting contact, they assure group members think alike. People in different age groups don't understand each other. It's not just a difference in fashion, it's a difference in thinking.

You First Think What You Feel

There is truth in speaking of the mind in terms of the brain's layers: the deeper you go, the more primitive things get. Our cerebral cortex is a thin layer on the outside of our brain, and this is where all of our human thought is said to be processed. Not that this can really be defined, but the things that humans do are done here. This includes language, logic, problem solving, and reason.

Every thought has some motivation, and motivation is rarely reasonable. We find reasons for our thoughts after some needs have directed us to think, but the origin is need. Even emergencies are situations of need, and we execute a particular kind of thinking in emergencies, but mostly we respond by reflex.

Emergencies Create Thought Tunnels

"Anxiety is dangerous, but it makes you think it's your friend."
— **Noah Baumbach**

In simple situations, like emergencies, our thoughts run along behind our actions. Even when we don't have an immediate response, we have reflexive thoughts. These are the associations we draw from similar situations. Sometimes we think about the present and make calculated guesses, but usually we remember the past and make assumptions. In threatening situations, most of our thinking is pessimistic, and it should be as avoiding trouble is a priority.

If there is anything that could be defined as the opposite of trauma, it would be a positive attitude in a troubled situation. I remember a long fall off the biggest mountain in the Canadian Rockies. During the fall, which extended 500 feet, I kept a continuous, positive attitude. As a result, I suffered no trauma. On another occasion, after two days of wet hiking through a trackless, boggy river valley, I was in high spirits. I was manically light-hearted, as I recall—in a transcendently joyful state under the conditions of a miserable adventure.

I could hardly claim logic was at work in either case, though perhaps my reactions were effective in those situations. I suppose that if being anxious would have been helpful, then the more rational response would have been to be anxious. But in both cases, there was nothing to be done other than to be positive.

Most Thoughts Are Reflex Associations

"Logic is necessary; since without it, you cannot even learn whether it is necessary or not."
— **Epictetus**

Thinking is mostly responsive. We think for several purposes, and the primary purpose is to ensure our safety. The second purpose to which we apply ourselves is to gain benefit.

Few of our thoughts result from careful analysis. One might say that few of our actions are thoughtful, but I think that gets us off the hook too easily. Most of our actions are thoughtful. They just are not very smart.

I have trouble with the word stupid. It seems like an important word that we use too casually in our efforts to avoid applying it to ourselves. By watching my neighbor James, I better understand what being stupid means.

If being smart is knowing the truth, then being stupid means believing what you think, regardless of the truth. That could mean you believe what's false, or that you're not concerned with the truth at all. It should be recognized that we never know the absolute truth, and this is where being smart matters. Because the smarter you are, the closer you can come to holding widely different versions of the truth in mind at the same time.

As a therapist, counselor, and coach, my skill is in thinking otherwise. Whatever you or I think, I perform the mental gymnastics to find alternatives. If you might find value in thinking differently, then I can help you.

We Hold People to Different Standards

We excuse the dumb actions of children based on their being unaware of the consequences, and that's true. A highly risk-tolerant person will also do dumb things, but we'll say they knew the risk they were taking, as if that somehow makes them smarter.

I think back on all the high-risk things I did in mountaineering and, while I may have known the risks, I didn't appreciate the consequences. The risk was I might die, but the consequence I overlooked was that my children would never be born. I have to conclude that I acted stupidly, but what were the alternatives?

Risk versus return is the usual refrain, but what if there are several widely different versions of the truth? In the case of my risk taking, the return might have been a healthier self-confidence. I believe I achieved that, and I gained without taunting fate too much. Still, I regret the degree to which I did taunt fate, and I blame my mother.

Blaming one's parents is a convenient reason available to all of us. I believe it was true in my case, and it was certainly true in James' case, but our responses have been different. I outgrew my behavior; James will not.

Learning to Change is Not Coping with the Present

"If anything simply cannot go wrong, it will anyway." — **Murphy's Fifth Law**

There is a difference between conquering and compensating, and a smart person will know the difference. Many of us are not smart enough to see this in ourselves. This is the origin of addictive behavior that's alternately referred to as self-medicating or as a coping strategy. In both cases, we justify it. We use the intelligence at our disposal, and we make a reasoned choice. In situations of stress, trauma, and anxiety, that choice may be wrong in retrospect, but it feels right at the time.

It is not intelligence that leads us to learn. It might be luck, the luck of seeing around a corner to which we're otherwise blind. Most of us go on repeating the same mistakes, following the same logic, and believing the same truth indefinitely. Learning doesn't require intelligence as much as it requires the ability to expand one's awareness.

It's almost ecological: negative situations continue to build on each other until the environment won't support them anymore. We build institutions to support our bad situations, and so extend bad thinking throughout the culture and the world. The mechanisms behind this are wrongheadedness, miseducation, and authority. Institutions create artificial ecologies. They are anti-evolutionary.

Authority Never Allows True Freedom

"The day you think you know everything is the day you become obsolete."
— **Evy Poumpouras**

I am an independent-minded, free learning, anti-authoritarian. I feel this is the smarter thing to be in the long run. In the short run, there is more reward in thinking what others think, believing what others teach, and following the instructions that others give.

James would be better off if he did what he was told to do, as half the time he can't even remember my name. He'll call me Lionel or Leonard. He'll introduce me to his new e-bike multiple times, make a nuisance of himself when he's smoked too much pot, and wash all his clothes twice a day because he thinks he has bed bugs. James' problems go beyond a lack of intelligence. He is a reminder of how the mentally ill can appear normal sometimes. He makes me wonder about other people.

James believes in his truth as much as you and I believe in ours. It's just that we have better minds. But our minds are not that great. I try, and I'm sure you try, but there are things we don't know and can't imagine. It's the imagining part that's especially important.

Stupid Is as Stupid Does, But Not Always

"Do not look down on nonsense. Nonsense comes to power. Nonsense murders millions. It prospers if we are too exquisite, too intellectually respectable to bother with it."
— **Leon Wieseltier**

Several people have called me stupid because I tried to do things I was not good at, but these were important attempts. Those who called me stupid did not, themselves, stretch beyond their comfort range, and as a result, their worlds were smaller than my own. They had greater skills in their domains, but I have more domains, and I continue to add more.

It's hard to rate what another person knows unless they tell you all they know. Even then, the smartest people will regularly go beyond what they know in order to learn more. There are many boundaries and you can't cross them all. Not all boundaries are safe to be crossed.

Seeing the edge of what you know is crucial. Seeing what you cannot see. This is why it's important to have a good imagination. It's important to be creative. It's not that you need to succeed—though perhaps you do when your life depends on it—it's that you need to find other truths. But if you believe what you think, then you'll never even look for them.

T3 - Black Magic and the Millionaire Mind

November 2012

T. Harv Eker's empowerment training is a pyramid scheme.

"Industrial (reality): Reality is external and knowable. Idiomergent (reality): Reality is constructed and negotiable."
— **Harold Linstone** and **Murray Turloff** (2002, 48)

Magic can be any act that causes change through unconscious effects. This includes using your unconscious to facilitate change in yourself. Saying that magic acts through the unconscious doesn't mean that it exists only in the mind, or that it is imaginary. Magical displays are common and are events the causes of which we are not aware. We see as magic any outcome that has no cause.

Magical thinking pervades our culture and is blamed for many poor strategies. It is given little attention in this "age of reason" because magical thinking is hard to predict and difficult to control. The subject is so large as to be approachable from many angles and circumscribed by none: religion, ceremonial magic, education, psychology, pop psychology, anthropology, politics, music, art, and theatre, to name a few.

Distinguishing black from white magic allows a narrower focus. The two are not opposites, but have different objectives. White magic involves a participation with the forces of growth, insight, and service to higher goals, entities, and abstract ideas. Black magic is controlling, self-centered, and extractive.

Black magic can be predatory or parasitic, but, in either case, it is intentional and exploitative in design, tactical in execution, and material in its goal. In contrast, white magic involves faith in a consciousness, design, and goal greater than oneself. Black magic extracts a near-sighted benefit at the expense of another, while white magic creates a far-sighted benefit for all involved.

Mythology is full of magical figures of uncertain intention, such as gnomes, dragons, and aliens. These figures are "real" but not in a scientific sense, at least not yet. The nature of their magic is determined by their effects upon innocents. The black versus white dichotomy is wedded to the dialectic of good and evil. Good and evil are manipulated categories, and an examination of intentions reveals shades of grey. It's useful when we can draw the line to say that a program or person is practicing one or the other.

My partner had been working with two marketing coaches when I first encouraged her to attend their free workshop. The issues she's dealt with have been pertinent to marketing and building a professional image for herself. When these coaches recommended a free weekend workshop 90 miles from my home, I took the opportunity.

I have 20 years of experience as a software consultant. I understand "marketing" to mean finding, creating, and maintaining an audience or following, building a brand, a following, or a tribe. In my experience, marketing is a poorly taught and unfairly maligned essential activity in any business.

Marketing

Wikipedia defines marketing as "the process of communicating the value of a product or service to customers." It says, "marketing might sometimes be interpreted as the art of selling products, but selling is only a small fraction of marketing." It's a mistake, though one that's overlooked, to confuse marketing with selling.

Marketing is also sold as an entity in itself—one buys the marketing—and I don't understand this. In this sense, the term means something like a confident self-image. This has as much to do with impelling people to act—getting them sold on something—as it does with the building of relationships for a specific purpose.

The 3-day workshop called "The Millionaire Mind Intensive" was offered by T. Harv Eker, a reputedly popular figure in the world of marketing. I looked forward to a new group of people and a new perspective on business and culture. Because I felt no financial risk, I did no research into Eker or his program.

Held in a New Jersey convention center, the cost of attendance was $300 for a VIP ticket and free for everyone else. The marketing coaches who recommended the event gave me their VIP upgrade, so I expected better seating, materials, and attention.

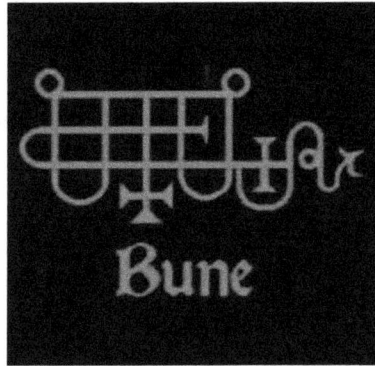

Figure 4: Sigil of the demon of wealth.

The Millionaire Mind

I arrived for the Friday evening presentation at 7 PM. It was scheduled to end at 11 PM. Saturday's training was to run from 9 AM to 11 PM, and Sunday 9 AM to 8 PM. There would be a few breaks for food. We were warned to bring snacks. Collecting my cheap VIP tote bag, raffle ticket, and T. Harv Eker 8-CD presentation series, I was waved into the coliseum.

The football field-sized, concrete-floored "conference room" was empty except for a curtained-off area of 300 folding chairs. This was not what I was expecting. There was a single presenter pacing a stage of make-shift risers. He was not T. Harv Eker, and this was not what I had been led to expect.

The speaker, whose full name I never learned and about whom no information was provided, began with a story about how he survived a natural gas explosion. He used this theme of redemption and transformation as he wove his myth of wealth and freedom. He showed pictures of a burn victim which might have been him, describing his transformation to success and wealth. His list of newfound powers flowed nonstop with evangelical chants of, "Am I right or am I right?!" The audience thundered its affirmation. Questions were not entertained.

You can get a good idea of the endless verbiage and thin promises at T. Harv Eker's website. There you will find no information about Eker or any of his trainers—or that there even are trainers. You'll find no information about the organization, the material, the program, or

135

anything else.

Manipulation

Manipulation of people arises from the manipulation of information. Black magic is embodied in a person's indifference to the damage being done. Management, control, propaganda, data, reports, and opinions are common themes of social discourse. Lies, deception, and exploitation have become impolite topics used to flag the disaffected and the paranoid. These tools are taught and used specifically for exploitation, but we're encouraged to overlook the implications of this.

> "Who is this person offering me some new cure-all, some religious, political, social, psychological, health-related, or other life pathway that he wants me to purchase and follow?... certain training programs use the same types of intense influence techniques that are identical with cults. Also, many of these programs are actually recruiting venues for certain cults. Cults have put on three-piece suits and come directly into the workplace, disguised as self-improvement management courses."
> —**Margaret Singer**, from *Cults in Our Midst*

The Delphi Method of group management was developed by the RAND Corporation in the 1950s to extract consensus from the opinions of experts. It relies on the psychology of groups in which members follow leaders. Groups of experts are more inclined to limit their thoughts than groups of people who are less invested.

The Delphi Method feeds group opinion back into the group in repeated cycles of refinement. The method is "a way of systematically analyzing, complex-value laden, policy-related subjects" (Alder 1996, 95). A good reference to the general method is the 600+ page book, *The Delphi Method: Techniques and Applications*, (Linstone and Turloff 2002) which can be downloaded for free.

Education or Mind Control

The system has been appropriated to manufacture consensus by seeding group opinion and insisting it is consensus. I am surprised to find so little analysis of or instruction about how the system is misused. Even a Wharton School analysis titled, "Methods to Elicit Forecasts from

Groups: Delphi and Prediction Markets Compared" (Green et al. 2007), has nothing to say about this. Yet variants of the Delphi method are being applied all around us in more or less refined ways.

> "The desired result is for group polarization, and for the facilitator to become accepted as a member of the group and group process. S/He will then throw the desired idea on the table and ask for opinions during discussion. Very soon his/her associates from the divided group begin to adopt the idea as if it were their own, and pressure the entire group to accept the proposition."
> —**Lynn Stuter**, from *The Delphi Technique, What Is It?* (Stuter 1996)

This method of controlled opinion feedback, or "reality shaping," is a standard tool for teacher organizers, public school programs, and areas where institutions want to limit participation.

> "School, city or county public meetings are led by so-called 'facilitators' who have been trained to turn the public to a pre-determined outcome and marginalize the final few they haven't 'rolled' to their position."
> — **Eagle Forum**, quoted by Copperhead Consulting Services

We're all on guard against obvious manipulation, illusion, and fallacy. But we are easily misled when these tools are skillfully used and the results endorsed by our peers. The alternative is to reject the consensus and be an outsider. A person trained in group manipulation will marginalize a solitary stand to preserve the group's crafted uniformity.

In chapter three of "Cults in Our Midst," Margaret Singer summarizes five organizational stages that range from empowerment to mind control:

- **Education**: openly presents many bodies of knowledge

- **Advertising**: focuses on selling and influence via biased information and legal persuasion

- **Propaganda**: aims at the political persuasion of masses of people. Authoritarian and often exaggerated.

- **Indoctrination**: designed to inculcate organizational values. Consensual and disciplinary.

- **Thought Reform**: changing people without their knowledge using a deceptive, hidden agenda. Unethical and disrespectful.

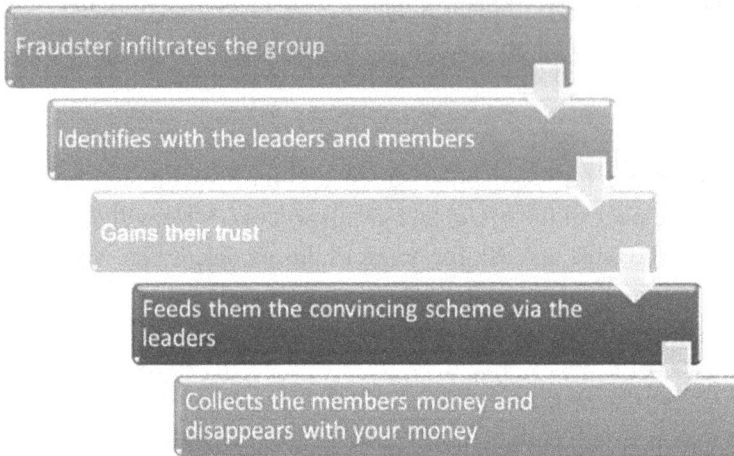

Figure 5: Steps in affinity fraud.

Affinity Fraud

If you research cult movements, you'll find many common ploys like Ponzi schemes, pyramid schemes, shell games, redefined language, withheld rewards, false authority, humiliation, bait and switch, and unsubstantiated claims. You'll also find "affinity fraud."

> "Mr. Madoff, whose victims lost perhaps $20 billion, perpetrated the largest 'affinity fraud' ever. The term refers to scams in which the perpetrator uses personal contacts to swindle a specific group, such as a church congregation, a rotary club, a professional circle, or an ethnic community. Once the scammer gains their trust, his scam spreads like smallpox."
> — from Fleecing the flock: The big business of swindling people who trust you, in *The Economist* (2012)

A method to extract consensus can also inject consensus that will lead people to act or allow them to be acted on. When used in this way, the Delphi Method, or some variation of it, is a manufactured consensus for a non-consensual action. It is used to derail action that the handlers of the group do not welcome.

Most employers manufacture an artificial consensus and then require its adoption by their employees. Therefore, the mind-reform espoused by the New Age movement, currently called WOKE activism, is easily sold to large organizations to improve their public image. Margaret Singer (1995) discusses this as a cult movement, and it is being exploited by businesses (Klee

138

2023; Dowell & Jackson 2020). Because two-party systems exist to manufacture consensus, election politics becomes another form of affinity fraud.

Peak Potentials Training

> "It all comes down to this: if your subconscious 'financial blueprint' is not 'set' for success, nothing you learn, nothing you know, and nothing you do will make much of a difference."
> — **T. Harv Eker** (2005), from *Secrets of the Millionaire Mind*.

At the start of the event, the presenter asked attendees to agree not to divulge information they learned at the seminar. The trust that we needed to build with the presenter and with each other depended on confidentiality. He further warned us that only by seeing this event through to the end would we show our ability to see anything through to the end.

We were told that wealth was born of a state of mind. We needed the courage to believe in our ability to make money work for us, rather than our working for money. "No one ever got rich working 9 to 5!" he told us.

> "Recognize that whether you are worthy or not is all a 'made-up story'... nothing has meaning except for the meaning we give it... There's no one who comes around and stamps you 'worthy' or 'unworthy.' You do that. You make it up. You decide it. You and you alone determine if you're going to be worthy. It's simply your perspective. If you say you're worthy, you are. If you say you're not worthy, you're not. Either way, you will live into your story."
> — **T. Harv Eker** (2005), from *Secrets of the Millionaire Mind*.

Passive income creation is a means of wealth creation that operates with little guidance. We can achieve that through income-producing assets, like rentals and royalties, or judicious investment. The secret to investing, we were told, is secret knowledge accessible only to the wealthy. We're told the measly return of our 401-K retirement programs was a scam by which the wealthy program managers earned 20% annual returns from our savings.

This is what we all need to learn, our speaker exhorted, as he showed us how much our savings would grow with compound interest. Coming to this training was to be the watershed event of our lives, so how could we even put a price on it? "Am I right or am I right!" he exhorted.

They had a special seminar just for this purpose called "Warp Speed Success," which asserts that "investing in the stock market is one of the fastest and easiest ways to earn money and build wealth." In this training we will:

> "Discover the Secrets to Generating Double-Digit Returns Managing Your Own Stock Investments in 15 Minutes a Day... Even If You Know Nothing About Stock Trading ... as Multi-Millionaire Entrepreneur T. Harv Eker and Veteran Stock Trader and Multi-Millionaire Courtney Smith Reveal the Surprising Secrets to... Stock Trading Success in Any Market."
> — from the T. Harv Eker, website marketing material.

To whet our appetite and establish his credibility, we were told that the stock market rose and fell in cycles. Recognizing this would allow us to get in at the bottom and out at the top. If we learned to manage our funds, their methods of skillful investing would have us all millionaires within the decade.

It was 11 PM when we were told the evening was to conclude. People were getting tired and gathering their things, but he was not through yet.

"This information is valuable, and it doesn't come cheap." Enrollment in their investment course–which ran for an undisclosed duration as a webinar, or a set of CDs–usually costs $7,999... but if we went to the back of the room right now, our promoter had special authorization to allow the first 21 people who signed up to pay only $999.

This program worked for him, and he guaranteed it would work for us. We were told that this was something we all needed, and everyone should get out of their seats and go to the back of the room to sign up. No one moved, so he chided us further: "How did we expect to move forward if we were not willing to invest in our education?"

Buying In

I was disappointed. T. Harv Eker espouses some basic truths that people need to understand: our self-image shapes the person we become. Our achievements are limited by what we feel we deserve. Fear marks the boundary of our ability, and our fears only get bigger as we approach them, but we must approach them if we're to get beyond them. And to succeed, we must develop faith in our intuition and the courage to transcend self-preservation.

Intuition is key. It's a glimpse beyond what you know. Intuition is the mind of Roger Penrose, the mathematician, who says to himself, "... and then I do this, and then I do this, and then I do this..." It's the exploitation of people's lack of intuition that paves the way for T. Harv Eker's black magic.

Their stock market "information" was garbage, as would be transparent to anyone with even minimal experience. That was in keeping with the parasitic tone of the entire program.

I've been managing my investments for 50 years. No one regularly beats the market by 20% or even 10%. High returns are achieved either by intense work or by illegal trading.

The world of finance is a world of insiders where power is traded and information is manipulated. Only the most crass and careless schemes come to the regulator's attention, such as the 2012 Libor scandal. In this scheme, major financial institutions colluded to manipulate the London Interbank Offered Rate. The LIBOR rate was used to set other interest rates for corporate lending, mortgages, and private lending.

The banks illegally manipulated the rate to create an economy in which they could buy low and sell high. This was done at the expense of investors, national economies, and world trade. The scheme, which had been going on for nine years, resulted in governments taking power away from the entire banking industry.

The Millionaire Mind training was a fraud in offering 20% returns and above. Their information was puerile, their methods manipulative, and their intentions criminal. I had come interested in learning the views of those attending and to observe their response. By the end of the first day, I was no longer interested, and I did not return. I trashed the CDs, but I kept the tote bag.

Here is another summary of the Millionaire Mind training posted on 6/23/2012 at the Cult Education Institute (2011) website:

> "We were provided with a bag which contained a packet of CDs related to the seminar and a workbook. I really do not know how to describe the workbook because I think most of the contents were idiotic..."

"Adam has a disturbing habit of calling the crowd to repeat after him phrases and keywords like 'Integrity,' 'Attitude matters,' and such. The crowd was repeating after him constantly throughout the seminar. And he has this habit also of calling people to hi-5 to each other and say 'You have a Millionaire mind'..."

"By 6 PM, it was evident that the crowd was getting tired and many were going to the toilets for a break. Adam now suddenly starts his forceful and fiery manner of promoting countless seminars offered by Peak Potentials. He wrote down the prices of each seminar and proceeded to cutting the prices each time in half for a couple of times. The crowd was going into a euphoric mood with people cheering and shouting... (and) he proceeded in blasting the crowd who didn't register by saying 'Stop being afraid,' and 'have the guts to finish the race!'"

"...people who still hadn't bought anything were asked to close their eyes and imagine their ideal lives... and many people awoke from the hypnotherapy with tears in their eyes. And when the people were at their most emotional, the selling continued. They told people how they couldn't afford not to purchase their products and how a real millionaire would do whatever it takes to purchase it..."

"The most disturbing part of the entire weekend is the way in which they marketed to a group of emotionally and financially vulnerable people. In sum, I didn't learn much about making money, but I did learn a lot about mind control and brainwashing."

Neither Black Nor White

Any system that extols personal gain over all else is nefarious. If that system employs mental subterfuge, then it is magical in a general sense. Black magic does not require occult curses or demonic evocations because consciousness is already supra-rational. There is no known mechanism of consciousness. We may be guided by reason and natural law, but our spirit is effectively built on magic.

A culture that recognizes only the deductive and material world ignores higher levels of consciousness. Such a culture accepts any means to its all-important material ends, accepting any color of magic that gets it there. As Adolf Hitler said, "I use emotion for the many and reserve reason for the few."

Two young men dream of being soldiers. They both use the same process of reason. One experiences the real world, speaks to no one but the voices in his head, murders his schoolmates and is considered a psychopath. The other lives in a virtual world, takes commands from voices in his headset, murders other people's schoolmates and is considered a hero. The difference lies in their intuition and their judgments. There is a place in society for even the most severe psychopath (Dutton & McNab 2014).

References

Adler, M. (1996). *Gazing Into the Oracle: The Delphi Method and Its Application to Social Policy and Public Health.* Jessica Kingsley Publishers.

Copperhead Consulting Services (undated). *Building Consensus AKA You've Been "Delphi'd"!.* https://www.rollbacklocalgov.com/building-consensus-aka-youve-been-delphid/

Cult Education Institute (2011 Jun 23). *Millionaire Mind Intensive "Training" by T.Harv Eker, Peak Potentials,* under the topic of Large Group Awareness Training, "Human Potential," at Cult Education Institute. https://forum.culteducation.com/read.php?4,101700,132743

Dowell, E., & Jackson, M. (2020 Jul 27). "'Woke-Washing' Your Company Won't Cut It." *Harvard Business Review.* https://hbr.org/2020/07/woke-washing-your-company-wont-cut-it

Dutton, K., & McNab, A. (2014). *The Good Psychopath's Guide to Success: How to Use Your Inner Psychopath to Get the Most Out of Life.* Apostrophe Books.

Eker, T. H. (2005). *Secrets of the Millionaire Mind: Mastering the Inner Game of Wealth.* Harper Business.

Green, K. C., Armstrong, J. S., & Graefe, A. (2007 Aug 31). *Methods to Elicit Forecasts from Groups: Delphi and Prediction Markets Compared.* Monash University Business and Economic Forecasting Unit. https://mpra.ub.uni-muenchen.de/4999/

Klee, M. (2023 Apr 8). "Companies That Get 'Woke' Aren't Going Broke—They're More Profitable Than Ever." *Rolling Stone.* https://www.rollingstone.com/culture/culture-features/woke-companies-broke-profits-1234710724/

Linstone, H. A., & Turoff, M. (2002). *The Delphi method: Techniques and applications.* http://www.foresight.pl/assets/downloads/publications/Turoff_Linstone.pdf

The Economist (2012 Jan 28). "Affinity Fraud: Fleecing the Flock: The Big Business of Swindling People Who Trust You." https://www.economist.com/business/2012/01/28/fleecing-the-flock

Singer, M. T., & Lalich, J. (1995). *Cults in Our Midst: The Hidden Menace in Our Everyday Lives.* Jossey-Bass Publishers. https://archive.org/details/cultsinourmidst00sing

Stuter, L. (1996). *The Delphi Technique; What Is It?* https://freedom-school.com/lessons/the-delphi-technique-what-is-it.pdf

T4 – Learn to Think

Thinking is a human instinct, but thinking well is not.

"Critical thinking requires us to use our imagination, seeing things from perspectives other than our own and envisioning the likely consequences of our position."— **Bell Hooks** (aka Gloria Jean Watkins), social philosopher

Consciousness

This is going to be quick, so hold on. Before I define thinking, I need to define consciousness.

Consciousness is being aware of what comes up in your mind. That means thoughts, perceptions, and sensations. Consciousness is not the control of these things, it's awareness of them. Control happens elsewhere.

We are not conscious of decoding perceptions, filtering, and assembling pictures and ideas. We are not conscious of storing and retrieving memories. We are aware these things are happening below consciousness, but we're only conscious of the result. Awareness regulates attention, it doesn't do anything.

Our unconscious assembles thoughts by habit, rote, pattern, and repetition. Computers can do this, but this is not thinking. Our subconscious recognizes imperfect patterns and builds novelty using inference, metaphor, and emotion. In doing this, it connects new mental structures with old ones. This is thinking, and no machine does this.

Thinking

The assembly of ideas happens in the subconscious, not the conscious or unconscious mind. We delude ourselves if we believe that being aware of our thoughts means we control them. Awareness and control could not be more different. You think while you're conscious, but thoughts come from a place outside your awareness.

Through awareness, you gather information. If you process information in a regular fashion, this fashion becomes a habit. This is not thinking, it's an automatic response. My son's first grade worksheets do not teach him thinking, and people are not taught to think. Thinking involves novelty and emotion. Since focusing your awareness does not lead to thinking, how can you learn to think?

Learning

Learning to think is gaining an awareness of where ideas are created—not how they're created—and then becoming involved in the process. Learning to think is learning to let go of what you think you know.

Most of what goes on inside your head has nothing to do with thinking. Doing what you usually do does not require thinking. Listen to people talking and reflect on how much thinking is going on. Then listen to yourself and ask the same question. Talking is for people, what grooming is for monkeys. Those lower on the social ladder aspire to talk with those higher on the ladder, but those higher rarely deign to speak with those lower. Much the same as grooming, you conduct these conversations in a kind of waking sleep.

Thinking happens when you do something new, like jumping out of an airplane. If you're not in an airplane, then create the experience by imagining it: be in front of the open, roaring door of an airplane flying. Take part in the experience: jump out the door. Do this and you lose familiar awareness of self and place. New ideas form when you experience emotions in new ways.

Learning Thinking

I would like to teach you how to think. I would like to take you in the airplane of your mind, open the door, and invite you to jump out. This cannot be done in your normal, conscious state of mind, the "watcher" state where everything is familiar and sensible. In this "normal state," everything happens "out there," while you are "here."

In a creative state, you feel the door is really there, and the airplane is more than a metaphor. The door may look familiar, but what's on the other side is nowhere you've ever been. Here's how you do it.

First, reflect on a situation that is important to you. Focus on what is meaningful. Next, drop into a deeper state and lose the conscious mind. Recall some animated scene, or assemble such a scene from memories, and simply watch it. Don't talk, just watch. And if you can recall some sensations: the heat of the sun when you walked on the sand, or the balance of your body as you walk a trail. Recall images and sensations, to dialog, attitude, or judgment. These are the first steps that lead to the open state.

The open state is the wellspring of your imagination, the place where ideas form. Move deeper into that state by letting your mind wander. Go off the rational path and catch associated feelings. Go to where the words form and shush each thought that starts. You won't be able to stop thoughts from starting, but you will take the wind out of their sails to leave them flapping like broken sentences. Let go of continuity and welcome the confusion of ideas and recollection.

In my dreamscape, I find myself on a cliff pushing a handcart, swimming in an endless ocean, driving down a mountain road without brakes. People need help here; it can get a bit nightmarish. There are many unpleasant thoughts that will pop into our minds if we let our guard down, and you want to let your guard down. You can still gently reject whatever unpleasant thoughts occur, but you want to be aware of them. You want to allow them to approach the gates of consciousness without letting them through.

Don't try, don't struggle. Give up and ask for help from a deeper part of yourself. You're in front of what you don't know... but something knows. That thing may not talk to you, but it can hear you and it understands you.

Go to the edge and ask for help. Speak into the void of your mind. You can practice this. Asking for guidance is important. Don't expect a spoken response, expect shape-shifting.

> "I was trying to choose between walking or crawling. Both seemed too risky... the real solution is to trust and let go. As I do so, leaping into the beautiful sunrise sky, I am overwhelmed with feeling and awaken with tears of joy."
> — **Stephen LaBerge** (2000), psychophysiologist, from *Varieties of Lucid Dreaming Experience*

"Thinking is the hardest work there is, which is probably the reason why so few engage in it."
— **Henry Ford**, industrialist founder of the Ford Motor Company

Conscious Thinking

The result of thinking is not thought, it is insight. You won't get answers until you understand this, and you might not get the answers you expect.

Do you recall the first time you mixed yellow with blue paint and made green? That's what thinking is like. You don't get out of it what you put into it, but something new.

Thoughts are not thinking. Thinking is a process that involves emotion that does not result in conclusions, it results in arrangements of values and ideas. Creativity generates possibilities bounded only by your tolerance to chaos. Your need to understand is what shuts off the tap of information. Each of us has our limits, but these limits can be expanded.

Not unlike our fear of drowning, being fully informed pushes our heads underwater. Thinking is what happens when we're below the surface, and it takes a change of mind to take in ideas, memories, associations, sensations, and emotions without their making sense or your being attached to them.

Unlike submersion in water, you can still think when flooded with information, but you need to learn how to experience things without making sense. You learn with practice, and practice involves going beyond what you think you're capable of. Crisis, struggle, and commitment can help us grow. There will always be change, but it will not be traumatic if you keep your integrity. This involves maintaining a sense of separateness while remaining fully aware of the experience.

When I fell 500 feet from the summit of Mount Robson, the highest peak in the Canadian Rockies, I had a detached state of mind. I watched the world spin around me while my tethered ice axe, torn from my grip, sliced at my clothes. I did not know where I was headed and I had no control over what was happening. I fell into a bowl of snow with nothing more than a tattered jacket and a sprained ankle. I didn't plan on being courageous, I just took in what the experience offered. I suffered no trauma because I had no fear.

Digesting meaningful messages is the last step in learning to think. It is a process of putting away for later all the rich confusion you cannot cope with now. This can take time, and I help people with this step as well. While colors mix immediately, spices take hours, and concrete takes days. You will take a lifetime. Don't object. Savor it.

Don't expect a stroke of insight, and too much examination won't help. Often, in impatience, I simply make up answers that look like Cubist paintings: reflections of what I see but do not understand.

> "I would rather live in a world where my life is surrounded by mystery than live in a world so small that my mind could comprehend it."
> — **Harry Emerson Fosdick**, pastor

The less said, the better. Knowledge is not in words, it's in feelings and relationships. Do not force knowing too soon and never force words. When I work with clients, I give suggestions and encourage confidence and patience. Learning to think is learning to see, and most of us have never been encouraged to think. It can be difficult, but it is life-changing.

Many of our personal and interpersonal frustrations stem not from a lack of trying, but from our inability to think. Reflect for a moment on how you know you can think at all. You don't know. You cannot even describe the process.

You will run through patterns, structures, and plans in your mind, shoring up the connections between ideas, adding vitality to adjectives and recognizing implications. For some people, this happens quickly, especially if the subject is emotionally charged.

For most of us, it takes some attention and, if we're too tired or distracted, our ideas come out half-baked. And in situations that are obscure, boring, or confused, thinking can feel like chewing gristle, as is often the case with problems we can't solve or situations that make no sense.

Forty years ago, I asked Jerome Bruner, a celebrated psychologist, where words came from. He didn't know and suggested I answer the question myself. These writings are my answer.

References

LaBerge, S., & DeGracia, D. J. (2000). Varieties of lucid dreaming experience. In *Individual Differences in Conscious Experience,* edited by R. G. Kunzendorf and B. Wallace: 269–307. John Benjamins Publishing Company. https://doi.org/10.1075/aicr.20.14lab

T5 – The Reality of Illusion

Thoughts generate things that are perceived, which are also in one's imagination.

"The unreal is more powerful than the real, because nothing is as perfect as you can imagine it, because it's only intangible ideas, concepts, beliefs, fantasies that last." — **Chuck Palahniuk**, author

… and the Illusion of Disease

This piece is about what we think is real and the difference between sensation and feeling. It is about the worlds of imagination and dreams, and making feelings into sensations. It's about making dreams real.

There is confusion about real and imagined disease, and it's just plain dumb. It is not true that imagination does not affect reality; imagination can have as much effect as any other perception. In fact, everything sensed through perception is an act of imagination. Perception is imagination that we all agreed on.

Actual diseases have an organic cause, while imagined diseases are malingering behavior. The symptoms of the first have a mechanical cause—perhaps yet unknown—while the symptoms of the second have none. At the same time, you can create a mechanical condition using the power of mind alone. But here's the thing: all systems consist of parts and relationships, and dysfunction can occur either in the parts or the relationships. You cannot extract relationships and put them under a microscope, but they are as real as the parts.

This is clouded by the unhelpful intrusion of clinical medicine—more an attitude than a science—that claims to distinguish reality from imagination; that it can distinguish the real from the imaginary using the objective methods of repeatable observation.

This is sleight of hand: first you see it, and then you don't. This deception works because people prostrate themselves before science, as before Jehovah. The unfortunate result is that

151

science is being made into a religion. The claim that "real disease" is what can be observed as separate—as something that is caused by something separate and external—is baloney.

A little microbiology is useful. According to the accepted endosymbiotic theory of the origin of eukaryotes, our cells evolved by aggregating simpler living organisms within a single membrane. Our body is the collaborative effort of many cells working together.

In this picture, three levels of disease are obvious: problems that occur within a cell, problems that occur in maintaining the integrity of a cell, and problems that occur in orchestrating cells.

So far in our young medical history, we understand something about the second sort of problem, problems of our cells' integrity. These are the problems caused by opportunistic bacteria. We can disrupt bacterial invasions using antibiotics. We know little about viruses, but we're learning. We know almost nothing about the two larger and more complex aspects of disease, the intra-cellular and systemic.

From our limited success, and because we overlook what we don't understand, we think of all diseases as pathogenic invasions. We have created a medical establishment that promulgates this point of view, and we follow this despite our better judgment. Our medicine works when it understands what's happening, and it fails when it does not.

Fixing this massive failure, says Dr. Mark Hyman (2014) in *The Disease Delusion:*

> "…requires a fundamental paradigm shift from medicine by symptom, to medicine by cause; from medicine by disease, to medicine by system; from medicine by organ, to medicine by organism… an ecological view of the body where all the networks of our biology intersect and interact in a dynamic process that creates disease when out of balance, and creates health when in balance."

It's great to talk about paradigm shifts, but talking does not make it happen. Better to just tell people what to do. And as any good educator knows, you can't teach anything to anyone unless they are ready to discover it for themselves. So, I hope you are ready to discover the obvious: you are a system.

The Software is Real

You consist of things that function, an environment, an awareness, and the ability to respond. And what's making you "alive" is the "software" that animates you, and software is real.

Somewhere in that mix is your sense of self. In fact, you're in all of those things, which is why separating what's real from what you feel, see, or think is dumb. Here's a picture.

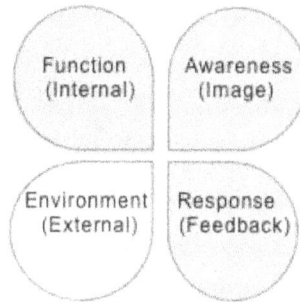

Figure 6: Forces affecting one's sense of self.

In this picture (Figure 6), the grey lobes interact to maintain balance. They each have a relationship with the environment depending on, responding to, and affecting it. Allopathic medicine considers only two of these lobes: function and environment. According to the mechanistic view, health is just a matter of function, and if you're not functioning, we'll fix it.

Hypnotherapy manages awareness and encourages response. Hypnotherapy recognizes that self-controlled function relies on self-awareness. Self-awareness triggers protective and restorative responses.

I take it further. Working with the brain's underlying networks, I increase self-awareness. I can train the autonomic nervous system using hypnosis and neurofeedback. I can teach you how to remix the frequencies of consciousness. These set the communication speeds for each of a host of simultaneous inner voices. Voices of joints, organs, tissues, and mind.

The connection between awareness and response is poorly understood. Medicine throws the baby out with the bathwater when it says, "Since we don't understand the mind, it isn't real." With the invention of new kinds of observations, new things have become real but institutional healthcare has not changed.

Molecular biology and genetics spawned the field of psycho-neuro-immunology. Genetic responses to environmental changes created the field of epigenetics. Brain science opened new views on how we regulate ourselves, showing "real" connections between body and awareness. Voluntary change in your autonomic functions, once considered impossible, has now been documented. But lacking a theory it is overlooked in standard healthcare protocols.

I'm reminded of the Yogi Berra-ism of astrophysicist Sir Arthur Eddington, who supposedly said, "Never trust an experiment until it has been confirmed by theory." He seems to have been responding to Yogi Berra's insight that, "You can observe a lot just by watching." It's unclear whose nonsense is more profound since medicine has scant theory and is entirely based on looking!

Awareness and Health

You are normally unaware of autonomic functions and, because of this, you assume you cannot control them. It would seem to be a contradiction to assert you had control over something you're unaware of. Yet there are channels of control below awareness, and here medicine has taken a blind turn. This is not a mechanical connection, but it is real. Subconscious control operates through synchronization, focus, inclination, intuition, imagination, and, perhaps, telepathy.

Awareness is not the same as consciousness. Awareness is feedback and self-regulation. We have some awareness of every aspect of our system, everything from muscles to the DNA in our big toe. We have some awareness of everything, without regard to our being conscious of this awareness. This awareness is not only real, but necessary.

The opposite is also true: much of what we're conscious of we never perceived but have invented. Almost nothing of what we see, taste, hear, or feel is a "real" perception. It's all created in the software of our brains. Much of it is guesswork, and much of it is wrong. We live in a world of constructed hallucination, as Dr. Anil Seth (2017) demonstrated in his popular TED Talk, "Your brain hallucinates your conscious reality."

And Everything Makes Sense

We are used to living in a causal world. We look for causes and we expect them, but we only see what we look for, and only look for a tiny part of what's there. Much of what goes on we don't see, and we don't recognize what or who drives these systems. Our blindness leads us to think we understand things when we really don't. Much of this magical thinking we call "science."

Science cannot supply the ultimate cause for anything, and it never claimed to. For our actions, we credit ourselves with "free will," a magical notion if there ever was one! We think we're completely rational, but it's unclear if we are ever rational. Instead, we're governed by what's habitual and socially acceptable, and what's worked before. We do what we expect others will understand. This comes to us as feelings.

Can you tell what's real apart from what's imaginary? What about the difference between imaginary thoughts of real things and imaginary thoughts of unreal things?

If you look carefully at why you behave the way you do, or why you feel the way you do, or at anything you feel at all, you'll hit a wall of silence. At this wall, everything fades into fog. You don't have words to go farther; no sentences come to mind. Free will does not explain itself.

At the boundary of the known, we feel ill at ease. Things don't work right there. It can be a place of chaos and malfunction. The dis-ease that we feel mirrors the dysfunction we perceive, a dysfunction we imagine.

At the boundary of the known, at that point where new ideas form, most of us run out of steam. In the territory of confusion, we turn around and head back to the comfort of consensus opinion. "Consensus opinion," I think, is what we call "free will."

... Until It Doesn't

How can we regain control if only to regain balance? One answer is to analyze, and this is our inclination, but on the edge of knowledge, where we cannot see and hardly understand, analysis usually fails.

Another answer is we talk, and this we do to extremes, ceaselessly, and without direction. We talk in circles, trying and retrying pegs in holes where they would not fit before. This is the understanding delusion, a particularly human predicament. It works sometimes.

Repeatedly attacking a problem in previously unsuccessful ways may eventually work. It will work better if we're sloppy and don't repeat ourselves. That's what we're really doing when we repeat ourselves: we're hoping some random mutation will lead to a better result. Beating on a screw with a hammer rarely does anything useful, but if you're careful, sensitive, and observant, you might see it turn just a little. At that point, a creative person might try to turn it.

We credit ourselves with being creative, but most of the time, we're just wrong. In quantum mechanics, prevailing through repeated failure is called tunneling. It involves random movements in a classically impossible direction. Tunneling is a fundamental mechanism of the universe. It is the mechanism by which most things are stable, and occasional change is achieved. It is how everything works. Without it, we wouldn't even have atoms.

If you're fast and determined, then you'll make progress, though it's hard to know how much. It's 100 monkeys at typewriters writing Shakespeare. They do it for the bananas. Through the repeated efforts of many, a new understanding may emerge.

Talking to Emptiness

How do you interact with what you're not aware of? By imagining it. Where do the words come from? From that place where our sensations connect with our awareness. In the realm of which we're unaware, or think we are.

How do you connect with the beating of your heart, the function of your liver, the intention of your disease, the chatter below your mind, or the voice of your ancestor? You imagine there is a connection, and you allow yourself to create a response. Is it real, or is it imagined? There is no difference!

That is why I like to work with sleep, sleep issues, and people who think they are rational. Sleep, of all our realms, is the least rational, and the most fertile. Sleep is a rabbit hole, and you won't be the same on the other side. You don't want to be.

References

Bland, J. S. (2014). *The Disease Delusion: Conquering the Causes of Chronic Illness for a Healthier, Longer, and Happier Life.* Harper Wave.

Seth, A. (2017). "Your Brain Hallucinates Your Conscious Reality." *TED2017.* https://www.ted.com/talks/anil_seth_your_brain_hallucinates_your_conscious_reality?

T6 – How I Seem to Be (Different)

November 3, 2019

The recent podcast I did has given me a chance to compare myself to pop–psychology celebrities and pundits.

"Psychology is the policeman of capitalism."
— **Dr. Bayo Akomolafe** (2022), psychologist and West African scholar

Pundits

This is not a comfortable topic. It's always uncomfortable to compare oneself. Does anyone like doing this?

I've recently been introduced to other people who seem to be on a similar path. My friends and the universe have put comparison in front of me, so it seems worth doing. The recent podcast I did with Bonnie Groessl gave me a chance to speak in broad generalities, which provides a basis for comparison.

I am moving toward the realm of celebrity academics because of my academic degrees, the constellation of my interests, and my marketing efforts. This doesn't mean I will join them or that I want to, just that I'm heading in that direction. I find myself compared to:

Steven Kotler (2018), Journalist, performance coach, and co-author of *The Rise of Superman* and *Stealing Fire.*

Moran Cerf, Neuroscientist, management advisor, and editor of *Consumer Neuroscience.*

Steven Pinker (2003), Psychologist and author of *Enlightenment Now* and *The Better Angels of Our Nature.*

Joe Dispenza (2013), Chiropractor and author of *You Are the Placebo* and *Breaking the Habit of Being Yourself.*

These are pundits of the New Psychology, a vortex I feel I'm being sucked into, like a river through narrows. I also work in therapy, research, systems theory, trance states, indigenous

158

culture, and education. These areas are all related, but this isn't being emphasized by these authors. I try to create bridges between these fields, but I find much resistance. Publishers understand only A or B, not A and B. My pitches fall on deaf ears. There is tremendous resistance to a unified understanding. This is a fundamental aspect of the ego, which struggles to keep itself separate and distinct.

Teachers

In mathematics, there is "proof by contradiction," and there are theorems most easily proved in this fashion. You complete a proof by contradiction by assuming what you don't believe, and then proving it isn't true. In life, such proof only applies to the case you've examined. But in mathematics, you can disprove the general case and learn a general truth.

Demonstrating the negative of an assertion rarely shows the positive to be true. For example, it's false that all politicians are liars, but it's also false that all politicians are not liars. But if you're careful, disproving a negative assertion can, if not prove the positive, at least make a strong case for it.

"Half the lies they tell about me aren't true."
— **Yogi Berra**, professional baseball catcher, team manager, and coach

I can't prove the teaching profession is a fraud, but I think it is. The only teachers I value are those who impart skills by mimicry, which is tool-using. You cannot teach insight. The only teachers who express an interest in my work on the fundamentals of learning are those who repudiate the teaching profession. I also base this on public education, which hasn't changed in the 50 years I've known it.

From this, I see there is nothing we cannot learn—or in his case, couldn't *be* learning—to better ourselves. Despite the enormous changes in what we know and how we need to know, school teachers haven't changed their attitudes toward learning. They still teach pliant behavior and intellectual weakness.

Blinded by pedagogy and elitism, school teachers believe their efforts are valuable. Every school teacher I've known feels they know more than those they teach. They're wrong, and they're *especially* wrong about children. Children, with their malleable brains, can understand new concepts difficult for most adults. Knowledge is not about what's in your head, it's about what you can do with what's in your head. What is currently being offered to children in schools is a complete waste of their time. It has zero value.

Mentors don't behave this way. Mentors don't tell you what or how to think, which is why mentors typically spend little time with mentees. A mentor's role is not to teach, expound, or direct, but to inspire and suggest. The future of humanity hinges on our ability to learn. This will be determined not by the details of things, but by their connections.

Researchers

I'm starting to feel the same way about research scientists as I do about teachers. We see this in the rise of celebrity scientists, and the descent of scientists into celebrities. These pundits are typically people who are not so much "doing" science as "teaching" it; following rules and not making them. Most researchers, like most teachers, work to establish old ideas rather than explore new ones. Shoring up old ideas is not a bad thing, but it's not what these folks are paid to do, which is to create new ideas and new idea makers. To create new connections.

From kindergarten through graduate programs—throughout my life in educational institutions—I have insisted on broader thinking. I have fought the closed-mindedness of teachers, researchers, and administrators and gotten nowhere. Not until I became a counselor have my suggestions been taken seriously, and with positive results. There are many science popularizers who make large profits selling false information. I consider Joe Dispenza to be one of the worst because I know the fields of which he speaks. I struggle to find any accurate statement in his writings. He exploits hypnotic techniques to mislead his audience, as was done by Anton Mesmer and Émile Coué in the eighteenth and nineteenth centuries. Dispenza is not a researcher, expert, scientist, or journalist, he's a showman. Like T. Harv Eker, he's a scam.

If you listen, watch, and read the performances and presentations of other celebrity scientists —such as my friend Neil deGrasse Tyson—you will hear more policy than science. With the pandemic of Covid-19, many researchers, doctors, and journalists endorsed mandates that were uncertain, unsafe, or unsound. Reflect on your visceral memory of these presentations and you will notice their effect is more directive than educational. They would like you to believe that being directed is being illuminated. What do you think?

The original goal of science was gnostic, to explore what was hidden, but the present effort is social, commercial, and political. This is the same trajectory taken by religions, and the comparison between religion and science has long been whispered. My attempts to engage research scientists in considering the personal context of their actions have fallen on deaf ears. My suggestion that researchers examine their own minds, if only to perform better, is met with disdain.

I am not claiming science cannot progress. I assert researchers are weakly aware of their direction. They are like teachers who do not question the educational paradigm or soldiers who do not question the program. Teachers are soldiers, and scientists are becoming soldiers, too.

Explorers

I advocate exploration. You don't need to be certified to explore, and exploration, almost by definition, is a field in which one is always self-trained. The desire to explore, like the desire to play, create, grow, and achieve, is in our blood. It is at its best when left alone. Explorers understand the territory in ways that teachers cannot know.

Consider this for a moment. When you know your way around a city, it's not only because you know how to go from A to B, it's because you know many ways from A to B. You also know all the paths that *do not* connect A to B. It's knowing all the wrong ways that makes up understanding, whereas knowing one right way is akin to a blind person who has memorized their route.

If you ever need learning, get it from an explorer. I learned some things about navigation from Fred Beckey, a great mountaineer. He taught me one simple thing that will save your ass if you ever need to navigate through difficult terrain. He taught me to always look behind me and to remember what it looks like when you want to go in the other direction. If you don't, you may never find your way back.

Here are what explorers say about themselves, taken from my book, *The Learning Project:*

Rites of Passage:

"Try to find your place in the world and make your mark in that world either through accomplishments or through your voice."
— The Phantom Street Artist

"I go about things in a way that has nothing to do with what universities teach… You make it up as you go along, and God knows how it comes out; you don't know."
— Jerry Lettvin, MD, psychiatrist and neurophysiologist

"I don't think I can tell you one thing that motivates me, but certainly, love motivates me, and also anger motivates me—all my life—and hope motivates me. Love, anger, and hope."
— Tom Hurwitz, filmmaker

"Chuck Strobel … said, 'You know, Nancy, you and I … we're really the pioneers of the field. We are the foundation…' And I'm thinking, 'Who, me? I don't even have a clue what I'm doing!'"
— Nancy White, psychotherapist

"Where does it come from? I don't know. Half the time, I don't even know what I'm doing."
— Lou Giani, wrestling coach

"I don't have any answers anymore. I've learned that answers are things you just make up… and until it falls apart, it's reasonable enough."
— George Plotkin, MD, neurologist

Explorers aren't teachers. They don't work with established knowledge. They're not pundits because they don't have a following. Explorers can be mentors, though that isn't their goal. To an explorer, celebrity is ridiculous because a person who only sees what they've achieved can never know what they've accomplished. What explorers achieve is not just new information, but new ways to understand information.

Prophets

People rise to stardom on paths of marketing, celebrity, and self-promotion. This seems to be part of our cult of technology, as anyone with the imprimatur of high-tech is seen as an expert in everything. Yet the definition of high-tech has increasingly more to do with how it is delivered than what it contains. High-tech used to mean science and electronics. It now means taxi services, grocery delivery, office rental, YouTube, and exercise equipment. Tech-stars have become the new salespeople.

As I watch the videos and TED Talks, which I referred to above, I feel that some of these people are more nourished by celebrity than by exploration. They are commodities unto themselves. It's unclear whether they're uncovering new knowledge, repackaging old knowledge, or just making it up. I'm not saying this is bad, I'm just asking if this is inspiration or direction. How much exists beyond the presentation?

Clearly, there are defenses for enthusiasm; the proof of the pudding is in the eating. We have made progress, as Steven Pinker argues. Helping to generate this enthusiasm is a pyramid of science-to-policy advocates who range—in descending order—from Steven Hawking (physicist) to Neil Tyson (Director of the Hayden Planetarium) to Bill Nye (The Science Guy), to Jamie Hyneman (Myth Busters), to Stephen Barrett (Quackwatch), to an army of lobbyists and informers.

Each of these experts has their audience, message, and social effect. Each of these agents has a progressive, evolutionary effect, but that does not mean their effect is positive. What is in the pudding?

Some of these folks have special knowledge, and their explorations have been essential. Others simply explain or fail to. People believe them not because they know them to be right, but because they like them. Their authority has a simple explanation: it is the cult of celebrity and the attraction of groupthink.

Prophets and futurists swing the rudder of investment. Will we plant trees or build spaceships? Fund research or house the elderly? Should we even be spending money at all? Shouldn't we be talking about what happens when we create money from nothing?

Investors

Now, you might think business endeavors are held to the lowest social standard, being entirely material and self-serving; but this isn't necessarily so. Stable businesses fulfill a social function and maintain the social structure. In every case and to varying extents, businesses not only adapt to change but create it.

I attended an informal gathering of private investors in 2019. This was an unusual economic time when asset values were at historic highs and interest rates were at historic lows. This boom had been going on for over a decade. An enormous quantity of cheap money, backed by no assets at all, was having an amphetamine effect on the economy. Economies on amphetamines become hyperactive, but, like people on amphetamines, they are impaired.

So much money was available that only the worst deals remained unfunded. Money was being thrown at ventures that didn't have an expectation of generating a profit in a reasonable time frame. So much money was available that venture capital firms were investing in creating more venture capital firms to hire more people and find more investments. There is something delirious about this. Economist Wolf Richter (2019) calls this "consensual hallucination."

> "If everyone believes stocks will go up, no matter what the current price or the current situation, or current fundamental data, then stocks will go up. They will go up because there is a lot of buying pressure because everyone believes that everyone believes that prices will go up, and so they bid up prices and chase stocks higher.
>
> "I call this phenomenon 'consensual hallucination'–'consensual' because everyone eagerly smokes the same stuff in order to be able to get the same hallucinations everyone else is having, and to be part of the movement, because they believe that this movement will make them rich, and if enough people have this consensual hallucination, and if algos are programmed to trade with it, then it works wonderfully... until it doesn't. The moment it doesn't is when this hallucination begins to fade. And what happens then?"
> — **Wolf Richter**, economist and author

"Progress" strains at the bit, fanned by pundits in every industry. And the more enthusiasm, the more need for enthusiasm, and the more funding for it. It's not that there is no reason for optimism, it's that the optimism is not fairly reasoned.

"The more it snows, tiddly-pom,
The more it goes, tiddly-pom,
The more it goes, tiddly-pom,
On snowing."
— **Pooh**, the optimist, on the way to build Eeyore's house, from A. A. Milne's
The House at Pooh Corner.

But it's not just the economy, it's each of us within it. We become engaged and optimistic; resonant circuits in a self-amplifying system. We want what feeds us and remember better those who assure it. No one is in direct contact with the final product, which is the entire system and the future. We believe in the flow of time, our position in it, and the reason things are the way they are. Living in the now, listening to what's ongoing, and aiming ourselves toward targets we believe in. We are the network.

Thinkers

There is something more honest about having direct control of your product, thoughts, reality, and mind. Moran Cerf, neuroscientist and investor, warns us not to believe everything we think. This surprises me. Are there people who believe what they think? I find that unfathomable. I thought such thinking was limited to lower primates.

Consider this: you have a feeling and it stirs up images and more feelings. Before you know it, thoughts have emerged and you have an opinion. Where does it come from? Is it even yours? How could anyone believe the ideas that arise in their minds? Moran Cerf warns that believing what you think makes you vulnerable to the bionic mind hackers, those who think for us. Isn't that the story of civilization?

As a therapist, my job is to examine the ideas in people's heads. I'm a mind expander. I do for others what I do for myself: I doubt what I hear. I will accept each message as the voice of someone speaking from somewhere. The very fact the message has appeared, having made it through our elaborate internal vetting system, means it has some importance.

The ideas promulgated by celebrities echo public and financial interests. They echo unquestioned thoughts in our collective heads. To be a celebrity is to be a spokesperson speaking from and to this group mind.

I don't like the group mind, it's schizophrenic: too many voices colliding without good intentions. I don't like to listen to or talk to it, and I certainly don't want to speak for it. The group mind has the power to approve, empower, and accept—not to mention enrich and authenticate.

I don't feel approved and I don't want to be. I used to want to be affirmed, but emotional abuse and disrespect by authority cured me. Affirmation forms a cyst around what you know that limits the uncertainty necessary for exploration. Don't trust voices that affirm. Take responsibility.

Shamans

I'm different from this roster of intellectual celebrities. I feel the intellect is a storyteller, not a truth-teller. The intellect is a perceptual amplifier, like a television. The intelligence that comes out of it did not originate inside it but is broadcast to it through the voices and structures around it.

The intellect is overreaching, self-centered, and egotistical. It may be the product of our more evolved brain, but that doesn't mean it understands anything. Your intellect is a well-meaning bungler. "Trust but verify" was Ronald Reagan's joke because it belied no trust. My dictum is simpler: never trust, always verify. You never know if the awakening you've just had has put you in another dream.

When you listen to celebrities, you are eating poop that's been digested by another brain, and already denuded of most of its nutrients. Go out and do it yourself, perceive it for yourself, perform your own investigation, and find all the mistakes to avoid.

You must alter your states and your network genetics: what you pass on. It's not enough to read about travel, foreign culture, or mountain climbing—you have to experience these yourself. It's not enough to listen to the pundits allowing your brain to be hacked in the guise of inspiration. Make the journey yourself. You don't have to be great, you just need experience. The integrity of a network is determined by the independence of the hubs. Are you a link in the chain or a hub of the network?

The pundits deliver thought-pizza. Neil, Steve, and Joe will lead you to the promised land of health, order, and potential oblivion. I'm more interested in that big hole waiting for you at the end of the road to nowhere, your next frontier. It's likely that you're heading right toward it. "X" marks the spot.

> "(Human beings) don't use the knowledge the spirit has put into every one of them; … and so they stumble along blindly on the road to nowhere—a paved highway which they themselves bulldoze and make smooth so that they can get faster to the big empty hole which they'll find at the end."
> — **Lame Deer**, Lakota Shaman

References

Akomolare, B. (2022). *Emergence, Self-exploration & Recovery, Episode 56.* Inside the Wooniverse. https://www.colettebaronreid.com/wp-content/uploads/2023/02/ep56_-emergence-self-exploration-recovery_.pdf

Cerf, M. (2020 Apr 17). *Free Won't.* TEDxAix. https://www.morancerf.com/videos?wix-vod-video-id=d4f2038eeb1f4da9aa33723c8aae72d8&wix-vod-comp-id=comp-k862g4g01

Dispenza, J. (2013). *Transformation,* TEDxTacoma. https://www.youtube.com/watch?v=W81CHn4l4AM

Kotler, S. (2018 Jun 29). *How to Open Up the Next Level of Human Performance.* TEDxABQ. https://www.stevenkotler.com/video/how-to-open-up-the-next-level-of-human-performance-steven-kotler-tedxabq

Pinker, S. (2003). *Human Nature and the Blank Slate.* TED.com. https://www.ted.com/talks/steven_pinker_human_nature_and_the_blank_slate?language=en

Richter, W. (2019 Oct 30). *What Will Stocks Do When "Consensual Hallucination" Ends?* Wolf Street. Retrieved from: https://wolfstreet.com/2019/10/30/what-will-stocks-do-when-consensual-hallucination-ends/

T7 – Who's Conscious?

February 5, 2020

Consciousness has neither the authority nor the ability to create us.

"The key to growth is the introduction of higher dimensions of consciousness into our awareness." — **Lao Tzu**, founder of Taoism

To Be or Not To Be...

Who are we and what's it all about? This silly question is the starting point for all our problems, questions, and issues in health, philosophy, and religion. You start on some foundation, and there isn't much lower that you can go.

Dictionary.com says, "'I think therefore I am,' was the end of the search Descartes conducted for a statement that could not be doubted." We might say that those who accept this become scientists, while those who doubt it become comedians. What better way to question the status quo than to make fun of it?

Terry Pratchett's Discworld is a series of magical stories about a flat Earth held up by four elephants standing on the back of a turtle. Rather than starting with what cannot be doubted, Pratchett starts with the untenable.

"I think therefore I am," makes as little sense as Discworld. They are both ridiculous and superfluous. The perception of being is just that: a perception. It does not need to be grounded in anything, because perception is a process, not a thing.

Processes are fabricated out of relationships; they are not made of anything. Emergent processes are the basic processes that have no prior explanation. The electromagnetic force is an emergent process that emerged in the early universe (LibreTexts), and atoms, molecules, and all of chemistry are based on it.

We get farther by embracing emergence as fundamental, than arguing for self-perception as something more basic. Your identity is built on relationships; why is it so hard for people to accept that everything else is too?

What's It Worth?

To believe that through the process of thinking, you will settle the question of your existence really means you will not think about it anymore. You are accepting the subjective point of view that self-perception is basic. You are taking your experience as something everything else needs to fit into.

To think there is one sense of being is a mistake. From this error arises confusion that leads us in directions that are never entirely right but can be entirely wrong. Religions avoid this closed way of thinking by positing higher levels that are inaccessible to humans.

In learning, the breakthrough comes when you realize there is more to the world than what you see. Learning to see more or more widely is an emergent process, and from it, new relationships emerge.

In almost every case, my therapy clients are looking for a different self, one that requires enlargement. Relationship counseling encourages breaking the constraints of one's previous world. Problems are not fixed, they're outgrown. Problems are not puzzles that need to be solved, they are elements of larger relationships. Growth is realizing that what you think is not what there is. Learning means finding a new being.

Our Choices

Being grounded means temporarily feeling permanent. It's being satisfied with temporality. Being healthy means being both permanent and impermanent, and also not permanent and not impermanent. There is something in between. This is not a simple state; it's a state of being close to wonder but not bewildered. If there was only one of you, what hope would there be? And if there is more than one of you, where are the others?

Consider reincarnation, which, in its radical form, says that lives accumulate outside of bodies. If we see our birth and death as endpoints, then reincarnation is an idea that has no support. But if we were to find that we inherent aspects of our identity and even memory, then the idea becomes plausible.

Other animals inherit knowledge. Insects appear to inherit almost all of their knowledge, and their societies are complex. You might say that a bird learns to fly through muscle memory, but how does a spider learn to weave a web?

The greater part of what is you is not built from your memories at all, but from the aptitudes and instincts you've inherited and which have naturally emerged. Our personalities are the identities we associate with ourselves, but these personalities are little more than a costume. We may be born without an identity, and our identity may disappear when we die. Our personality feels like everything, even though it contributes little to who we are.

Our personality is a house of mirrors. We can't see outside it while we're within it. To be stuck in one's state is a problem, but so is not having a state to be in. Being able to change requires having something to change, and something to change into. Your internal voice is just a voice. You might feel aligned with it, but it might say things you don't expect. You are the publisher, not the author; your voice isn't you.

You cannot be only what you think. After all, words are just symbols. To have meaning, your voice must be more than just sound. You must have a personality, and a flat and toneless voice has none.

Imagine that the words you speak are just thoughts. Not your thoughts, just thoughts like the writings on the billboards you pass on the highway. What I'm saying is that thoughts are not all there is. You can have a personality without speaking or thinking anything. You can just listen. All that's necessary is awareness.

This self is the primal being. It does not need to think or speak. If you can understand this inner self, then you can communicate with yourself without words. As would seem obvious, telepathy certainly exists in the realm of communications going on inside you. This communication encompasses all of who you are, no matter how many voices you contain.

Who Speaks?

Why have any voice at all? If words need a mouth, and a mouth implies an identity, and an identity desires to be singular, then would it not be better if we had no speaking self?

One answer is yes: having a sense of self beyond words is a step toward transcendent self-knowledge. But, at the same time, no. We tried that. That was us as nonverbal animals, and our power was limited. We need a voice that uses words and ideas. We need to master the egoistic, self-limiting reality that ideas create.

I know two paths to get beyond the limited thought of who you are. As Dante said in *The Divine Comedy* in 1321, they are the guide and the void.

Be at a loss for words or—even better, a loss of self—and find your way into a lost space. This could be a space of total emptiness, or a space of such chaos that you are overwhelmed: the void. A place beyond the world that you know.

Connect with another voice. This voice might have a viewpoint that you recognize or not. We do have several voices based on recollections of ourselves from earlier times, and maybe later times. We create these voices to introduce us to things that we don't yet know. These are our guides.

The Void

There are more voids than there are real worlds, or so it seems. Void-ness exists outside the bounds of our emotions. When anger goes beyond words, you enter a space of feeling, and also when enraptured with love and connection. These are not empty places, they are full of emotion. They are empty only because speech is inadequate. These spaces can be mysterious, despairing, ecstatic, or of any emotional texture.

Voids are memorable. They can be sparse or overwhelming; I've been to both. They are extremely emotional. In fact—as voids lack words and form by definition—emotion is the most memorable thing about them. The emotions they elicit are unique. They are unlike any other situation in their strength and composition. They are visions of new worlds.

The Guides

I recently spent some time with my mother in a dream. She was not a guiding force during her lifetime, but an important personality, of course. Now, she was livelier than usual and, as our conversation wound to a close, I asked her where she was. She brightened and declared with certainty, "Oh, you're silly. I don't exist!" Shocked, I woke up.

If thinking is existing, then my mother existed simply by virtue of her thinking, but she denied this. Maybe she was wrong; maybe she did exist. What are we to think when a part of us tells us it doesn't exist?

This was certainly the deepest thing she'd ever said to me, ever, and I believe she spoke directly. She addressed the idea that something needs to exist in order to be real and she refuted it.

Learning and healing exist because we can be led or otherwise moved in an orderly manner to create something that does not yet exist. There is some preexisting state of knowing or health; a primordial state that we're aware of. Perhaps it's simply the blueprint of a thought-structure that's talking to us.

We think in ideas and we hear in words, and if the blueprint is going to communicate with us, it must do so through the mechanisms of ideas and words. Or, perhaps, it's us who clothe the ineffable message in a speaking form. The form of the message is not important.

Lucidity

Reality is a diversion. What we call real is consciousness perceiving itself. Looking for consciousness is definitely a looking-under-the-streetlamp sort of phenomenon. It involves looking for what's not there in the realm of what can be seen, because it isn't anywhere else. It's not in the brain, of the brain, or outside the brain. Awareness is an active state of energy, not a stable state of matter. Like one of those inflated air structures, it's got to have constant pressure holding it up or else it deflates.

Who became lucid in the dream with my mother? Did I become lucid that my sense of existence was only in my mind? Or did my subconscious become lucid that my conscious mind had strayed into the kitchen? Who was aware of whom?

I am amused by encounters of this sort. They change who I am. You can deny the reality of your mother in a dream, but you cannot deny the feelings that accompany the experience. It's feelings that change us, not facts.

172

This is the message I offer to lucid dreamers and to all dreamers: your dreams are the kitchen of your mind, the subconscious realm where reality is cooked up. If you have integrity, respect, and act responsibly, then you may be allowed to witness the chef at work. And, if you can demonstrate your maturity, you might be allowed to do some cooking.

When this happens, you will not be awake in your dream, nor will you be conscious in your subconscious—it will be something else. You will be in the kitchen mixing belief, memory, and experience to bring to the table a dish of reality. We are not aware enough to be brilliant chefs, but we might aspire to pancakes.

> "Life isn't about finding yourself. Life is about creating yourself."
> — **George Bernard Shaw**

References

LibreTexts, "Evolution of the Early Universe." In *OpenStax CNX, University Physics III: Optics & Modern Physics*. https://phys.libretexts.org/Bookshelves/University_Physics/Book%3A_University_Physics_(OpenStax)/University_Physics_III_-_Optics_and_Modern_Physics_(OpenStax)/11%3A_Particle_Physics_and_Cosmology/11.08%3A_Evolution_of_the_Early_Universe

T8 – The Fundamental Question

September 16, 2020

Do fundamental questions make any sense?

"You only live once, but if you do it right, once is enough." — **Mae West**

The Beginning

What would you say is the most fundamental question? Would it be the origin of the universe or the meaning of life? What about, "Does God exist?" or "Is there other intelligent life in the universe?" I suggest there is a deeper question that underlies them all. I suggest the most fundamental question is, "How do we understand anything that we don't already know?"

A person who is blue-green color blind cannot distinguish blue from green. They can see both, but they cannot tell them apart. How can you describe the difference between blue and green to a blue-green color-blind person? If you said, "It's like the difference between pink and orange," would that make any sense?

What if there was someone who knew the answer to some tremendously important question —let's call them a prophet—and they gave answers using words we didn't know? Would we call that an answer? What if they explained it in words we knew but couldn't make sense of?

Let's say the prophet is a mathematician. They gave you formulas that answered the important question. These formulas were mathematically correct but exceeded your understanding. Would that be an answer?

The answer in each of these cases is no because to ask any question presumes you will understand the answer. It presumes that you could see what you're looking for if you only knew where to look. All questions make this presumption.

In fact, they are not really questions in the sense of looking for a new understanding. All our questions only make sense as questions of location or arrangement. They are questions in the same form as, "Where did I leave my keys?" or, "Which one of these choices is correct?"

The fundamental difference between physics and mathematics is that physics is based on observation, while mathematics is based on consistency. These two approaches are independent. There are an infinite number of logically consistent mathematical expressions, and there are an infinite number of things that can be observed. Most of the expressions are not observable, and most observations have no mathematical expression.

Both physics and mathematics have criteria for accepting novelty. They accept innovation because there are always new observations and proofs. Physicists accept new observations, and mathematicians accept whatever can be proved.

The Middle

We don't live in either of these two worlds. No one but a physicist or mathematician is satisfied with an explanation grounded entirely in one of these fields. When we ask fundamental questions, we're expecting something personally meaningful. What is our basis for accepting an answer?

What is personally meaningful depends on whether we're offered an answer we already knew but didn't think of—such as locating our keys—or whether we're offered an answer that we can't understand. Of course, it's the conflict between the kinds of answers we'll accept that makes all the difference.

If we're given a tangible answer, then we're in the physics camp: we can touch and test the answer, and it satisfies whatever need generated the question. We're satisfied.

If we're given an intangible answer, we could go either way. Usually, if we've got something we can apply to a problem, then we might call it an answer, even if it doesn't always work. If it doesn't work at all, then we're clearly in the market for a different answer.

If you want to know how to make it rain so the crops will grow, then you might accept a solution that entails performing a ceremony that sometimes works. Seeding clouds with dry ice and farming with nitrogen fertilizer might work better. You might call those better answers to a different question.

What do you do if you're offered two answers, one that you understand and one that you don't? Let's say you've got a disease and you want a cure, and your religion says pray, and your doctor says there's nothing you can do. What then?

Well, naturally, you pray. What else could you do? Perhaps you'd abandon the whole question and go out and have fun, but that would be cheating because it doesn't answer the question.

The issue lies here: is an answer something you do or something you know? Those two paths have formed the warp and woof of the fabric of human history. And it's because we have those two elements—and no other animal seems to have gotten as caught up in them as much as we have—that makes our species special.

This doesn't mean we can answer fundamental questions. It means humans create new foundations on which we can build things. We create foundations to support certain kinds of answers.

The insightful approach to the fundamental question is to recognize how we structure answers and to consider how this defines what an answer can be. It turns out that no matter how robust and inclusive we feel in our ability to find answers, there is an infinite area beyond this foundation. We might call this area "the sacred."

I take it as proved that there are an infinite number of logically consistent possibilities that we cannot observe. There are also an infinite number of things we can observe that we cannot logically explain. It's the intersection of these two domains—those things that we can both observe and explain—that satisfy our demand for answers. The number of explanations that meet our criteria, compared to the number that don't, is infinitesimally small. In mathematical terms, we say this is a space whose size measures zero.

This should be somewhat deflating. It certainly casts doubt on our search for the ultimate answer. Worse than that, it casts doubt on our ability to find any fundamental answers. But I don't think things are as bad as all that.

The problem is this: what are we to do with answers we don't understand? Or, to put it another way, how are we to come to new understandings? I have answers to both questions.

Consider answers we don't understand, such as, "There is a God," or, "The universe is a hologram." We accept these as answers, at least some of us do, so what does this tell us? It tells us that sometimes, and for some people, a fundamental answer lies along a dimension that has two extremes. The answer can mean nothing or it can mean anything.

"There is a God," which is an answer similar in form to the statement, "The purpose of life is to be happy," means nothing in itself. It's actually the name of a program, and it's the program that provides a practical answer to a fundamental question. This program does not provide a logically consistent answer. Some fundamentalists might disagree, but they are out of their territory.

Religion is not logically consistent, and it's a fraud to claim it to be. It can never win the logic battle and, as far as its adherents are concerned, it does not need to. Religion answers the practical side of the question of existence. It provides a useful answer in the domain of behavior. Unfortunately, religions don't patrol their practicality well. Enforcing behavior is a different problem.

At the other end of the nothing/anything dichotomy lies those answers that we cannot understand, and we cannot even think we understand. Here lie the logically consistent answers that we cannot observe, or we might observe but cannot understand what we see.

The statements such as "the universe is a hologram," or, "before the Big Bang time did not exist," or, "everything exists because of fundamental equations," may all be true. There may exist logical demonstrations of them. But do these statements answer our fundamental questions?

They do not. They answer their own questions or questions that only have meaning within the mind of a holographer, astrophysicist, or mathematician. Actually, holographers, astrophysicists, and mathematicians who speak with integrity won't claim their answers apply to you.

These two forms of an answer to our fundamental questions—the no answer and the anything answer—are two forms of the same answer. A no answer leaves space for anything, and an anything answer gives no direction, which also leaves space for anything.

The End

This brings us to the conclusion that unless you can phrase your answers in terms that are practical, you don't have a valid question. All you've got is a program that can amount to anything or nothing at all.

This focuses us on the practical: a useful answer must have practical meaning. Practical meaning refers to something that you have experienced, something that has told you something about how the world works, and shows you how to work in the world. Neither God nor equations fulfill this requirement. It's the program, prescription, algorithm, or instructions that make up the answer.

But we're not quite done. There's one small path we need to traverse: the path of learning. Whenever we learn something, we expand the range of what we can do. This expands what we can admit to our program, the range of our algorithm, and the instructions we can follow. If we never learn anything, then the limits of our program are circumscribed. That may still leave a large domain of possibilities, but, from a practical point of view, we're constrained to think and act within a limited range.

Important kinds of learning provide new options. How do we achieve that? How do we learn something that we don't know?

> "Recent decades have revealed that social learning and the transmission of cultural traditions are much more widespread in the animal kingdom than earlier suspected, affecting numerous forms of functional behavior and creating a secondary form of evolution, built onto the better-known primary, genetically based form."
> — **Whiten, Ayala, Feldman, & Laland** (2017)

We have watched other animals of every species encounter novelty, overcome obstacles, and learn new skills (Whiten 2000). But in the wild, animals only seem to learn what other animals of the same species have learned before them. This applies even to our closest animal relatives. It seems humans are the only exception, and the scope of what other animals learn is circumscribed by their genetics.

"The intellectual abilities supporting learning by imitation, teaching, symbolic language, etc., may have developed to the point where culture could develop only within the hominid line." — **Bennett G. Galef, Jr.** (1992)

In 1952 and 1953, primatologists studying troops of Macaque monkeys on Koshima Island, Japan, introduced a novelty in the form of sweet potatoes left on the beach. The monkeys discovered they could make the potatoes more comestible by washing off the sand in the seawater. This behavior was seen to start with a single individual and then spread throughout the troop.

These observations became the foundation of what was later heralded as "the hundredth monkey theory," in which new behavior telepathically jumped—whatever that means—to monkeys on other islands once enough monkeys adopted it. Subsequent examinations of field reports show that this "jump" did not occur. Instead, the new behavior was taught from one monkey to another (Rensberger 1985). These observations show how unusual it is for a species of any kind to learn anything new.

The question of what is learning is a fundamental question closely associated with the question of what is knowing. Is learning to do something by imitating another the same as conceiving a new thought for yourself? Is imitation just following along, or is it thinking ahead?

> "To understand how another works as a goal-directed agent, an observer must understand not only his goals but also his perceptions because what he sees and knows helps to determine what he does."
> — **Josep Call** and **Michael Tomasello** (2008)

When I was taught calculus by memorizing answers, I behaved correctly but understood nothing. Yet when calculus was explained to me, I understood what was being done and where to apply it, but I didn't know how to solve as many problems. In the first case, I had learned mimicry, in the second case, I had insight. When I complained that the first learning program was lacking, I was punished by being given a poor grade: I had failed to "understand."

Learning something new, and being aware of knowledge in others, can be important. But if you don't know how to use a new idea, then it can have no significance at all.

"Reactions to the death of companions and recognition of the self are phenomena that may also relate to a general capacity for empathy, which has similarly been identified in the great apes and in elephants."
— **Richard Byrne** and **Lucy Bates** (2010, 822)

The social pressure and the individual need to learn are different for all social animals. The meaning of learning and knowing likely differs between these two circumstances. And while most of human learning is social, it's learned from communicating with others, most inspired acts of learning, human or otherwise, occur in isolation. What you learn from others telling you is not of the same epistemological quality of neural structure as what you learn yourself.

" 'Species intelligence,' by analogy with usage of the term intelligence in differential psychology, refers to the innate potential for cognitive power of every individual of the species; but the extent to which that potential is realized may depend on an individual's social network… Some particular skills such as insightful cooperation or deception, perception of intent, imitation of novel skills, and mirror self-recognition, signify a qualitatively different representation of mechanisms and minds."
— **Byrne** and **Bates** (2010, 824).

Defining the realm of answers brings us to the question of how we enlarge the realm of answers. This returns us to the question of what we knew before, and how we add to that.

I assert it can be proved the set of answers is infinite, and that expanding out from our limited domain of understanding is a recursive process. We find answers; we discover the answers are inadequate; and we look for new answers. There can be no answer to how we learn because we can never define what it is to know in the first place.

In summary, all those who want fundamental answers are doomed not to find them. Fundamental answers never made sense and, while we now have terabytes of answers, they only amount to instructions for orienting ourselves in an increasingly large house of facts. Our answers are still some combination of nothing and anything, and no combination of that form meets the requirement of practicality.

Perhaps I've performed a sleight of hand, and all of this has been a shell game. The truth of the matter is that none of the fundamental questions make sense.

References

Byrne, R. W., Bates, L. A. (2010 Mar 25). "Primate Social Cognition: Uniquely Primate, Uniquely Social, or Just Unique?" *Neuron, 65*: 815-30. https://www.cell.com/neuron/pdf/S0896-6273(10)00181-9.pdf

Call, J., Tomasello, M. (2008). "Does the Chimpanzee Have a Theory of Mind? 30 Years Later." *Trends in Cognitive Sciences, 12* (5): 187-92. https://doi.org/10.1016/j.tics.2008.02.010

Galef, B. G. (1991). "The Question of Animal Culture." *Human Nature, 3* (2): 157-78. https://doi.org/10.1007/BF02692251

Rensberger, B. (1985 Jul 6). "Spud-Dunking Monkey Theory Debunked." *The Washington Post*. https://www.washingtonpost.com/archive/politics/1985/07/06/spud-dunking-monkey-theory-debunked/20866773-cf8f-44ed-a801-1c1323064460/

Whiten, A. (2000). "Primate Culture and Social Learning." *Cognitive Science, 24* (3): 477-508. https://doi.org/10.1207/s15516709cog2403_6

Whiten, A., Ayala, F. J., Feldman, M. W., & Laland, K. N. (2017 Jul 25). "The Extension of Biology Through Culture." *Proceedings of the National Academy of Sciences USA, 114* (30): 7775-81. https://doi.org/10.1073/pnas.1707630114

T9 – The Time of Your Life

November 6, 2020

If time is so valuable, why are you so unaware of it?

Come fruit flies once fruit is wasted; time flies once time is wasted.

We all have the experience of being aware while we're awake. We feel that we're self-aware all of our waking lives. Sometimes we space out, but even then we feel we were somewhere, even if in our own world.

Most likely you're only here half the time, depending on the situation. The most dramatic example that we're familiar with is doing something that doesn't require our reasoning mind. Driving comes to mind.

In almost every case, while you feel yourself to be aware while driving, you can remember almost nothing about the drive. You may remember a few notable sights, events, or ideas, but often you can't recall much. Maybe you remember that first turn as you exit your home street. That memory is ingrained more by repetition than intellectual engagement.

This is common, and we give it little thought. We tell ourselves, if we even bother to think about it, that there were better things to think about then, and more useful things to remember now. We assume we were aware during our drive, but we choose not to dwell on it. Driving perceptions do not make it into long-term memory.

The truth seems to be that little of us is present during events where we act automatically. Our sense of self is a deception. We have little sense of time. Like a tablecloth, time lays over our experience, creating an even texture of highs and lows: it provides the perception of peaks of high attention and valleys of scant attention. Little of us is engaged in self-awareness at any moment. Time passes like the flutter of the leaves on a tree. In a few moments, we lose awareness of it.

Keeping Time

"Time may change me, but you can't trace time."
— **David Bowie**, pop singer and songwriter, from the song *Changes*

There are several ways to look at this. The most common way is that this doesn't matter. We are as present as we are, and that's the end of it. One might even claim that if we were more present, we'd quickly become exhausted. This might be true, but if it is, then it reflects more on what we're used to than what we're capable of.

I look at this from a subtle perspective, exploring my thinking and that of my clients. By watching brainwaves, I've gained some ability to sense my frequency of awareness. It's an indirect thing similar to watching the scenery: you focus more on how you're seeing and not what you're seeing. I keep track of how much I feel is happening, and keep a tally of how aware I am as the day goes by.

I awoke with a dream that irritated me, and I recalled the scene and the feeling. I was left with more of a mood than a memory, as I couldn't recall the topics of the dream. Nevertheless, I thought about it as best I could. Then I read some articles, and this resulted in one thing I have resolved to remember. I made breakfast and, while I can recall what I ate, I recall nothing more. My sense of time is proportional to how much I can recall.

This is not "the power of now," such as many are enamored with. "The Now" is whatever is happening now, which may be a lot or nothing. If you are too narrowly focused on "the now" then you're watching a window of time that more reflects your awareness of what's around you, rather than your awareness of what's inside you. This can add up to a lot or it can add up to nothing. Being in "the now" is looking at the beans without counting them.

What's Happening

Perception and awareness are exclusive. You can't do both at the same time because it takes time to convert what you perceive into what you're aware of. You might think that we've got different systems that act at the same time: the eyes perceive and the brain reflects all in a continuous stream. This does not seem to be the case.

It's like digestion: there are waves of input, consideration, interpretation, and reaction. Some things are done in sequence, such as receiving stimulation from our senses. But the consideration, interpretation, and reaction parts are all done in our brain, or somewhere in our nervous system. The brain does not have separate mechanisms for every input.

Self-awareness is distributed throughout our brain, and this produces various forms of cognition for different events. It does a kind of task sharing in which dissimilar elements of awareness are prepared at different rates, with the more important elements getting higher priority. Then it puts these back together in time for our consideration. Experience is like betting on a horse race: we're constantly moving back and forth from watching the race to changing our bets.

Experience is like the kitchen of a busy restaurant preparing many meals at once. Different parts of different dishes are cooked at different stations, some in sequence and some in parallel. Some components are prepared ahead of time, others are done just in time. The components are assembled and the dish—which represents our whole perception of something and not just bits and pieces—is delivered to the customer who, in this case, is some aspect of ourselves, "hungry" for action.

The time between ordering our meal—encountering the situation that needs our response—and receiving our order can vary from minutes to microseconds. Sometimes, we have to sleep on it. There are some problems I've been working on all my life, and you've got these too. Much of who you are constitutes a dish that may never be finished cooking.

Who's Counting?

As in the kitchen metaphor, managing your world requires coordination. A kitchen isn't dominated by managers with stopwatches only because those who work there have learned to manage themselves. The kitchen is run with precision timing. It comes with experience and becomes part of the skill of cooking. But even though no one in the kitchen is holding a stopwatch, there are stopwatches ticking everywhere inside people's heads.

Your head is filled with stopwatches too. They are your brainwaves, and there are different brain waves to coordinate different tasks. The clock speed of your visual cortex is 8 to 12 cycles per second, which is rather slow if you think about it. It's the jagged frame rate of an old movie or a poorly responding video game. This is not the speed of your discrimination, which is three or four times faster.

Your ability to discriminate is set by the basic length of the "measure" counted by the metronome in your visual cortex. Electrical waves sweep over your visual cortex. Your cell membranes are cyclically receptive to changes at this frequency. You might compare this with the boiling of pasta: the bubbles are rapid, but the cooking takes place over minutes.

The clock speed of your motor cortex is 12 to 14 cycles per second, and the clock speed of your auditory perception is higher still. Compare this with the braising of meat or vegetables, which occurs over a twenty-second time span. These clock rates, which we can see in our brainwaves, are not the speeds of our actions, they are the metronomes that synchronize our actions. Just as in music, the tempo can differ from the length of the measure, but the measure holds the musical structure.

As with music, you can speed things up or slow them down, but only to a point. You can learn to act and think more quickly, or be more relaxed and think at a slower pace. Beyond some point, you can't hold it all together. If you tune your speed down to a rate that's too slow, some things just won't "cook" right. Slow your brainwaves down enough and you'll first lose self-awareness, and then you'll fall asleep.

Amphetamines will raise your brainwave frequencies, and that will make you more engaged. You'll process shorter perceptions and execute faster brain processes. You can do this with a computer too: you can goose up a computer's clock speed and, as a result, get improved performance. This comes at a cost. In a computer, a faster clock generates more heat and, with overheating, you'll burn out the motherboard.

People overheat too, but it's not the heat that causes problems, it's the discomfort of continuous rapid response. This generates irritation that can lead to anxiety and rage. These are high-energy states that raise your pulse, trigger your hormones, and sap your strength. If sufficiently stimulated, you'll go berserk.

The fact remains that if you boost your clock speeds, you'll accomplish more, remember more, and have an expanded sense of time. You will have more time in your life. Here's the challenge: can you be more aware without expending more energy? I'm not asking whether you want to; I'm asking whether you can.

Flying Cars

Flying cars are right around the corner, so to speak. The technology is almost here, but you will not be driving one. That's because you don't have the neural hardware for it. Our brainwaves are not fast enough; they only to go up to 100 cycles per second. You can become more adept, but it will cost you in terms of energy and personality.

We're built to survey a horizontal plane, to see what's in front of us and to either side. Flying requires a three-dimensional awareness of things coming from all directions, and we don't have that. This is why the Federal Aviation Administration has created "streets" in the sky, and segmented the airspace into horizontal planes. You're not supposed to move from one plane to another without announcing your intention or getting their permission.

Birds have the required brainpower. Their brainwaves go up to 300 cycles per second. Their visual processing power is much faster than ours. Just watch songbirds at a feeder, or hummingbirds chasing each other, in order to get a sense of just how much faster their response time is than ours. They can fly through foliage at 30 miles per hour without hitting a leaf. This is all the more amazing when you appreciate that air is a sloppy medium. Changing your direction when flying takes much more planning than when you're driving a car. In the air, you're always skidding.

If you train as a pilot, you'll learn to boost and manage faster brainwaves, but that won't be enough to fly cars in the numbers and speeds that commuting requires. A pilot does not want to be within a mile of another airplane. A highway of cars flying next to each other at 200 miles per hour is far more than humans are built to handle.

We'll be flying in cars soon enough, but they'll be autonomous cars: they'll pilot themselves. It's easier to design an autonomous airborne car than one that drives on land because the only thing you need to watch for in the air is other flying objects. Remote sensing can do that.

The Hands of Time

I don't much care how you spend your time. You can waste it if you want. My purpose in writing this piece has nothing to do with what you choose to do. While it's true that you can become more aware by modulating your various clock speeds, I'm more interested in you in theory.

I suspect your nervous system eats time in discrete bites and does not experience time as a continuous flow. This is an active issue in computational neurology. Different parts of our nervous system take bites of different sizes—of time, that is—and we're only really aware of our biting-off pieces and not the time to chew them. Similar discrete-time theories can be found in ancient Buddhist texts.

Imagine strobe lights illuminating the temporal landscape with many flashes. Each of these flashes only illuminates a part of the landscape, not the whole of it. Some of these flash faster and others flash slower. What would your eye perceive?

Your eye, which has a narrow field of view to begin with and registers changes slowly, would see your field of view as continuously illuminated. But how much of what's out there would you really be seeing at any one time? Not much; almost nothing.

You would hardly be aware of the duration between flashes. You would see momentary flashes and you would process them all rather slowly, only interacting with things that move slowly enough to follow. We will not be piloting a flying car any sooner than we'll be texting while driving along a country road at 200 miles per hour, or catching flying bullets in midair.

Your brain takes a snapshot. You process it, and then you go back for another. You hope you can fill in the gaps with a continuous sense of change because you need to perceive the direction of things. That sense is what you use to predict where things will be next. If you can't do that, then you'll be caught flat-footed and trip over the sidewalk. Similarly, you struggle to feel continuity in a movie whose images are presented too slowly.

Your reality—all our realities—is like a mechanical clock. We "tick" along. The ticks are rather brief, around a tenth of a second for most of our functions, and between these ticks we're "thinking about it." Our brain goes somewhere to figure things out, and we are put on

187

automatic pilot.

When out of nowhere, someone demands an answer, what do you do? You say, "What?" What if the universe jumped out at you and demanded that you account for where you've been for the last nine-tenths of a second? That might be a sensible question for a bird, but not for you. You'd say, "What?"

Try being aware of your surroundings every second. Try being in "the now" every second, continuously for a minute. It's exhausting, but it's a good exercise in practicing what's ridiculous. With practice, you'll stop caring.

I would guess that you're aware half the time, and I think that's generous. If you live to be 90, then you've amassed about 45 years of awareness. Except, you slept for one-third of the time, so that means you were only half aware for 60 wakeful years, and aware for half of them. This cuts the time you were aware down to 30 years. That is the amount of time during which you're perceptive: 30 years of a 90-year-long life. We consider that perfectly natural.

Some people need more life and they struggle to get it. Speed yourself up with amphetamines and your teeth will fall out. Expand your mind with hard drugs and you may be dead before you're 40. These seem like poor solutions to the problem of leading a larger life, but you cannot dismiss them. There is an undeniable attraction to living more fully, and, for some people, whatever the cost, it's worth it.

T10 – It Comes From Space

December 3, 2020

The notion of distance in a network theory of thought processes.

"Those, however, who assert the absolute reality of space and time, whether they take it to be subsisting or only inhering, must themselves come into conflict with the principles of experience."— **Immanuel Kant** (1998, 166), philosopher

Distance

Of the many things we take for granted, space may be what we take for granted the most. Not only do we take it for granted, but we don't examine how much we apply it to things to which it doesn't apply. We project our notion of distance onto things that don't have distance, and we don't think about it.

For example, we recognize emotional distance, which has nothing to do with space or measure. We categorize people by their movements and how close they are to us. But it's their attitude, not their location or mobility, that matters. We need to attend to those who are right next to us, but it's the jet setters, homebodies, good neighbors, urbanites, car campers, and road warriors that we need to keep an eye on.

We describe space by quoting distance, but we experience space subjectively. Space is not so much a matter of distance as it is the time or effort required to traverse it. We're constantly distorting our subjective experience of space but overlooking these experiences. When we unconsciously drive to our destination, we consider the short time elapsed to be unreal. When we endure an unexpected period of walking, it dominates the recollection even though it took up no mental space. We write off as illusions the dreams we have of spaces that make no sense.

Humans experience space as something uniform in all directions. Distance is a measure that does not change when pointed in another direction. We carelessly take these objective notions of navigation—which are not what we experience—and apply them to all manner of experience. We understand distance and depth instinctively, but not accurately.

These preconceptions are wired into our brains. They're built into our bodies and have nothing to do with our abstract notions of space. We use our instincts of distance, speed, and momentum in learning to move and balance, and then we apply them to everything.

I want to talk about space for two reasons. First, because there's more to it. And second, because our preconception causes us to ignore what we should see.

Thinking About Space

We don't navigate physical space; we navigate mental space. When we think about motion, we apply a subjective meaning of distance. Physical space is something we abstract but largely ignore. In fact, we don't see physical space—we construct a projection of it. The distances and depths that we perceive are things we create in our minds based on the movements of light and shadow.

We guide ourselves using paths, not distances, measuring paths in terms of risk, reward, time, and cost. We might use the measured distance as a shorthand to express the separation between us and our friends, but distance plays no role in our decisions. In some sense, distance doesn't even exist because we're always in the same place; wherever we go, we're always "here."

The simple and fundamental understanding of space is that it's the same in all directions. We apply this notion to many other "territories" that should not be described in terms of space at all, such as growth, maturity, aptitude, and emotion.

We are full of measures like I.Q., sociability, wealth, and happiness. We apply these measures to ourselves and to everyone else. Wherever we describe something as being more or less, we create a map of equal spacing and place ourselves on it. You have placed yourself on such a map now; you are judging yourself according to your distance to your goal. But this is nonsense: there is no such "distance."

You may be described as being happier than I am, but who is to say that our notions of happiness can be compared? You may think you have a long way to go to make your life meaningful. You may think you are close to achieving your goals. These distances are deceptions.

What's measured by an I.Q. test is not intelligence. The many things that stand between you and happiness are not "there." Just because you have one hundred childhood traumas does not mean you have one hundred issues to resolve. Just because something can be measured, named, or enumerated doesn't make it real.

> "The problem is not that our perceptions are wrong about this or that detail. It's that the very language of objects in space and time is simply the wrong language to describe objective reality." — **Donald Hoffman** (2019), cognitive scientist

Space as a Network

We don't really think of our movement through space in terms of distance. We don't map our thoughts on a graph. Our thoughts form a network—like our movements. It is an organic network that grows and shrinks with our mood and to which new links are frequently added, but we don't bother to map it. We should.

In this thought network, there are dominant thoughts that occupy us most of the time. These are our thought network's main nodes. Connected to these nodes are less common thoughts. There are paths between thoughts, and these connections can be rich or impoverished. These paths are strange and we leave them unexplored. The network of our thoughts is filled with passages—doors we've passed a hundred times but prefer not to see. We've taken some of these passages a hundred times, but we overlook their significance or prefer to.

Most intermediate thoughts lead in several directions, leading to differences that depend on how you approach them. Approaching thoughts of your parents from the perspective of money will take you to a different conclusion than what you'd reach if you were thinking about mortality or childhood.

Compared to the network of your thoughts, the network of your paths in space is far simpler. Your spatial network is a series of maps, each for a different mode of travel. There will be one map for walking, and others for driving, flying over the landscape, and puttering around the kitchen. Your thoughts are not so simple.

The network of your thoughts is made complicated both because of the connections you ignore and the way your thoughts combine. You don't combine paths on a travel network—you either take one or the other; but when you build thoughts, you often pursue several lines at once. You set up resonances where thoughts bounce back and forth between paths, and what you do will depend on when you act more than what you think.

It's hard to imagine your thought network, but you can build it area by area. A complete map might be possible, but you'd never need it. These maps are not stable. They change over time, and they change just because you look at them. You can always rebuild a thought network when you need it.

Imagine that you understood yourself as a network of thoughts. Different nodes of your map might represent different thoughts or points of view. They might represent different people. You might map your personalities as if they were other people—other people who you might be rather than the person you are.

Imagine you could see the map for other people you know, even if you could see only a small portion of it. More usefully, what if you could choose to look at particular parts of this map for certain people? Isn't this what you're doing when you try to understand someone?

There is good evidence that chimpanzees can understand something of what we are thinking and what other chimps are thinking. They understand goals, intentions, perceptions, and knowledge. But what it seems they cannot understand is false beliefs, the knowing of things that are not true (Call & Tomasello 2008, 191). For us, truth and untruth are inseparable. For our closest relatives, untruth, or false knowing, does not exist.

Consider the consequences. Armed with untruth, we can make conceptual enemies, people with whom we'll go to war based on their false beliefs. Chimpanzees only go to war based on territory or resources. They can dislike another individual, but only because of what they've done or threaten to do, not because of how they think.

With our power, we can demonize races and dismiss traditions. Our range of thought is more powerful, but are we using this power to positive ends?

Using the Network

In a post titled "How the World Changes" (Stoller 2020) I mentioned there is a "force of mind" that determines what thoughts emerge in our consciousness. This idea related elemental thoughts that work together to activate our ideas. These form a network of salient links connecting familiar territories.

Force of mind is a measure of distance. It measures what gets you from one idea to another. You reach related thoughts by understanding their strengths, what supports them, and where they lead. Every thought has a context in terms of what it accomplishes and where it comes from.

When you are depressed, you inhabit an unhappy network with few paths out of a dismal valley. Within this network, you will notice inner conflicts, odd connections, and strange conclusions. You don't need the entire map, as mapping your critical nodes will be sufficient. Your map's instability is not a failure but the whole purpose of the exercise: you're seeing how you're thinking in real time, rather than rationalizing how you should be thinking.

If you're fearful, trace your thoughts as they turn from possibility to panic. This is partly rational, but it is also the actual path of experience. Understanding the progression could stop the runaway train of fears.

I had a client who was facing a trip to Southeast Asia and who was afraid of air travel. We followed the thoughts and discovered it wasn't the conclusions that were the problem, but the powerlessness of the situation. It was not airplanes of which my client was afraid—although that thought instilled panic—it was powerlessness and captivity.

Your thought networks show the details of your thought patterns. This is far more useful than a label. Labels don't give any sense of direction between states of mind or differences between people, and they don't provide insight into how to change. My client's label was "fear of flying," a kind of paranoia, but that said nothing of the origin of the situation.

We take space for granted and, because of this, we employ simple notions of how we think. There is no "space" in mind-space. There are no linear distances or dimensions in your thoughts. These measures don't exist.

Mind-space is something that emerges dynamically from the way thoughts build themselves. Without a theory of our mental network, psychology is sterile. With such a theory, who knows how far we can go?

References

Call, J., Tomasello, M. (2008). "Does the Chimpanzee Have a Theory of Mind? 30 Years Later." *Trends in Cognitive Sciences, 12* (5): 187-92. https://doi.org/10.1016/j.tics.2008.02.010

Hoffman, D. (2019), *The Case Against Reality: Why Evolution Hid the Truth From Our Eyes*. W. W. Norton & Company.

Kant, I. (1998). *Critique of Pure Reason* (1781). Cambridge University Press. https://rauterberg.employee.id.tue.nl/lecturenotes/DDM110%20CAS/Kant-1781%20Critique%20of%20Pure%20Reason.pdf

Stoller, L. (2020 Nov 12). "How the World Changes." Mind Strength Balance. https://www.mindstrengthbalance.com/2020/11/12/how-the-world-changes/

T11 – Independent Thinkers

December 13, 2020

Independent thinking is not an alternative because dependent thinking is not thinking.

"In economics, the majority is always wrong."
— **John Kenneth Galbraith,** economist

Stereotyping

Stereotyping makes it easier to categorize thoughts and behavior. The danger is that it's incorrect. This opens the issue of critical versus collective thinking, where to draw the line, and what are the advantages of the two.

The following thoughts were stimulated by a *New York Times* article titled, "Why Do So Many Americans Think the Election Was Stolen?" (Douthat 2020). I'm not concerned with the vote count, I'm focusing on the way the author, Ross Douthat, stereotypes people. Douthat defines a category of "outsider-intellectuals" this way:

> "The next category of believer consists of extremely smart people whose self-identification is bound up in constantly questioning and doubting official forms of knowledge."

The New York Times, a cautious bastion of liberalism, seems to blow a smoke screen to cover its editorial prejudice. It certainly is not logically consistent to lump into one group all people who question anything, regardless of whether they're smart or self-identifying. To do so is to consider them all identical to a large degree.

What does it mean to be extremely smart and have one's self-identification bound up in constantly questioning? This is not a statement, it's a judgment. I constantly question things. Does that mean that I'm bound up in it, and does that mean that I invalidate myself?

195

Official Knowledge

There is a big difference between doubting official knowledge and doubting knowledge that claims to be official. To doubt official knowledge is to say, "There's something wrong with the official reasoning." To doubt officially endorsed knowledge is to say, "Officials can't justify knowledge." People who have difficulty discerning the difference between knowledge they justify themselves, and knowledge justified by decree will have difficulty recognizing reason from prejudice.

Most people are poor critical thinkers and do not distinguish between what they've heard and what they say. Putting "outsider-intellectuals" into a separate camp and then setting up critical thinkers as self-identifiers—which isn't defined but sounds bad—is preparation for dismissing alternatives entirely.

The New York Times defines East Coast liberal bias, although no one authorized them to play that role. Nothing good will come from a biased group that does not recognize their bias and, instead, puts the onus of narrow thinking on other groups. Several "logical fallacy" alarm bells should start to ring as you read Ross Douthat's piece.

> "Conservatism has always had plenty of this sort in its ranks, but the consolidated progressive orthodoxy in elite institutions means that more and more people come to conservative ideas because they seem like a secret knowledge, an account of the world that's compelling and yet excluded from official discourse.

> "This, in turn, instills a perpetual suspicion about anything that seems to have too much of a liberal consensus defending it, especially any idea that gets mocked and laughed at more than it gets rebutted. And it creates a strong epistemological bias toward what you can only find out for yourself, as opposed to what Yale's experts or Twitter's warning labels or *The New York Times* might tell you."

Following this argument, we've gone from collecting independent thinkers to implying they reject the views held by *The New York Times*. He has gone from expert opinions being opinions that reflect expertise, to expert opinions being opinions put forward by experts. That is a conflation of what's true with what's proclaimed. He has seen the enemy and, it seems, they are all those not in his camp.

"In many cases, the outsider-intellectual's approach generates real insight. But it also tends to recapitulate the closed-circle problems of the official knowledge it rejects."

Do you do that? Do you recapitulate your rejection of the closed-circle problems of official knowledge?

"Thus, the outsider-intellectual type looks at the no-voter-fraud consensus and immediately goes out in search of cracks in the pillar of official truth, anomalies that official certainty elides. A lot of the supposed evidence of fraud that circulates online comes from these efforts—not from grifts or lies (though grifters and liars do pick them up) but from sincere analyses of election data, which inevitably turn up anomalies here and there, which confirm the searchers' assumptions, which closes the circle and convinces them that the official narrative is false and voter fraud is real."

This is not what every skeptical person does. He has created a "straw man" argument.

"To the outsider-intellectuals fascinated by anomalies in ballot counts or ballot return patterns, I've argued that anomalies indicating fraud would have to show up in the final vote totals—meaning some pattern of results in key swing-state cities that differ starkly from the results in cities in less-contested states… but where claims for those kinds of anomalies have been offered, they've turned out to be false. So until a compelling example can be cited, anomalies in the counting process should be presumed to be error or randomness, not fraud."

Logical Fallacies

This author begins with the fallacy that those who deviate from any norm make up a type. In the above paragraph, he adds two more fallacies: the "straw man" and ignorance as corroboration.

The straw man fallacy is when you surreptitiously divert the argument to a different subject upon which you can give a compelling argument, and then, have reached a compelling conclusion, you redirect this conclusion back to the original issue. Whether fraud would show up in the final vote totals is an entirely different issue from whether voting fraud exists. It is a specific case. You cannot argue generalities on the basis of specifics.

T11 - Independent Thinkers

Acceptance of ignorance occurs when you argue that not knowing is equivalent to there being nothing to know. Here, he argues that not knowing of fraud indicates there is no fraud. It may be that there is no fraud, but our not knowing about it in no way implies that it does not exist.

Consider crime. There is a lot of crime we don't know about and of which we see no evidence. It still exists.

In the end, as is so often the case in passive-aggressive confrontations, we feel we're being helped to see more clearly. Neither this author nor myself believe significant voting fraud was perpetrated. He rejects the notion as unsupportable because he can't see it. I simply believe it was insignificant or so deeply embedded in the system as to be invisible.

He rejects the concept, whereas I reject the conclusion. He implies that if you are not confused by self-identification, then you should accept the general conclusion based on the specific example. This is not super smart, it's dumb.

Evidence can never prove a theory, it can only limit a theory to a realm within the evidence. You can disprove the theory that the moon is made of green cheese, but you can never disprove the lesser theory that some of the moon is made of green cheese. Implausibility is not disproof.

This is no small matter. A theory is just a construction; it is never the complete story. Every theory can be adjusted to fit the evidence. You can never know the ultimate truth because there is no such thing. Ultimate truth is a human concept.

There is no unassailable truth, but some people insist there is. This underlies the prejudice against independent thinkers. Those who hold this prejudice are the real self-identifying thinkers, and Ross Douthat is one.

Every advance sprouts from the cracks in the old truths. If you are not an independent thinker, then you're not thinking. I am of the independent-thinking tribe, and you should be too. Join me. There is only room for one in the group that always agrees with me, but you can start your own group.

Ivermectin

The "wonder drug" Ivermectin (Crump & Omura 2011) has been explored as a treatment for COVID-19 since the summer of 2020. The results of six large clinical trials now appear in a preprint presented by the Front Line COVID-19 Critical Care Alliance (Kory et al. 2020)

Dr. Pierre Kory, MD, the leading author, appeared on December 8th before the Homeland Security Committee imploring the government to pay attention to these results. His testimony can be read here: https://www.hsgac.senate.gov/imo/media/doc/Testimony-Kory-2020-12-08.pdf. Almost no legislators attended.

The study reported a 90% improvement in COVID-19 case outcomes, averaged over the six studies. All studies showed improvement. Improved outcomes were seen in all stages: pre-infection, infection, and post-infection viral fatigue.

The NIH last issued a statement of uncertainty regarding Ivermectin in August and has said nothing since. None of the US mass media outlets have reported the hearing, the studies, or even Ivermectin at all. These outlets are waiting on unresponsive government institutions to issue their opinions.

My December 10th search—using the *New York Times* home page search tool—for articles on Ivermectin yields no mention within the last 10 years. This is despite Ivermectin's current use in worldwide trials. These trials can be found and followed through the U.S. Library of Medicine. To follow the story in the media, you'll have to go to *The Daily Star* (2020), from Bangladesh. They published the December 8th story, "Ivermectin Effective in Treating Mild COVID-19."

If the government agencies respond as slowly as we've seen, it may be two or more months before they offer an opinion. At the current rate, a two-month delay will cause 200,000 deaths. If Ivermectin is 90% effective, then its use now could prevent 180,000 of these fatalities.

Institutional thinking favors vaccination. Vaccination is entirely different and independent from treatment. Vaccination is expensive, has many risks, takes time to implement, and has no curative effect.

Treatment and vaccination are complementary; they are not alternatives. They can and should both be pursued, but this seems to be beyond the ability of current institutional thinking. Because of this, hundreds of thousands may die. Such is the result of failing to think independently.

References

Crump, A., & Omura, S. (2011 Feb 10). "Ivermectin, 'Wonder Drug' From Japan: the Human Use Perspective." *Proc. Japan Academy, Series B, Physical Biological Sciences, 87* (2): 13-28. https://www.ncbi.nlm.nih.gov/pmc/articles/PMC3043740/

Douthat, R. (2020 Dec 15). "Why Do So Many Americans Think the Election Was Stolen?" *New York Times*. https://www.nytimes.com/2020/12/05/opinion/sunday/trump-election-fraud.html

Kory, P., Meduri, G. U., Varon, J., Iglesias, J., & Marik, P. E. (2021 May/June). "Review of the Emerging Evidence Demonstrating the Efficacy of Ivermectin in the Prophylaxis and Treatment of COVID-19." *American Journal of Therapeutics, 28* (3): w299-e318. https://journals.lww.com/americantherapeutics/fulltext/2021/06000/review_of_the_emerging_evidence_demonstrating_the.4.aspx

The Daily Star (2020 Dec 8). "Ivermectin Effective in Treating Mild Covid-19." *The Daily Star*. https://www.thedailystar.net/city/news/ivermectin-effective-treating-mild-covid-19-2007697

T12 – Where Thoughts Come From – I

June 30, 2021

Knowing the origin of your thoughts can tell you who you are.

"The sea drowns them out with its wide sounds, cleanses me with its noise, and imposes a rhythm upon everything in me that is bewildered and confused."
— **Rainier Maria Rilke**, poet and novelist

This series on the origin of thoughts presents a constructive answer. I'm not sure why others are not answering this question, or why other approaches to understanding thought don't provide us with more opportunities to ask the question. The topic is large and this series could become fairly long, but I will not let it get too complicated. I want to focus on the basic ideas.

The Question

We're built not to ask, not to care, and not to see where our thoughts come from. Because we don't see where thoughts come from, we have the illusion they don't come from anywhere. Because they seem to be spontaneous, we believe they are our own. We have a similar illusion that our identity has not come from anywhere, which we interpret to mean that it has come out of ourselves, that we have spontaneously arisen. This is the user illusion. It is the illusion of free will. Not all free will is an illusion, but this perception supports a false impression of free will.

We are built to act with a sense of autonomy. If we felt we were governed by rules, situations, obligations, and consequences, then we might have trouble responding to situations. Feeling responsible only for the thoughts of the moment allows us to act in the moment. We feel we are free to act within a context we understand and in accordance with the rhythms we perceive. Our minds play a simple game.

The Analogy with Vision

Our circle of visual acuity is small, a circle of 1-degree diameter, the size of your thumbnail held at arm's length. Our visual awareness is built by moving this circle over areas of interest in order to create a map of what we see.

Outside of this circle, our vision is peripheral and our acuity is poor. We scan our environment by moving our circle of acuity, but create nothing more than a small amount of detail. Our eyes see the world through a fogged glass, and our circle of acuity traces lines of detail like a finger clears tracks of transparency through condensation.

We automatically create a full visual map built on our fuzzy, unresolved peripheral vision. This low-resolution peripheral map is crisscrossed with lines of acuity created by our small circle of focused vision. Our brain interpolates details in these peripheral areas so that our visual map is consistent with our general blur in conjunction with the thin lines of focused vision.

We design buildings, houses, paths, roadways, vehicles, and speed limits to support our limited peripheral vision. The design of objects seen in our peripheral vision—from roadside vistas to storefronts to household wallpaper—is repetitive. And they are of less importance. Repetitive patterns support what we infer but do not see and allow us to relax. Repetition is calming, and an environment with too much information makes us anxious.

Our visual map of what's in front of us is uneven and fragmented. It's a tangled weaving of past details, perceived, remembered, and largely empty of the detail that our brain tells us is there. We are hardly aware of this map's deceptive structure or the effort we put into creating it.

We think we see everything, and persist in this belief despite being unable to describe more than a few details. We think we see, but, in fact, we perceive little. Presuming most of what we see, we cannot comprehend that our sight might not be true. Optical illusions endlessly fascinate us.

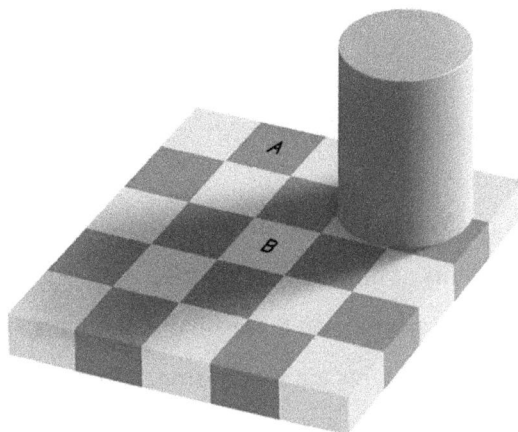

Figure 7: The squares at A and B are the same shades of gray.

Try these simple experiments. Right after you navigate through a familiar environment, your kitchen or bedroom, take a moment to reflect on what you saw. What you remember you saw is a combination of a small amount of what you really saw and a large amount of what you assumed from familiar peripheral details.

Now walk through an unfamiliar and detailed environment, such as through a wooded path or a busy street. A place where you're not able to stop and examine what's around you. After you pass through this environment, you'll realize that the only details you recognized were those that helped you navigate.

You may remember seeing nothing at all beyond what was in front of you. If you do remember any detail, then you'll probably have a fairly static memory of it, like a snapshot or a cameo. You may think that you only remember a few things, but, in fact, these are probably the only things you bothered to identify. The rest of your surroundings, the vast majority of it, you saw only vaguely and didn't think about at all.

What you're aware of in the picture of what you see are the elements that make some impression on your mind. You are not aware of the indistinct elements you actually saw. From what you saw, you inferred other objects and created a map of the location of the objects you recognized. You may remember that you saw these reference objects when, in fact, you hardly saw them at all. You saw a few parts of them and filled in the rest using your memory and imagination.

Threshold Theory

This models how you think. You're only aware of the thoughts that you recognize. You've assembled these from smaller bits of thought that are too small, brief, or elemental to be memorable. You are not aware of having had these smaller thoughts, as they don't correspond to images, words, or ideas. Your thoughts are woven from a loose tangle of what I call "oughts."

In analogy with the cells at the back of our retina, these oughts are triggered by small acts of conception. These would be memories, associations, impressions, reflections, and perceptions, none of which make it to consciousness. We are only subliminally aware of them.

In the same way that our visual cortex recognizes patterns in our visual field, various parts of our consciousness recognize patterns in our "cognitive field." However, our cognitive field is not planar, it has many dimensions, limited only by the depth of our awareness. In both the visual and cognitive cases, we do not consciously recognize an object or a thought until we have recognized a pattern.

In my threshold theory, our minds are full of "oughts." Below our consciousness is a churning mass of impressions and associations. These thought bits change with new information and create new associations among themselves. We throttle down what we take in to avoid being overwhelmed. We also restrict how we react in order to maintain our focus and to build thoughts of some coherence and duration.

The breadth of this coherence is the extent of the associations we can consider. The duration of our attention is determined by the rhythms of our brains. Some people's attention is brief and focused, while others are broad and enduring.

Not only could a person have other combinations of awareness, such as short in duration but broad in scope, but our breadth of awareness differs by subject. Some people are good with numbers, others are good with words, others are good with images, and still others have a refined body awareness.

Each of us has particular content-related skills. Positive and negative life experiences have made us more interested, attentive, perceptive, and responsive in certain areas.

We build our identity on certain preconceptions of ourselves, such as being smart, funny, insightful, or attractive. We are particularly attentive to events around us that relate to these aspects of ourselves. We pay attention to things before we know exactly why or what we're paying attention to. The events that might apply to us attract our attention. We are responding to the evocation of "oughts" that are not yet fully thoughts. Subconscious awareness leads us through our environment before our conscious awareness knows what we're looking at. This is the basis of the stage performance of mentalism, in which mentalists predict what members of their audience will see, say, or do. The audience members are "primed" with these thoughts without being aware of it (Corinda 2011).

Bigger thoughts come from smaller thoughts. Not really smaller in size, but less consequential and thought-like. We have to take our external awareness somewhat offline in order to apply our minds to the construction of larger thoughts from smaller thoughts. While we're thinking, we become less situationally aware.

Small thoughts come from indiscernible oughts. These small thoughts emerge subliminally, but they still require some investment. Because we can't put together all of our ideas at once, we exert a level of subliminal focus. We do this by letting our minds range over relevant associations while we await the assembly of an idea.

You may have had the experience of trying to remember a word or a name. While you're trying to grasp that memory, your mind ranges over associations similar to it, such as images of a face or locations where something took place. These diversions in our attention help us get our bearing on the retrieval of memory and the assembly of thoughts.

Oughts

Distracted and incomplete thoughts are made of oughts that are not quite whole thoughts; they are aspects of memories and ideas. These emerge as incomplete images, gesticulations, or verbal expressions. Parts of words, expletives, inchoate utterances, like parts of a feeling; inklings, presentiments, glances, and unconscious movements.

Imagine these oughts populate our minds like a dense garden filled with wind chimes. When ideas or perceptions strike us, these chimes ring. We don't hear them clearly, as our minds put a damper on the noise, but we are aware of the sound. Our attention is drawn toward the themes these elementary thoughts create.

Some of these oughts connect to each other through reason; we believe there are cause-and-effect relationships between them. Others are related to memories or sensations in our body, things that have been wired into us through experience. Where these connections are "hard-wired," we don't have to think at all as the thoughts arise without our intention. This is the case with muscle memory, such as learning to play a musical instrument. These associations can hijack our thoughts involuntarily, such as the incessant musical jingle that annoys us.

T13 - Where Thoughts Come From - II

July 7, 2021

What can you make from the pieces of yourself?

"The great thing about falling apart is that you get to decide how to put yourself back together." — **Stacie Hammond**, author of *Wild Horses and Mistakes*.

In the previous piece, I presented the contrast between what we see and what we think we see as an analog to how we think. I explained how our mind creates the illusion of a well-formed vision, and we do not question this. The components of this are:

- Perception is a mental illusion.
- We guess at the appearance of what we don't perceive.
- Memories and assumptions fill in what's uncertain.
- Always believing what we see, we justify it regardless.
- We trust what works, and work with what we trust.

This is the normal, ongoing process of vision of which we are unaware. Many things in our pre-conscious, imaginary field of vision are handled in this fashion. Most of them never reach our consciousness.

We see before we know what we see, and we accept what we see without judgment. If something that we see changes, then we change what we think without judgment. If a cat becomes a shadow or a shadow becomes a cat, we don't question it. We not only believe what we see, but what we believe can change instantly without disturbing us.

A few ideas and images become important enough to enter our consciousness. These are the ideas and images we think about. Things that require further thought. Once we start thinking, we become more attached to our beliefs. We remain unaware of the many images that do not pass this threshold.

Time

Unlike vision, which we can stop by closing our eyes, there always seems to be thoughts in our mind. Our mind is aware of the passage of time, whether or not we're seeing things. We can compare the length of time during which we have sight with the length of time we don't. This is not the case with thoughts.

Thoughts clock our sense of time. In order to sense time passing, we need a flow of thoughts. These thoughts don't have to be cogent, focused, or precise. They can be nonsense, repetitive, or hallucinatory. They can be quiet and observant. But when our thoughts stop and stop completely, so does our sense of time. Training yourself to accurately judge the passage of time requires carefully controlling your flow of thoughts. I used to watch my father do this with the exposures he made using his large-format camera. He timed the exposures of his world-famous images using a thumb-operated shutter release. Nothing was automatic.

As sleep lacks thoughts, sleep lacks time, and we cannot sense sleep-time passing. A hypnotic trance lacks the normal duration of thoughts and a hypnotic trance is perceived as lacking the normal duration of time. The perception of shortened time during hypnosis is called time dilation.

We have a limited ability to be aware of thoughts, and we automatically throttle back our sensitivity to new thoughts when our minds are active. We can't have too many thoughts or we become confused. When we don't have conscious thoughts, unconscious thoughts enter our awareness. Our flow in time requires them.

We are addicted to the flow of time in the same way we're addicted to air. The compulsion to think is like the compulsion to breathe. Practicing mindless meditation is like holding your breath. After a short period, regardless of your intention, new thoughts arise. We equate time with life so that a fully mindless meditation—no thoughts, sensations, or sense of awareness—feels like a suspension of being alive.

Mind

Our minds are severely limited in the rate at which we can process information. We've all had the experience of having our train of thought disrupted by outside issues. When this happens, we cannot perceive, process, or respond effectively. We need to focus our attention on what we see and eliminate outside distractions. When that fails, we struggle to organize our thinking.

We do this internally as well, even if we're not seeing anything. We shut out the cacophony of elemental ideas and associations and only recognize an idea when it reaches a threshold of form. Sometimes ideas come fully formed as phrases, images, or recognizable feelings. We're clearly aware of much in our environment subliminally, though we are not aware at a conscious level. Magic tricks work by manipulating what we're consciously aware of.

Rarely do we recognize what does not have an expression. Without a clear impression, all we have are suggestions and possibilities. In such a state, we are uncommitted to our perceptions and we are suggestible in our thoughts. If you're listening carefully, then you'll be aware that you hold your judgments until you understand what's being said. Before that point, you might be aware of several ideas forming.

Oughts

In the previous piece, I introduced the notion of oughts, bits of mind, memory, and ideation that comprise a thought, similar to how letters comprise words but with more meaning. They are the consequential elements that make up an idea. Oughts are not abstract symbols or phonemes, they are bits of meaning. We don't recognize the oughts, or thought elements, until their assembly reaches a critical point. Oughts are fleeting references until they are concretized into a meaningful structure.

Anxiety is partly the inability to reach closure with thoughts that feel important. Anxiety is reduced when you feel you understand your choices and their outcomes. This differs from being fearful, which is a state where you feel certain of something threatening.

Being undecided is the same as having multiple lines of thought vying for primacy. Being chronically indecisive comes from lacking a fundamental criterion of purpose, safety, or self. Some ought elements add the glue to hold things together, or the fiber to which elements attach. We can see certain syndromes as lacking the thought elements needed not to find solutions, but to state them.

You may recall having half an idea, having the urge to speak a sentence that you couldn't finish. This would be rare, as even people who speak gibberish finish their sentences. This would be a type of aphasia that is localized to language, but I want to think more broadly in terms of something below language.

Sometimes, we lose track of our thoughts, getting ahead of ourselves and having a second thought distract us before a first thought can be completed. This gives the strange sensation of having something to express, but the idea is gone and the emotions have nothing to attach to. We'll work ourselves up to make a presentation, feeling the emotion that motivates us, and then admit, "I forgot what I was going to say!"

Dreams

One reason dream images feel disconnected is that the oughts in the dream do not form complete thoughts. We can learn to perceive these oughts similarly to the way we recognize feelings evoked by images before we think about them. Dreams-thoughts are not so much strange as unfinished.

Elements in dreams map onto full or partial thoughts—that is oughts. We don't have these visual oughts during waking consciousness because in waking consciousness we suppress partial thoughts. In this way, the dream presents us with our thought-assembly process. In dreams, we "see" thought fragments and experience their incomplete assembly. The result leaves us confused if we're aware of it happening. This inclines us to forget our dreams.

I recently awoke from a nap in which I was dreaming of an elaborate escape strategy. At the end of the dream, I was in an uninhabited skyscraper and an office with locked cabinets. I found one whose lower latch had not caught. I jimmied it open by bending the door open enough to reach far in and manually unhitch the top, inner catch.

In my dream, I had opened the door, and I was examining the contents of this cabinet: a tennis racket, a beach ball, and party supplies. I considered stashing the two books I was carrying but decided against it. As I struggled to put the contents back and re-latch the door, I realized this was all pointless. I didn't care about the cabinet, the contents, or anything about the office. The dream had become self-referential, a fixation on details that was a waste of my dream time. What began as an escape from a meaningful situation ended as wasting time with unimportant objects in a meaningless office. I woke up annoyed.

We have trouble rising to self-awareness in our dreams because dreams don't make sense. We sink into them like quicksand in the same way that I obsessed over my dream cabinet's useless contents. Without sense and meaning, our self-awareness is hog-tied. How do you become self-aware when part of you is absent? If you can become aware of your truncated self, the result is often unpleasant: a sense of being unresponsive.

Our conscious mind expects full thoughts because those are the things our conscious mind trades in. But we can learn to accept and even take part in the incomplete thought process. We can do this by experiencing dreams as a witness rather than a participant. Participation is a prejudice we apply to dreams from our normal, conscious state, a state whose comfort requires thought completion. Being a witness relieves our anxiety, and reducing our anxiety is crucial for remaining lucid in a dream.

This is how you learn to lucid dream: not by becoming fully self-aware in a world of half awareness, but by becoming half-aware in your waking world of full awareness. You do this by developing an autonomous sense of half-self that thinks half-formed thoughts. It's not the dream that's difficult to enter, it's the half-formed thought processes of it. Until we construct for ourselves a half-formed identity, we won't have a self that can be lucid in dreams. Of course, it's not a full lucidity either, it's a dream lucidity. I discuss this at greater length in my book *Becoming Lucid; Self-awareness in Sleeping & Waking Life* (Stoller 2019).

By gaining awareness of oughts as they pass through our minds, and by establishing a sense of self that can survive the amputation of its parts—a process that's constantly happening in dreams—we gain the ability to be relaxed dream participants.

What Is Lost

If you compare your self-created identity with a finished film, you'll recognize that there are other ways that you can be put together. The "finished film" version of yourself is something you've created for general viewing. The viewing audience is not just other people but includes you. You adopt the story that you tell and you identify yourself with it. Your identity is a thought about yourself that you believe in.

You would like to have more options. You'd like to be more of a filmmaker than a film viewer. To do this, you need to go back to the original material. You need to consider the pieces left on the cutting-room floor. These are the bits that were removed from the final version.

In a larger sense, these could be whole narratives that don't fit comfortably into your story. But on a smaller scale, they could be elements of timing or meaning that you've trimmed from your self-awareness. They are distinct tones and timbres, and different rhythms of attention and expression. These little bits are oughts of fragments of your identity. They may be small, but they can make big changes. Like broken bits of pottery, together they may fill in large holes.

If you can focus your mind on things smaller than thoughts, then you will recognize similar unexpressed parts in the identities of other people. You will notice what isn't there, or what could be understood in different ways. This is most easily seen in another person when they're going through a decision-making process. We often sense when another person is forming ideas. It's in these fertile times when you have the most leverage to change the outcome of another person's thoughts.

These are the opportunities I try to create as a therapist. They are often signaled by expressions of emotion in my clients or their stories. In contrast, clients whose reality is rigidly assembled are defensive and close-minded. Their narratives are regimented like soldiers.

I try to dissolve their attachments and lubricate change. I might exhort them to surrender or bombard them with contradictions. Without the flexibility of alternatives or the options of indecision, such clients retreat into the maze of their original confusion. I can call to them, telling them what turns to make and promising safety in crossing the battle lines, but I cannot loosen their grip and I cannot drag them out. The warfare analogies may sound harsh, but that's the level of fear and anxiety these changes elicit.

While threatening parts of ideas are not verbalized, they may be expressed unconsciously. I can see them in the face of a surprised person as they filter through various impressions, searching for understanding. I try to adduce positive idea fragments to create attractive opportunities. As a client, you may have to imagine these parts to sense them based on fragmentary evidence. You might be wrong and the positive may be more fragile than is expected, but that doesn't mean that you didn't see something positive. Anything you imagine, you can build on.

Numbers and Pictures

Let's put some numbers on this by building a network-picture of oughts. I think these oughts are persistent things. They are like some physical mode or excited state. They might even exist in a place in your brain. Like thoughts themselves, oughts might be complex assemblies of many aspects of perception; combinations of many sensations and impressions stored in various locations in your brain.

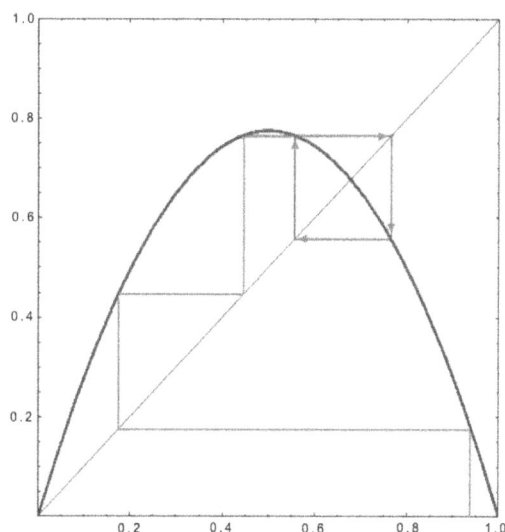

Figure 8: Cobweb diagram: the sequence of corners of the crooked line describes the states through which a system progresses. Here, the line ends in the repeating cycle at the top square. The x-axis is horizontal, the y-axis is vertical.

We can build simple mathematics using the logistic equation. That's the equation that describes processes of growth and decay, as happens with populations in nature. Our oughts behave like the population of a species. When they elicit a reward, they grow in power and number. When they have a negative effect, their strengths and numbers are reduced. The ones

213

that are rewarded are linked and emerge as thoughts. The ones that are inhibited remain unexpressed or fade away.

The dynamics of these thought fragments follow the straight-line paths in what's called a cobweb diagram (Texas Instruments 2008). This diagram's was originally used to relate the population of a species at one time to the population at another time. In this earlier context, the path that's traced in the construction of the cobweb diagram is the changing value of the population over time.

In this case, I'm equating the members of a species with the strength of an ought. The ought's strength grows at its inception, has a peak strength, and then becomes exhausted if it grows too strong.

This cobweb diagram starts with a simple, balanced parabola standing with its feet on the horizontal x-axis, and its nose pointing up, like a nose cone, in the direction of the y-axis. The cobweb diagram can be confusing because it's the combination of a function y of x, which is the parabola, and a progression through time n, which is given by y(n) and x(n). The graph superimposes both on top of each other.

The parabola is a function that shows how the population changes as it grows or shrinks. The parabola's left foot is planted on the origin, at the left side of the picture. Its peak rises in the middle, and its right foot is at the right edge of the picture. This indicates that the population grows fastest when it's small, reaches a peak when its numbers grow larger, and then collapses if it gets too large.

A separate, diagonal line is also needed. This starts at the origin, coincident with the parabola's left foot, and goes up and to the right along a straight line angled at 45 degrees.

Where it starts on the left, the parabola has a slope that's greater than 45-degrees and begins by rising above the diagonal line. The curve reaches a crest, turns, and heads back down to the right, passing through the 45-degree line and then coming to rest, on it's right leg, on the x-axis below, to the right of the straight line, at the x value of 1.

To create the cobweb path of lines and angles, you can begin anywhere on the x-axis between zero and one, and you travel upwards until you hit the parabolic curve. At this point you stop moving straight up. Your line turns 90-degrees to travel either to the left or to the right.

You travel horizontally to the right if you've met the parabola on the left side of the arched peak. You travel to the left if you've met the parabola on the right side of the arched peak. In either case, you continue horizontally until you reach the 45-degree straight line that angles from the lower left to the upper right.

This process generates two straight line segments: one going up from the x-axis and the next going left or right to meet the sloping line. In figure 8, I've drawn a line upward from the x-axis from the point x = 0.94, and reached the parabolic line at a vertical, y value of about 0.2. Then I traveled straight left to meet the sloping line at the point at approximately x = 0.2 and y = 0.2.

From this point, I created the third line segment by traveling straight up to meet the parabola. In this diagram, this creates a vertical segment that connects the point on the sloping line at x = 0.2, y = 0.2, with the point at x =0.2, y = 0.45. There I stop, turn 90 degrees clockwise, and draw a horizontal line segment that reaches from the parabola back to the sloping line. I have now drawn four line segments.

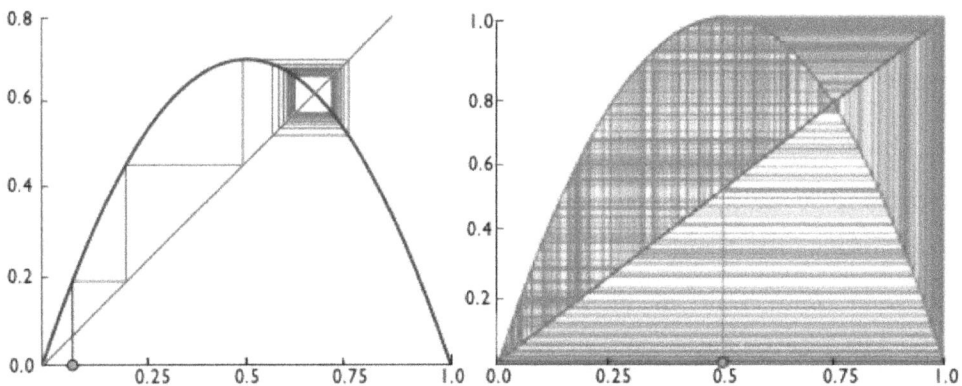

Figure 9: Convergence and divergence: the first pattern starts at x = 0.05 and converges to cycle around a point. The second starts at x = 0.50001, tends toward a point, and then wanders away from it.

Continue moving horizontally from the sloping line to the parabola, and then vertically from the parabola to the sloping line. I travel either left or right, or up or down as required. We're looking for a pattern, and this pattern could display infinite variety.

One property, as shown on the left side of figure 9, is to converge to a repeating square. Another pattern is a spiraling square that shrinks not to a square, but to a point. A third pattern is the alternation between two squares centered on different points, or multiple squares centering on multiple points. And a fourth pattern is chaos, shown in the pattern on the right side of figure 9. This chaotic pattern first converges to a point, but then moves outward, traveling all around the parabola, irregularly tracing lines, and never settling on a repeating pattern (Gershenson 2003).

Cobweb diagrams represent the changing population numbers of competing species, such as owls and mice, or coyotes and rabbits. As the food supply rises, the population of the predator rises. As the food supply dwindles, so does the predator's population. There might be a balance, an alternation, unpredictable chaos, or a complete collapse of both populations.

The possibilities that result depends only on the shape of the parabola and the point from which you start. It's from this that I offer a model of how we think. Our thoughts are represented by the parabola, and the starting point is the idea that triggers it. The vertical line segments map our feelings of reward or inhibition. Greater reward corresponds to higher points on the graph and inhibition is shown by lower points. The horizontal line segments represent how that outcome triggers us again.

If the cobweb diagram leads us to settle high on the parabola, then the thought becomes conscious and we consider it. When it leads us to a point low on the parabola, the thought is suppressed and does not disturb us. If a pattern of regular alternation develops, our thoughts alternate. And if chaos results and the cobweb pattern fills an entire area, then we are indecisive, uncertain, confused, panicked, disengaged, or anxious.

References

Corinda, & Rauscher, W. (2011). *Encyclopedia of Mentalism and Mentalists.* 1878 Press.

Gershenson, C. (2003). "Introduction to Chaos in Deterministic Systems." Carlos Gershenson. https://arxiv.org/ftp/nlin/papers/0308/0308023.pdf

Stoller, L. (2019). *Becoming Lucid; Self-Awareness in Sleeping & Waking Life.* Mind Strength Books. https://www.mindstrengthbalance.com/becominglucidbook/

Texas Instruments (2008). *TI-nspire: Getting Started with Chaos.* Texas Instruments Incorporated. https://compasstech.com.au/TNSINTRO/TI-NspireCD/mystuff/webplot/webplot.pdf

T14 – Where Thoughts Come From – III

July 15, 2021

The better you understand of what you see, the more you see in it.

"The only thing that makes life possible is permanent, intolerable uncertainty."
— **Ursula K. Le Guin**, author

I was going to go into mathematical detail, but before I describe how thoughts might be formed, some additional background will make it more recognizable.

We assemble our image of ourselves from what we've learned and what we've seen. Our thoughts emerge from pieces of ideas I've called "oughts." Oughts are elements of meaning, pieces of thoughts that do not appear in our minds until we have a context for them. Oughts have tone and inclination, but they are not enough to visualize or verbalize by themselves.

We know little about the mind beyond rudimentary chemistry and physiology. We know little about the workings of the brain, and we know virtually nothing about the connection between mind and brain. Your ignorance does not handicap you. Everybody's ignorant.

On the other hand, to connect with what we know, we've got to reach beyond the obvious. We've got to grasp loose ends that are far from making a good connection with anything we're trying to understand. The yawning distance between what we do and don't know puts us firmly in the land of conjecture.

Neuroscience

Neuroscience is segmented into areas of specialization. The most active areas are those where new observations are being made. Importance is directed to the new machines that are creating new images. We like pictures, especially when we have nothing else. Researchers are creating lots of pictures that conclude nothing but generate a lot of interest. This is more about making bets and designing machines than it is about understanding the brain.

Psychological neuroscience approaches the brain along research and therapeutic lines. Here you'll find studies of injuries, exceptional symptoms, and behaviors. This is the realm of Oliver

218

Sacks (*The Man Who Mistook His Wife for a Hat*) and Norman Doidge (*The Brain That Changes Itself*). People love odd stories of the mind, but it has little effect on the field.

Pop psychology presents poor science as anecdotal evidence instead of providing methodical observations. Clinical psychology has been obsessed with "evidence-based" practice for the last 40 years. This is an improvement over methods that previously had no evidence at all, but, as most of the evidence is poor, the result is poor therapy. Practice follows what's in popular demand, and popular demand follows what's advertised.

Clinical neurology concerns itself with explaining and addressing disabilities. This pragmatic field is less concerned with what's causing things and more concerned with what works to fix them. It's a field influenced by money and politics surrounding public policy, government support, and managed care.

Neuropharmacology provides psychiatry with pharmaceutical interventions. Pharmaceuticals are a multi-billion dollar industry that has captured much of government, institutional, and healthcare policy. Pharmaceuticals are part of the military's new biological weapons programs. These private corporations take a leading role in pharmaceutical research. They install their subcontractors in academic positions and on editorial boards. Corporations have allegiance to neither the objectives of science nor the health of patients. Their first legal responsibility is to their shareholders.

Neurophysiology is a laboratory neuroscience. It studies the nervous system in vitro: examining nerves, vivisecting animals, engineering genetic sequences, and testing chemicals. This is the most complex area because there is no limit to the theories or tools that can be employed. Laboratory neuroscience can pose any question and employ any means to address it. Jerry Lettvin, one of my mentors, was a laboratory neuroscientist (Stoller 2019, 55-68). He didn't move into this field until he was adept as a poet, psychiatrist, and electrical engineer. His skill lay in combining these fields.

Computational neuroscience concerns itself with abstract models that have little connection to observations or practical applications. The field builds off the axon-nerve-synapse model, which makes it appear mechanical and computer-like, but it is not necessarily so constrained. Unusual models of the brain can be found—models that don't rely on nerve impulses or digital analogies—and unusual computational models can be advanced from these. What I'm proposing is such a model. Finally, there are electromagnetic models of brain function. These models range from the microscopic, looking at the electrical behavior of individual nerves, to the macroscopic, looking at the fields produced by the brain. We can easily, painlessly, and cheaply gather data by observing outside fields generated by processes inside the brain. Even electric fields inside the brain can be explored without putting probes inside the skull. Invasive observations can also be done. When performed on humans, these programs are of a medical rather than a theoretical nature.

Spirit

Neuro-imagery, psychology, physiology, pharmacology, computational, clinical, and electro-magnetic neuroscience provide scientific approaches that encircle the Western question of the mind. The Western notion might not be right. The "circle" enclosed by these programs may not contain the answers we're looking for.

In a somewhat macabre analogy of Christians and lions, science throws questions of the mind into this arena, where they're torn to pieces. As far as I can tell, nothing comes out alive. The Western model consistently collapses into reductionism because it has no connection to a higher goal. In the mind's province of subjectivity, reductive thinking is a vine that has nothing to climb on.

Spiritual traditions reject purely intellectual notions of the mind. Instead of starting from the smallest parts, typical of reductionism in science, spiritual traditions start with the highest power, a universal principle. Spiritual traditions presume spirit to avoid a spiritless universe or a universe of spiritless objects. If you presume God, then you never need to prove God's existence.

Spiritual traditions object to the hubris of modern science, of which little is said in intellectual circles. Intellectual arrogance is a larger problem than most people realize. Arrogance rests on authority, fuels the devaluation of others, devalues truth, and accepts a predatory mindset.

The model that I'm suggesting is self-organizing. It isn't reductive, and it doesn't presume a higher power. It reduces larger structures to smaller structures, but every stage keeps its connection to the whole. One starts with relationships, rewards and inhibitions, and structures emerge from this. The "ecology" that results seems to have a sort of ineffable wholeness. In fact, the meaning of the whole is just the relationships of the parts.

These structures say more about how we create ourselves than they say about the atoms we are composed of. I'm not reducing spirit to mechanics, I'm reducing bigger meanings to smaller meanings. We are not spiritual beings having a human experience. We are self-aware agglomerations of thoughts, memories, and perceptions: neither no thing nor some thing, just the structures of self-awareness.

Measure

In my model, there are physical structures at some level, but we're still too far from an understanding of the mind to observe them operating separately. We don't know what a thought is at any level, though I imagine thoughts as having the properties of networks.

The most important property of networks, which distinguishes them from physical objects like cells or fields, is that they don't require the notion of dimension. You may think of networks in terms of drawings you have seen, but you cannot physically picture a general network. Every network that you've seen pictured is misleading. Networks have nodes and branches, but the measure of the distance between them is not spatial, it's procedural. It's something that is internal to the network itself.

The networks you've seen pictured are dead things. If you think of a tree as a network whose nodes are the branching of its limbs, then the essence of the tree lives in the forces in the limbs. The tree's network is the internal, living dynamic that exists within its structure, not its physical structure. This dynamic is defined by gravitational, cellular, chemical, solar, seasonal, hydrostatic, and symbiotic forces. To picture the tree geometrically overlooks almost everything it embodies.

Whenever you measure something, you take something out of it. If it's sufficient to take only a little, then you can leave the object mostly intact. But if you violate the object's integrity by interfering with its essential action, you destroy it. At the current time, we cannot observe a

221

thought without destroying it. That's because we don't know the structure of what we're looking at. We are workers with hammers, either crushing things together or smashing them apart.

The model I'm working with involves us with psychology and computation. It's interesting to incorporate other approaches, but simpler is better at the start.

The result is a tool useful for reflection, therapy, and self-exploration. I think there is physical truth to the model, and that aspects of thoughts will be measurable someday. Once that is possible, many extensions will emerge.

Psychology

A deeper understanding of thinking follows from a study of emotion. Most studies of emotion focus on neuroanatomy, asking which areas of the brain contribute to particular emotions. The consensus is that emotions are not localized in the brain. This is complicated by the vague distinctions between emotions.

Some emotions are more localized than others. Fear seems to be mediated by the amygdala, a small central organ that's part of the limbic system. A complex emotion like happiness is harder to define and localize. Complex emotions like love are not considered emotions at all because they lack a clear definition.

For my purposes, emotions are higher-order constructions. They are thought-complexes. I'm more interested in how emotions are built, as that sheds some light on how thoughts are built.

> "Putting into practice a workable computational system can also demonstrate which parts of psychological theories are coherent and reassure the appropriateness of the undertaken directions of further studies."
> — **Zdzisław Kowalczuk** and **Michał Czubenko** (2016)

Emotions are not built consciously or intentionally, and they're not subject to logic or reason. Unlike thoughts, emotions are not intentional. When we try to control our emotions, we often do it by first trying to control our thoughts. There are therapy models that manipulate emotions, which work with the connection between thoughts and emotions.

Anger is an example of an emotion that people often think of as intentional. I have clients with anger issues who think that I can give them a different reasonable understanding. They believe this will make them less angry. Anger is only weakly intentional. It is a combination of fear, anxiety, sorrow, and vulnerability. We justify these with logical explanations, but, upon examination, our explanations are neither logical nor powerful. They're excuses. Until these clients are ready to examine the roots of their emotions, no one can help them gain control.

Emotions are being constructed for artificially intelligent systems. The field of artificial emotions is essential for the development of human-like artificial intelligence. And while we don't have an organic theory of mind, we do have computer models of artificial minds. In this context, people are trying to build artificial emotions. So far, they have been unsuccessful (Jentzsch & Kersting 2023).

> "The primeval proteinaceous soup of comedy… requires a lightning strike of inspiration, and then out crawls a joke. Nine times out of ten, the joke expires feebly on the edge of the pond… Part of this task is undoubtedly computational: extracting and categorizing data, combining variables, and inverting values. Without these mechanics, however subtle, there'd be no comedy at all. There's no ridiculousness without logic."
> — **Tony Veale** (2021), computer scientist

Electricity

Two electrical properties relevant to this model are the brain's electrical waves and the electrical discharges of individual nerves. The harmonic properties are brainwaves: changing patterns of rhythmic excitations that move through areas of the brain. We can measure these to varying degrees. We can correlate changes in brain waves with gross changes in behavior. Training a person's brain waves will change their behavior.

We cannot identify the source of these waves, which originate in the collective discharge of synapses. The subtle aspects of their creation, synchronization, propagation, and absorption are unknown.

Electrical waves are shaped not only by what creates them but also by the medium they pass through. The brain is a non-uniform conductor whose properties can change faster than the currents that travel through it. A good part of the brain's operation is likely modulated by the brain's ability to shape these electric fields. The brain does this through the action of chemical gradients, membrane potentials, and phase boundaries. Science is only at the earliest stages of making sense of this. The implication is that the mind lies somewhere in the physics.

Different parts of the brain are subject to waves generated by local and remote parts of the brain. We know these field changes correlate with cognition. We believe these frequencies play the role of pacemakers for enduring, plastic changes in brain structure. In my model, these rhythms simply "clock" the step-wise evolution of our thoughts.

> "There is increasing evidence that low-frequency (2–25 Hz) neural oscillations are not simply epiphenomena, but reflect an essential mechanism for coordinating brain function."
> — **Kai Miller**, MD et al. (2012)

Computation

My model is computational, but it's unlike any computational model I know of. It's simpler because it correlates with the psychology we observe rather than physiology, whose mechanisms we don't understand.

There are bottom-up and top-down types of computational models. Bottom-up models attempt to derive behaviors from neural structures, while top-down models try to derive structures from observed behaviors.

This is a top-down model except that I'm not even trying to connect to neural behavior. I want to understand how the brain creates more complex information from less complex information. That makes this a conceptual rather than a physical model.

Digression on Foundations

Most people think the building blocks of a model must be physical, and that's a mistake. The tendency of people to believe more in what they visualize rather than what can be conceptualized makes them vulnerable to various forms of manipulation, including sleight of hand. We are prejudiced in believing our perceptions and distrusting our thoughts. This is a reliable bias because most of us think poorly.

All "building blocks" are conceptual things. All models are conceptual. That some of these "concepts" can be measured does not make them real, but we think so. We "believe" what we can see, but sight is an illusion. It is useful but not essential. It's repeatability that's the foundation of prediction, not visibility.

Most cognitive models are deterministic. They aim to create a method that either maps onto neural structures or simple behaviors. Deep learning models apply filtering and pattern recognition to large databases of information. They result in an ever-growing algorithm that extracts plausible answers from previous examples.

I am not satisfied with deterministic models because an essential aspect of the mind is its non-deterministic behavior. More advanced brains display less deterministic behaviors. We call this learning, adaptation, or intelligence. This distinguishes brains from machines. It is essential both for creative thought and adaptive behavior. I am proposing a chaos-based model that is both simple at its core and infinitely complex in what it can create.

Simplicity

My first concern is with simplicity. I want you to see the basic structure and quickly match it with your thinking processes. My next concern is that the model can grow but keep its original structure. I want the model to grow in a way that enlarges but does not destroy its simplicity. One way to make that happen is for its basic structures to be reiterated in its larger structures.

These requirements are met by systems that scale through iteration. Such structures are said to be scale invariant. This is typical of fractal systems, systems that display complexity based on simple, underlying patterns. This model is of the scale invariant type. Its instability leads us to explore its general properties rather than any particular predictions.

Consider how a snowflake grows. They all grow based on the physics of freezing water, and, while many snowflakes start from identical seeds, no two resulting snowflakes are the same. Snowflakes are scale invariant because the physics of their formation is the same at every stage of their growth, yet the result of their growth process is not predictable.

This is consistent with what we see when we observe our thoughts. Introspection leads us to see patterns in our thoughts, not the mechanisms of them. We are more aware of our thoughts billowing like clouds than we are of chemical gradients and neural structures.

Next, I'll generate a simple model of oughts creating thoughts. Because this model builds on the well-known logistic equation for population growth—these populations are thoughts rather than animals—we can make several predictions of how thoughts should behave. We can compare these with what we observe in ourselves.

References

Jentzsch, S., & Kersting, K. (2023 Jun 7). "ChatGPT is Fun, But It Is Not Funny! Humor Is Still Challenging Large Language Models." *Preprint: arXiv:2306.04563v1.* https://www.semanticscholar.org/reader/d962b6772dab0ce2573370e72a477665dfe5ab08

Kowalczuk, Z. and Czubenko, M. (2016, April). "Computational Approaches to Modeling Artificial Emotion – An Overview of the Proposed Solutions." *Frontiers of Robotics AI, 3*: 21. https://doi.org/10.3389/frobt.2016.00021

Miller, K.J., Foster, B. L., & Honey, C. J. (2012, 25 Oct.). "Does Rhythmic Entrainment Represent a Generalized Mechanism for Organizing Computation In the Brain?" *Frontiers of Computational Neuroscience, 6*: 85. https://doi.org/10.3389/fncom.2012.00085

Stoller, L. (2019). *The Learning Project: Rites of Passage.* Mind Strength Books. https://www.mindstrengthbalance.com/learn/interviews/jeromelettvin.htm

Veale, T. (2021 Sep 7). *Your Wit Is My Command: Building AIs With a Sense of Humor.* Random House. http://haddock.ucd.ie/Papers/wit_sample.pdf

T15 – Where Thoughts Come From – IV

July 22, 2021

A basic explanation of a new mathematical model of thinking.

"Nature is pleased with simplicity. And nature is no dummy."
— **Isaac Newton**, physicist, alchemist, and theologian

Little psychological work has been done on the question of how thoughts originate. Perhaps the question of justifying a thought cuts too close to the bone in the psychological field where the division between normality and deviance is taken for granted. Psychology is a field based on prejudice that masquerades as insight, as any exploration of its foundations will reveal.

I find more useful work in computational psychology, otherwise known as artificial intelligence. Here, one starts from nothing. An idea must work in practice for it to be taken seriously. In AI, the concept of a frame defines all that's needed to decide a given question. The frame is like a thought, and the constituents of it are the oughts, the data, associations, and instructions necessary to answer a human question.

Just as I decomposed thinking in analogy with sight, the concept of frames also emerged from Marvin Minsky's reflections on vision.

> "The frame-system idea also (applies) to problems of linguistic understanding,
> memory, acquisition and retrieval of knowledge, and a variety of ways to reason
> by analogy and jump to conclusions based on partial similarity matching."
> — **Marvin Minsky** (1974)

I assert thoughts are built of oughts: elements of meaning that don't appear in our minds until we have a context for them. Minsky would see the thoughts as frameworks. Oughts, by themselves, are not enough to verbalize.

In this final installment in the Where Thoughts Come From series, I describe how thoughts are formed. I offer a basic model that yields interesting results. But first, I need to address the problem that people are averse to math. I hope you can endure this description in order to see its potential. I will go slowly and coax you along.

Numbers are like words, and formulas are like sentences. A mathematical statement is like any other statement. It's just that it rests on the logic of numbers rather than experience.

The good thing about math is that you can add complexity without sacrificing clarity. If things make numerical sense at every step, then the whole thing makes numerical sense. You can't say the same with reason, because extending one line of reasoning usually weakens another. This is also the downside of math: you'll have a hard time adding additional steps not because they don't make sense, but because they make the total story more difficult. In order to combat creeping complexity, I'll start as simply as possible and sacrifice some rigor in putting the ideas together.

Math

First, exit the math trauma of your childhood. Math was used as one of several paddles to make you feel stupid and inadequate. As children, we were made to feel inadequate in order that we learn to obey authority. We were taught to accept the model of mental, material, and spiritual scarcity our society rests on. The lesson is: you don't have enough; you are not enough; and by yourself, you will never be enough.

Math is taught as something that must be done exactly right. You're given ideas you don't understand and problems you can't do. Girls are more affected than boys because girls mature sooner and see more nuance. Math was used to force you to abandon your natural insight, so of course you learned to hate math, but that's not what math is.

There is no "right" math, only math that's put together right. You can no more be wrong at math than you can be wrong at blocks. Of course, your blocks might fall down, but that's all part of learning. There is no wrong math, only math that falls down.

We use math to build things, and maybe they stand up. That doesn't mean they're right, it means they're consistent. Get over your math phobia. It's all about the abuse of your childhood. Reclaim your right to build with numbers.

Oughts

We're building a theory of oughts, bits of feeling and elements of ideas. Bits of images that mean little on their own. They are the red of a sports car, the flash of the sun in our eyes, or our first impression when we step into a room but have not yet seen what's in it.

Each ought has positives and negatives. The positives act as a seed to see it more clearly and hold the germinated idea in our mind, realizing what grows around it. The negatives repel us and cause a reflexive reaction to shrink it in magnitude, implication, and direction. Some oughts are all positive, like the suggestion of a kiss, others are all negative, like the suggestion that you've sliced your finger.

When oughts grow in strength, they entrain similar oughts, and through this process, ideas form. Eventually, if this collection of oughts gains enough strength and substance, it emerges as a thought, something with a vision, implications, and perhaps a story.

Some oughts fade away. They are not engaging, not because they're repulsive but because they're irrelevant. Like my whole diatribe on mathematics, which, for most people, will be forgotten. You might reflect on it for a moment, but little is brought to mind.

Other oughts become inflamed: lust, hunger, anger, grief, and depression. There seem to be more negative triggers than positive ones. This is actually true: we are more vigilant of threats than we are expectant of rewards. When ideas grow to dominating proportions, we are motivated to act or have the desire to. If our thoughts get away from us, we can act rashly, in frustration, or later have regret.

Time

We're told and we believe that time is continuous. Do you experience time continuously? Do you have a continuous memory of events? Does your sight grade continuously from one image to another?

Imagine the clock's second hand: it moves in a graceful and continuous arc. Imagine yourself falling: you pitch forward in a graceful and continuous arc. Aside from a few experiences such as these—which are more figments of your imagination than a real, temporal experience—we feel time move in steps. We experience time in waves, or pulses, like everything else in our bodies. The waves in your brain determine the resolution of your notion of separate events in time.

In this model, our experience of time is discrete, and our awareness proceeds in steps, much like the frames of a movie. By stringing them together, we get the sense of continuous motion. Unlike a movie, however, the intervals between our steps can grow longer to slow time down or occur more rapidly to give the impression of time speeding up.

Numbers

In the spirit of numbers that can say things, let's say an ought has a strength that's given by a number we'll call y and a time we'll call n. Think of time as a ladder with numbered rungs. So, $y(n)$ is the strength of this ought at time n.

Because we're modeling time in steps, we can say that after time n comes time n+1. We don't care what time n is, and we don't care how much time has elapsed between steps n and n+1. It could be anything. All that matters is that things happen in steps, and first, the strengths of our ought are $y(n)$, $y(n+1)$, $y(n+2)$, and so on.

In this formula:

$$y(n+1) = y(n)$$

y persists unchanged at time n+1 and, if this keeps going for all values of n, then it stays the same forever.

In reality, all our thoughts degrade over time and sink from consciousness unless something keeps them afloat. They might be kept afloat externally, as when a situation persists, or internally, by a process of reflection and rumination. This is also common but, without reinforcement, thought fades out fairly quickly. However, some thoughts do not fade out, and we'll consider that later.

If our ought grows in time, then it will eventually overwhelm our thinking. Here, the power of the ought would grow and we could write $y(n+1) = A\, y(n)$ where A is a number greater than

1. We call A the growth rate. At every step, the strength of the subsequent ought is greater than it was previously and, after enough steps, we are overwhelmed.

If A is less than one, then the ought degrades with each step until it eventually fades to a strength of zero. None of these three cases, A < 1, A = 1, or A > 1 is particularly interesting. Also, my proposal is that oughts are just little pieces of thoughts, and they are not enough to have full meaning no matter how loud they are. We need to combine the oughts, and we'll do that shortly.

At the moment, we have just one ought and it either grows, stays the same, or shrinks. We can draw a graph of the change in the strength of an ought over time, as illustrated by each of the three lines, as shown in figure 10. The time is given on the horizontal axis, and the strength of the ought at each time is given on the vertical axis. The graph shows three straight lines emanating from the origin, each moving up and to the right with three different slopes.

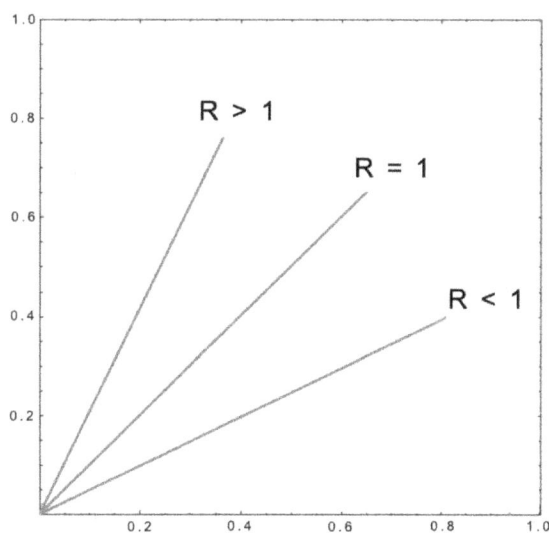

Figure 10: Different rates of growth. R=1 implies no growth.

In an auditory analog, the strength given by y would be the volume of a tone. The passage of time would be measured by beats. The tone would repeat at an even beat and either stay the same, diminish in volume to nothing, or grow without limit if the growth rate was greater than

1.

Many of our oughts fizzle out on the boundary of our consciousness. It's only through combination and reinforcement that oughts generate ideas that attract our attention.

Inhibition

Let's next say that the power of an ought grows in time. That means that the value of A in the equation $y(n+1) = A\, y(n)$ should be greater than 1. But the model would make no sense if oughts overwhelmed us. We need a balancing force that stabilizes their growth.

Here is the next term in our equation: $-B\, y(n)\, y(n)$, otherwise written as $-B\, (y(n))^2$. B is the inhibition term. The larger the value of B, the more negative the value of $-B\, (y(n))^2$.

Adding our inhibition term gives a more realistic equation for the power of the ought in the future. This equation is a combination of growth, given by the A term, and inhibition, given by the B term:

$$y(n+1) = A\, y(n) - B\, (y(n))^2$$

Now we can perform a simple bit of magic that's easier to do with math than with reason: we can simplify the equation.

We don't care about the time between time steps n and n+1. We can add in that detail later. The time scale doesn't change the general behavior.

We also don't care about the values of A and B. We only care about their difference, which can be given by their ratio: the ratio of the enlarging to the diminishing effect. Is the growth rate twice as large or half as large as the inhibition? That sort of thing.

We can simplify further. In order to get the general feel for the behavior described by this equation, we can set A equal to B, setting the growth rate equal to the inhibition. This is simpler because now there's only one variable determining the rate of growth.

We'll explore different rates of growth compared to rates of inhibition at some point, but the special case of A = B is simpler and has been studied in great detail. By defining R to be equal to A and also equal to B, we can write the equation as:

$$y(n+1) = R\,(y(n) - (y(n))^2)$$

The Logistic Equation

I think you're still with me. You may think we have accomplished little. It's true that we've come to no conclusions, but our little equation is called the Logistic Equation, and it's famous. It describes how populations grow and shrink using two variables, x and n, and one parameter, R.

From this modest equation, you can derive the behavior of many of the systems that you'll find on Earth. It's that powerful. If you don't believe me, watch the Veritasium video (Muller 2020) titled, "This equation will change how you see the world (the logistic map)." You can find it on YouTube. I'll give you a taste of it.

The following graph of growth rates (Figure 11) extends the first graph to include the effect of our inhibition term. The lines are now curved because the effect of the inhibition gets larger as the strength of the ought gets larger. I've also included the straight line that is the graph of y(n+1) = y(n), which is the diagonal line, because it represents that static case where nothing changes.

This graph of dynamic growth rates shows three parabolas, each starting at the origin where the horizontal and vertical axes are zero. From this point, one parabola rises faster than the diagonal line, peaks at the center of the graph above the point x = 0.5, and then falls back to cross the horizontal axis at x = 1.0.

A second parabola rises from the origin tangent to the diagonal but cannot keep up with it. This line also peaks at the center and falls back to the horizontal axis at x = 1.0. And last, a low-angled line emanating from the origin describes a shallow parabola, whose peak is lower than the other two and which also falls back to cross the origin at x = 1.0.

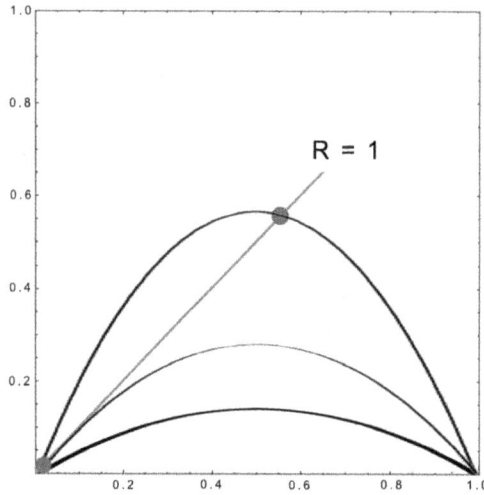

Figure 11: Different rates of growth and inhibition. The dots are locations where the system settles.

These are dynamic situations. You start with one value, x at time n, which is a value on the x-axis. From this, following the cobweb diagram construction, you locate the corresponding value y(n). The cobweb algorithm then tells you how to generate a new value for x at the next time step, at n+1. As you continue to iterate this construction, you get new values at each time step.

You'll generally get a different value for x and y at each time. Drawing lines between these points gives the web pattern. The values depend on the last x-value you got, which ultimately depends on the x-value at which you started. And as time goes on, the behavior of x(n) and y(n) will fall into various classes.

One possibility is that the strength of the ought will vanish. This happens when the amplification is less than 1, in which case the "amplification" term is not amplifying, it's leading to a diminution. The additional inhibition terms make the net strength only go to zero faster. The ultimate point toward which the strength of the ought moves over time is given by the dot at zero.

When the amplification value exceeds the value 1, everything changes. Now the system may move to a balanced state that is not zero. Over time, the ought moves toward the point where the diagonal straight line crosses the parabolic curved line. This is shown by the higher dot in Figure 11.

As the amplification increases, the height of the parabola increases, and the location of this fixed value shown by the dot increases as it climbs up the diagonal line, but it does not increase indefinitely.

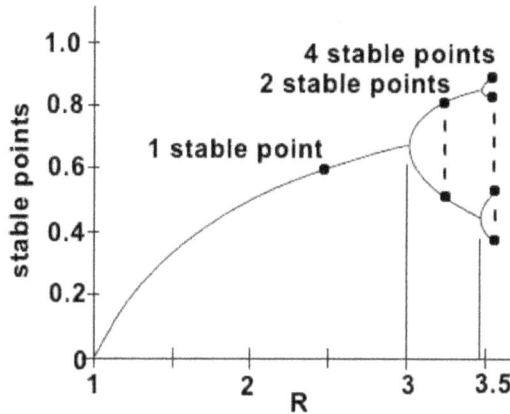

Figure 12: The population begins to oscillate as its rate of growth exceeds 3. The lines show population levels. The dots locate where the system settles, or points between which it alternates.

When the value of R gets larger, the system starts oscillating between values. When R exceeds 3, the system alternates between two points. This isn't evident in the inhibited rates of growth shown in figure 12, but is from the calculated behavior. As the amplification increases further, the system oscillates between four values, then eight values, and so forth, continuing to double with larger values of R.

Return to the analogy of sound, where the strength y is the volume of a note and the passage of time generates a beat. The volume of the note would repeat at an even beat and either grow louder or softer to stabilize at a fixed volume, or the volume would cycle between louder and softer.

As the growth factor grew further, the note would alternate between four values: softer, soft, loud, and louder, repeating this cycle indefinitely. With increasingly smaller changes in the strength of the growth factor, the number of distinct and regularly repeating volumes would continue to double. Then, at a certain point of increasing R, the regularity would cease and the volume would change chaotically.

The Model of Thoughts

This is not yet my model because this is just a single ought. An ought is not an idea and is not enough to become one. An idea is a combination of oughts that reinforce each other or, in other cases, diminish each other.

The simplest model is two oughts coupled to each other so that the action of one affects the other. If the strength of the first ought is x, then the strength of the second ought can be y. Here, x and y are no longer the x-axis and the y-axis, but the strength of oughts x and y over time, where time steps are measured by n. Separately, their strengths would evolve independently:

$$x(n+1) = A\,x(n) - B\,(x(n))^2$$

$$y(n+1) = A'\,y(n) - B'\,(y(n))^2$$

Where A can be different from A', and B can be different from B'. These differences would clearly have an effect on how things developed, but the general shape of things will survive their simplification to $B = B' = A = A' = R$, that is to say, we'll set them all to the same value of R.

Returning to the analogy of sounds, the addition of a second ought corresponds to the addition of a second tone. In this case, with each beat, there are two tones. Given the two separate equations, these two tones will behave independently, moving to find their own separate equilibrium volumes.

Now, it's time to leave what's simple and move to what might be real. To do this, link these two equations so that each depends on the other. We do this by coupling them together, by putting the effect of one into the equation for the other.

I make this addition using a multiplier "T," which can be any value, and which I can lower to zero in order to recover two independent equations. At this point, it's hard to speak the equations so that you can see them. It's much easier if you see them written down:

$$x(n+1) = R\,(x(n) - (x(n))^2) + T\,y(n)$$

$$y(n+1) = R\,(y(n) - (y(n))^2) + T\,x(n)$$

We can vary T between 0 and 1. When T = 0 we recover the two separate equations. The coupling between the values of x and y increases as the value of T gets larger.

Where the single logistic equation looked simple but generated complexity, the coupled equations no longer look simple. I would like to say that now we have great insight into the structure of thought, but it rather seems that we've traded what was before opaque with what is now complex.

There is extensive research on the features of the logistic equation and equations like it. There is little research on coupled logistic equations, and what research there is rarely goes beyond the coupling of two equations. I would like to couple many together, so I'm going to have to do this work myself.

One thing we can see is that the additional "T" term has the effect of raising the curves. With this additional term, the strength of x(n+1) does not vanish when the previous strength x(n) vanishes. That is, the effect of the other ought continues to stimulate its partner and vice versa.

As a result of this coupling, we expect to see new behaviors and new thresholds of behavior. We also expect to see aspects of the original behaviors. The strengths at which the oughts stabilize should be higher, that is to say, the effect of the stimulation will increase the magnitude toward which each ought settles. This is what we want: the effect of coupling oughts is to enhance each other.

Using the analogy of sound, we now have two notes in which the volume of one depends on the other. The volumes could stabilize at a constant value or they could cycle, or one could stabilize and the other could cycle. One might become soft while the other becomes loud.

If the combined strength of the oughts surpasses some threshold, then we expect thoughts, or a thought, to emerge in our minds. Over time, these strengths will fade, and our model needs to account for the fading of thoughts. Before that happens, we expect to see new structures, such as similar or opposing oscillations in the strength of the oughts.

In a 1998 paper in the journal *Theoretical Population Biology* (Kendall and Fox 1998), the authors explore similar equations for two coupled logistic systems. I've put in bold the similar components.

$$x(n+1) = (1-T) R (\mathbf{x(n) - (x(n))^2}) + T R' (\mathbf{y(n) - (y(n))^2})$$

$$y(n+1) = (1-T) R' (\mathbf{y(n) - (y(n))^2}) + T R (\mathbf{x(n) - (x(n))^2})$$

They use the coefficients T and (1–T) so that when T varies from zero to 1 the equations are either fully coupled or uncoupled. When T = 0, the equations for x and y are the same, and x at one point in time depends only on x at the previous time. But when T = 1, what happens at x at one time-step n depends on what happened at y at the previous time-step n-1.

The case that interests me is in the middle, where T is between 0 and 1. In particular, in this middle range, where T is small and the coupling between x and y is weak.

At the simplest level, Kendall and Fox find the two parameters x and y either rise and fall together, or rise and fall in opposition. There are stable and unstable configurations. In stable configurations, the system settles into unchanging values for x and y. In unstable configurations, the values of x and y fluctuate chaotically.

Applications

I suggest that when enough thoughts resonate in synchrony, we experience something like an emotion that gives us direction. When opposing thoughts alternate, we are emotionally upset and lose direction. At some point, there might be chaos, where we lose our minds completely.

These equations lead to fractal behaviors, as this is typical of these structures. Similar patterns would emerge at higher rates of growth and more complex thoughts. This would be like the chords on a keyboard that can be transposed to higher and lower octaves.

As we add more oughts in the equation, we add more notes in the sound analogy. All the notes are playing at each beat, but their volumes differ. Those that stabilize at a single volume will continue at that volume. The volumes of those that cycle will rise and fall, while those that are unstable will change volume in a chaotic fashion, seeming to swell and dissipate at random. The behavior that prevails depends on the growth rates of the various oughts and how strongly they affect each other.

I will be interested to find out if this supports the idea that dreams have a fractal structure. Dream narratives reiterate their themes, so that positive dreams unfold with positive details of varying depth and size, and negative dreams unfold into a spectrum of negative details. This is why dreams affect us so strongly, why we have a difficult time following them, and why our conscious mind prefers to forget them. Dreams allow us to find what we're comfortable with by exploring the many combinations of things that we don't like.

Finally, if we can identify oughts—our fundamental thought elements—then we could simplify and better manage our thoughts. We do that now to a rough degree, but we have no underlying theory and nothing to explain how this works. If we could identify which oughts contribute to particular states and behaviors, then we'd gain a general understanding of how our thoughts evolve. We would experience free will at a deeper level.

All of this will have to wait for me to put these equations into a computer program to see what they generate. I am interested in the simplest behavior that persists as we make this system larger. I'm not looking for detail, I'm looking for patterns; visualizable patterns that reflect thought.

I don't expect to find anyone who's done this work before, and I don't expect to generate much interest amongst other researchers. They should be interested, but until I generate opportunities for others, others pursue their own opportunities. Even so, working with the elements of thoughts has already helped me understand myself, my clients, and my dreams.

References

Kendall, B., Fox, G. (1998). "Spatial Structure, Environmental Heterogeneity, and Population Dynamics: Analysis of the Coupled Logistic Map." *Theoretical Population Biology 54*, 11-37. https://escholarship.org/uc/item/359696wj

Minsky, M. (1974 June). "A Framework for Representing Knowledge." *National Technical Information Service*. https://apps.dtic.mil/sti/pdfs/ADA011168.pdf

Muller, D. (2020 Jan 29). "This Equation Will Change How You See the World." *Veritasium*.

T15 – Where Thoughts Come From – IV

https://www.veritasium.com/videos/2020/1/29/this-equation-will-change-how-you-see-the-world

T16 – Beyond Sight and Feeling

September 23, 2021

The more you imagine, the more you learn.

"Imagination will often carry us to worlds that never were. But without it, we go nowhere." — **Carl Sagan**, astronomer and science popularizer

Sight

Sight teaches us that cause precedes effect, and that many things affecting us can't be seen. Observation teaches rational thinking when we can see the reasons for things. It also allows for irrational thinking when we cannot. "Seeing is believing" is a statement of the limitations of how we think.

By expanding our perception, we build a larger reality. Most people equate rationality with science, but in addition to reason, science requires repeatability, a foundation of belief, and the existence of alternatives. A theory may have laws, but science never does. Science, like every other theory of reality, rests on belief.

Sight teaches us to think beyond what we observe, and to expand our sight to what we can imagine. When we imagine, we start seeing what we're thinking and we start to believe it. It would be a mistake to think this is a rational process. Seeing is not perception but a process of recognition. Recognition is something we manufacture.

There are people who believe they've been abducted by aliens. But something need not really happen for you to think it has. There are people who believe they've seen flying saucers, and they may have. But seeing something does not mean it was ever there. Your eyes perceive. Your mind apperceives. And then, to complicate things further, you think you remember.

You don't need perception in order to have apperception. When you apperceive things it seems they really were there, and then you'll say you perceived them. Consider your dreams. You believe a dream while dreaming. You feel the images are real even though you are not perceiving anything. You feel you are real and that's the basis of the illusion. You are not real.

Reality is whatever things feel to be. You are absolutely convinced of the reality of the dream, even though, in retrospect, the dream meets none of your conditions for reality. Belief underlies reality: if you believe it, then it is.

Belief

"Seeing is believing" tells us that reason serves belief. No one believes everything they see. We hesitate when experiencing déjà vu, a mirage, or an object out of place. You're more likely to see what you believe. This form of sight does not stand up to scrutiny, but we rarely scrutinize. We don't care to and we don't have time.

When we see something that we don't believe, we are at a loss. It can cause us to become unglued, to lose our ability to think. We are designed for the evolutionary purpose of thinking straight. It's a survival trait. We are also designed to presume the greater evil, to be pessimistic. This is also a survival trait.

If you're afraid of walking alone on a dark street and you walk alone on a dark street, then you'll see things that support your fears, and this will support what you believe will keep you safe. We respect the curious scientist and the heroic explorer because we recognize that the person who sees more knows more, but this is not our inclination.

Sounds and Shapes

Where speech has vocabulary, images have shapes. We limit speech to what makes sense and build it out of words. We limit what we see to lines and edges and build these into shapes. In visual memory, we store recognizable shapes and textures. We put together what we see, similar to the way we put together what we say. If you can't verbalize something, then you can't say it. And if you can't imagine something, then you can't see it.

A creative idea is an idea that has an element of novelty. It differs from all its antecedents. A creative idea is not an error or omission, though it may look like one. A creative idea feels like something more.

Getting to something more requires making more space. You cannot say, see, or think of something outside your existing repertoire of statements, sights, or thoughts unless you have some mental space that is unoccupied.

The mind "space" is not a place or a thing, it's a construction. Novelty requires unoccupied thoughts. This either follows from expanding one's awareness or removing preconceptions. What does this feel like?

Thoughts

We often think we understand linearly, causally, and through association, but these are only slices of reality. Our reality is like a crystal and these linear thoughts are slices along its fault lines. Each of us has our own set of crystals, each of a different structure, and each of us is looking at the world along slightly different orientations of a crystal.

I'm giving you the image of cleaving through a crystal, but this picture is too small. This picture is no bigger than there are angles with which to look through a crystal. It is more accurate to say that many parts of our "crystal picture" of reality contribute to anything we imagine. Remote associations, metaphorical connections, and connections learned through experience can all contribute to how we understand what's going on at any moment.

Rather than a set of simple reflections, our understanding is a diffraction pattern, which is what makes a well-cut gem glow and sparkle. The sparkle comes from the facets on the outside, but the glow comes from the planes of reflection on the inside. And this is how we think: not just based on what we see on the surface, but also on the deeper connections layered inside us.

Dreams

Dreams are a language of associations that explore the plausible and implausible. Dreams explore our mental constructions in order to determine what fits, how to make things fit, and how to arrange our preconceptions, perceptions, and apperceptions. They explore confusion in order to assemble pictures of what perplexes us.

We speak of dreams as visions, but they're usually a scrapbook of images and feelings. It's not clear whether the dream feelings create the dream visions or the other way around. If the dream was just spoken, then we wouldn't feel much of anything. Dreams are richer than words.

Notice that dream images have little detail. They feel richly detailed, but they're not. They have dramatic detail regarding the topic on which they focus, but they lack detail in areas where they lack implication. This is not too much different from normal apperception, which feels thorough and complete because sight is detailed, but which actually contains little detail. We recognize little and record even less.

Dreams are a form of nonverbal, right-brain thinking. Sometimes dream characters speak, but they rarely say much or come to conclusions. I occasionally find written material in my dreams, but I can rarely read it. When numbers appear, such as the keypad on a phone, I'm helpless to do anything with them.

The desire to speak, read, or enumerate is left-brained and greatly underpowered in dreams. On some occasions—such as when you are deeply immersed in speech, words, or numbers in waking life—you can find symbolic meaning in words or numbers. But in a dream, these analytic expressions are inert. They lack a larger sense, feeling, or relationship.

In no case have I ever found numbers to have meaning in a dream, and I cannot even recall a dream in which they have appeared. On those rare occasions when I hold a lucid conversation with a character in my dreams, I'm astounded. Such conversations are break-throughs to another thinking mind.

Feelings

First we feel, then we imagine, and last we think. We can change this order by an act of will, but without the support of a new feeling our thoughts will lose momentum, and we will return to what we felt before. When thoughts and feelings are in conflict, feelings direct us.

There are parts of you that cannot express themselves in words. These parts use images, sensations, and emotions. These parts are not verbal or analytical. By themselves, these aspects of your personality don't have the power to separate things or choose one thing over another.

We relegate many of these parts of ourselves to our subconscious. We might call them "right brain thinking," or creative insights. They lead our conversations, but they don't speak directly. They don't verbalize well. Instead, we express them through attitude, emotion, posture, energy, and opinion. Our parts have power and we underrate them.

We spend our waking life in the realm of speech, words, and numbers, and our sleeping life in a world of sense, feeling, and emotion. When we enter a trance world, we are in-between the two. In a trance, we can think in one mode, both modes, or neither.

As overly thoughtful beings, we are awake for 16 hours and asleep for 8. What we encounter in 16 hours of wakefulness takes 8 hours of sleep to put into perspective. The world is complicated, our sleep is stressed, and time is at a premium. As things get more complicated, there is more to figure out. We need more right-brain thinking.

Thinking with both sides of our brain puts us between reason and emotion. As our actions have more implications, we need more associative thinking. We need greater mastery in visual, emotional, and sensual modes of associative thinking.

Awareness

Imagine an image with pictures embedded in it: a landscape with many vistas or layers of suggestive detail. These parts can be literal, symbolic, consonant, or dissonant. We can broaden our thinking to encompass multiple pictures at once. We can't do that with words. Using words, we have to jump around.

When we think abstractly, we think in symbols. Compare the narrowness of what you say in words with the breadth of what you can express using symbols. Each of these two forms says something different and, ideally, you can express yourself in both in slightly different ways.

The attraction of using words is their narrowness and specificity. What we gain in definition and exclusion, we lose in associations and relationships. Many of the misunderstandings in today's social and political topics stem from a conflict over their expression using narrower words or broader symbols.

We can enhance our thinking by taking a dual track: expressing ourselves using words and again, symbolically. We must do this if we aim to understand because the truth, if it exists at all, exists somewhere between words and symbols.

Consider anger and affection. Both can be expressed literally, and a literal expressing is entirely inadequate. It's taken for granted that words spoken without emotion are insincere. You must add inflection, expression, tone, rhythm, and body language, and you require the same of those with whom you communicate. These are not optional add-ons, they are essential. In fact, the symbols are not only more effective; they are more important. The words you assemble in your mind are more for your benefit. Beyond the invitation to talk, they add little to communication.

Don't reject the words even though none are satisfactory. Don't erase the symbols even though they're too vague. By embracing the conflicts that neither resolve, we find deeper relationships between them. As we experience our thoughts differently, we become informed. Words invite a safer dialog than actions.

Frequency

We have dimensions of reason and feeling, and we have a dimension of frequency. The dimension of frequency is the rapidity with which our ideas and associations form. The rhythm of your speech reflects the connections between your ideas.

Our physical and verbal rhythms interact with the frequencies of our actions and the objects we engage with. Physical sensations arise slowly, ideas travel quickly, and patterns appear in an instant. Think of yourself as a musical structure.

In the realm of reason, one reason affects another, and we rank them. In the realm of feeling, we create a network of associations and we relate them. The changing frequencies of things expand and contract our sense of time, narrowing and widening our definitions, and focusing our attention.

We see common and disparate relationships in things, remembering more of what we classify along familiar lines. The enemies we see now look like enemies from our past. Our friends and allies resemble those of our childhood.

Your awareness flows along patterned channels like the aisles of a library, with attitudes grouped like books arranged by subject. You engage the world using the associations at hand and miss those ideas shelved elsewhere.

The correspondences you find are neither real nor unreal, it's just the way they're cataloged. To perceive the world more accurately, be a librarian in cataloging what you see. The different frequencies of history reveal those patterns that repeat themselves. You don't need to remember everything, just where to find things and how to navigate your mind.

It takes a moment to recall a fact, longer if the context is confused. Switch an animated conversation from current events to family history and the conversation will pause, relocate, and pick up speed again. Topics changed across greater distances create greater disruptions.

In the library of frequency, there are sections containing memories of your childhood. In these memories, time passed at a different rate and we linked observations to feelings in a manner that's now unusual.

There are aisles of memory you rarely revisit, and when you do, it's as if the volumes are too thin, the type is too small, or the titles too strange, and you can't read them. We don't lose old memories as much as we lose access to them.

You often need a special state of mind to access these unusual materials. You'll find such different states in trance, reverie, exertion, contemplation, or emergency. To navigate flexibly through your mind is to remain oriented as new visions come into focus, to be acrobatic.

Altered States

When flexibly is detached, you can switch from one state to another, seeing from either without constraint. This is a form of channeling where multiple states of awareness coexist at the same time.

Without the ability to navigate, you get lost in the woods, or perhaps you never leave your spot. Without the ability to navigate, you forget what you saw in one state when you move to another. If you can't remember the irrationality that seemed rational in a dream, you'll have trouble remembering it when awake. The same occurs in a foreign language: if you can't remember the words, you'll get lost in the sentences.

T16 – Beyond Sight and Feeling

Move between your different states without losing your sense of self. Learn to navigate different states in order to access different thoughts, feelings, and frequencies. If you want to realize your dreams, then return to your dream state and recognize what things mean in that reality.

This is the challenge and the promise of letting go of who you've become convinced that you are. The process is challenging because the landscape is unfamiliar, progress is slow, and there are many new mistakes to make. These new landscapes offer more than different combinations, they offer unfamiliar elements, people, attitudes, and personalities. You must let go of yourself before you can get a better grip.

T17 – Thinking

September 29, 2021

Of all the things we do, thinking is the least understood.

"Whenever you find yourself on the side of the majority, it is time to pause and reflect." — **Mark Twain**

Few think about thinking. It isn't direct, and it has many levels. Here are a few of the levels that go on all the time when you're thinking.

Images

You use a kind of sight to visualize what's in your mind. Sometimes you will see things in the first person as if they were memories and other times you'll sense distances between things. You may see ideas and relationships expressed in images.

Words

Words are the teeth in the gears that turn our minds. We both recognize their importance and dismiss the degree they control us. It is as if we are an assembly of dust held together by the attraction between the particles. We ascribe little importance to them because we don't believe they have a mind of their own, but if it were not for them, we would fall apart.

> "A chance word, upon paper, may destroy the world. Watch carefully and erase, while the power is still yours... once it escapes, it may rot its way into a thousand minds, the corn become a black smut, and all libraries, of necessity, be burned to the ground as a consequence."
> — **William Carlos Williams**, poet, from *Paterson*

Thoughts

We often overlook thoughts as being things in themselves, independent from the words and images. When we're confused, we cannot tell under which shell our ideas first form, the image, the word, or the thought. It doesn't seem to matter, and we don't care. As a result, we think that wherever our thoughts came from, they're ours now, and they always were.

Disjointed thoughts, which can grow into daydreams, range from a single word to an elaborate fantasy. They can provide inspiration but need space in which to incubate. Some of us can allow our minds to wander a wider pasture while others are more corralled. We rarely speak or even have the words to discuss the pastures of our minds.

> "The quietest people have the loudest minds."
> — **Stephen Hawking**, physicist

Mind

The truth, in as much as there is truth in the mind's realm, is that the harder you look for your independence and free will, the less of it you find. If your words are the teeth of the gears that are your thoughts, then your brain is a clock, and your mind is the time it keeps.

We construct thoughts involuntarily. If you assert your intention to think about your childhood or a summer day, then you'll wait for the thought to arise. You can make a more detailed request, but you play no role in retrieving the memories or constructing the thought. That level of control would just slow us down and offer no advantage.

At the other extreme, even the most thoughtful and aware individuals play a minor role in forming their thoughts. The most we can do is guide our thoughts or derail them. Guidance plays a big role in what we think about, but a smaller role in the thoughts themselves.

The genesis and content of our thoughts are dictated by the patterns of our mind, the state of our body, the contents of our memory, and the situation in which we find ourselves. What rises in our minds are waves on an ocean of awareness. Surf them.

You can pick the waves and you can navigate skillfully. You can block waves as if you were a breakwater. You affect the weather, and the weather makes the waves bigger or smaller. The shape of the waves is the texture of your emotions. But the waves themselves, which are the contents of your thoughts, have an origin that's outside your control.

I try to be thoughtful. I try to be aware of as many simultaneous events, emotions, and perspectives as possible, and to avoid thinking any more than necessary. Thinking is to experience as talking is to listening. I try to limit my thinking to problems that require solutions, and perceptions that require focus and attention.

> "Listen more than you talk. Nobody learned anything by hearing themselves speak."
> — **Richard Branson**, business magnate

My thinking feels successful when I'm on the border of overload, aware of as much as I can hold. My thinking fails to create insight when it repeats itself. I try to limit my interactions to those people who are similarly thoughtful, but not identically thoughtful. As a result, I interact with few people.

To summarize this project, I am attempting to convey to you the means by which you can better influence your thoughts. This involves being more aware of what you're thinking, feeling, and perceiving, as well as what's going on below your thinking, feeling, and perceiving. This is complicated by the many things you are only partially aware of.

Rationality

Rationality is based on continuity. Events follow from other events because they are functionally connected. If events were not connected to the things that caused them, the world would not make sense. We need sense. It's how we protect ourselves, so we manufacture continuity. We manufacture a continuous experience and we call it time.

Let me suggest there is a circle of awareness around where you are now. There is a universe of events occurring at this moment, wherever you are, and you're aware of an infinitesimal amount of them. You are, at this moment, literally receiving electromagnetic radiation from the entire history of the universe. Sights and sounds are impinging on you from all directions. You are mentally experiencing an infinitesimal amount of this. What we call "reality" is based on this minuscule perception.

251

Making sense is not a sensation. Being sensible and being sensitive are unrelated. The similarity in the word structure between perceiving sense in the world and having senses to perceive the world is not a coincidence. We take both sense and senses equally for granted. We should not.

We project sense as perception on the world and believe we sense the world. We do not recognize that our mind must construct senses from sensations—as apperceptions from perceptions—and that, in fact, the real world is not what we perceive it to be.

"Making sense" is rational thought. As we project sensations on the world, so we project the sense we make on the world. We believe the phenomenal is real. Why? Because it works, but here is our mistake: there are other, radically different ways of seeing the world that work too.

Things don't have to make sense, and things don't have to appear to make sense. Much of what makes sense is fiction. You are literally making the sense you see in the world around you. How do you do it? You fabricate sense from the illusion of continuity.

We don't know if the world is continuous or not. Depending on what we examine, the world appears both ways: sometimes smooth and other times disconnected. We experience the world as continuous, yet it only takes a little reflection to appreciate that our experience is not continuous. Neurologically, there is no question of this. We are aware only a tiny portion of the time, much less than what we think we're aware of.

Our sense of continuous awareness, and our sense of the world as being continuously unfolding, is a guess, an extrapolation. This is what we do to paper over the infinity of holes in our perception, and it works well. We absolutely believe the world is continuous even though we struggle to keep up with it.

Internal Dialog

Please stop talking to yourself, if only for a while. You are not accustomed to a quiet mind, but if you try it, you'll like it. Don't you know how annoying it is to be in a room with someone who announces everything they think? If you could hear all the thoughts that go through your head, it would drive you crazy.

You have more than a single voice inside you. You could think along other lines besides the narration of your loudest thoughts. Imagine how those other voices feel having to listen to you verbalizing your one repeating narrative. It is the genesis of frustration. Can you not be yourself without gushing like an open fire hydrant? It's unnecessary!

The purpose of our mental dialog is not to hear anything, but to drown out a larger awareness and the democracy of our emotions. In the interests of the perception of continuity, uniformity, and reason—all illusions of our construction—we bark like dogs in heat, reiterating our one-track minds.

Through this process of constantly reminding ourselves, we draw our attention back to a narrow ledge of continuity. This ledge leads through a dizzying multiplicity of events, attitudes, and perceptions. As if we were traversing a ledge, we keep our eyes focused on the path ahead. To look around is disorienting. To look down is frightening.

We navigate life as if we're traveling a risky path, which life is, and we much prefer the comfort of security to the amazement of all the possibilities that would require a different frame of mind and might put us in danger. Because we are averse to confusion, we create confidence by committing ourselves to what's likely. We hate the vulnerability of the unexpected.

> "The brain evolved to be uncertainty-averse. When things become less predictable—and therefore less controllable—we experience a strong state of threat... [This] leads to decreases in motivation, focus, agility, cooperative behavior, self-control, sense of purpose and meaning, and overall well-being. In addition, threat creates significant impairments in your working memory: You can't hold as many ideas in your mind to solve problems, nor can you pull as much information from your long-term memory when you need it."
> — **Heidi Grant** and **Tal Goldhamer** (2021), social psychologists

Social Bonding

What you say to yourself is the story you would like to hear. It's childish, ego-centered, defensive, and weakly aware. This story is a protective container for your actions and decisions. This protects you from the specter of your own weakness and distracts you from doing better. You would do better if you discarded the fear, kept silent, and kept watch. That is how opportunities develop.

Our personal narrative is to our social narrative as our personal presentation is to our social presentation. We present ourselves socially in order to support both our story and the stories of others. These stories are strands in a social web that makes up a consensus reality. The aim is not truth, it's agreement. These narratives become social gossip whose function is much the same as grooming is for primates.

Social bonding is important; it creates a safe space in which we can relax. Without social bonding, there would be no social fabric. Without a social fabric, we'd be in a constant and debilitating state of vigilance and stress.

You can decide how much of your time, energy, awareness, and intelligence needs to be taken up with social bonding. For most people, socializing is more about bonding and less about discovery. You express a different social identity in your family from your identity at work. Bonding plays different roles in these environments.

To better identify yourself, recognize your different social, family, and work personalities. Reconcile their differences and unify their virtues. You are different people in these different environments. If these people are not working together, they are holding you back.

We question our sanity, family, or workplace only when things are not working. We do this when in distress. It is unlikely that you would rock any of these boats simply out of curiosity. You might if you were seeking wisdom, but others are unlikely to welcome any tinkering with the rules of the game.

We all need social affirmation. Acceptance is affirmation, but rejection is affirmation too. Either can support self-exploration and your authentic self. You want confirmation that your explorations and revelations will reward you. Consider your friends, family, and work environment in that light. Change your relationships to get more support for your personal evolution.

Volition and Control

Volition means having a desire to act; control is your ability to guide this desire. These two are not the same. What we want to do is rarely under our control. Most of us say one thing and do another. This "bait and switch" happens at the limit of our awareness, as we think we're consistent when we are not. Our typical deception is to convince ourselves that we are as we think ourselves to be, regardless of any evidence to the contrary.

> "People will do anything, no matter how absurd, in order to avoid facing their own souls."
> — **C. G. Jung**, psychiatrist

The best way to have one effect while believing that you're having another is to dull your awareness so that you cannot see the difference. Your desire to be unintentionally self-deceptive nurtures your lack of awareness. A huge obstacle to your becoming self-aware is your resistance to seeing yourself honestly.

You say you want to be more aware, but you don't want to see what you're afraid of. You cannot have it both ways. Call it courage or call it foolishness. One way or the other, you must become honest, first with others, and then with yourself.

References

Grant, H., and Goldhamer, T. (2021 Sep 22). "Our Brains Were Not Built for This Much Uncertainty." Harvard Business Review. https://hbr.org/2021/09/our-brains-were-not-built-for-this-much-uncertainty

T18 – Kinds of Thinking

October 6, 2021

Science, psychology, stupidity, and many others all have a place.

"Many highly intelligent people are poor thinkers. Many people of average intelligence are skilled thinkers. The power of a car is separate from the way the car is driven."— **Edward de Bono**, MD, psychologist, author, and inventor

There are many ways of thinking: deductive, inductive, reductive, analytical, emotional, literal, lateral, metaphorical, free, expansive, positive, negative, restricted, or shut down. Your personality emerges from the ways you think, which are built on ideas outside of your control.

Thinking is not just executive function, it includes inclinations, prejudices, triggers, memories, and associations. Ideas that emerge unintentionally define your personality. With effort, you can effect a measure of control, but this is not intellectual; it's control of your mental state.

Each of us has a personality that more or less exerts itself through attitude. If I were to read to you a detailed history of your life, a history that contained all of those sensitive things you told no one, you would recall past actions out of step with your current personality. At different ages and under different circumstances, you were a different person, even though you remember yourself as you are now.

You could not reconstruct the ways you thought then unless you could re-experience those moods and emotions now. You would find that you could recall some of those moods and emotions, but it would take time and lead you into unfamiliar mental spaces. Those spaces might be more comfortable or less.

We sandbag the foundations of our positive memories with objects, photos, and friendships. We clean up our mistakes with explanations, excuses, and dismissals. These are the intellectual things we do and they partially work to maintain our intellectual image and presentation of ourselves. Although we can clean up our conscious, social presentation, we cannot clean up our deeper subconscious, emotional, and traumatic memories. We naturally shun them. Without intending to, we are pressed into living ever more intellectual, social, and superficial versions of ourselves.

As we pad our memories with the good and distance ourselves from the bad, we paint ourselves into a corner. This is a corner where the sun always shines, but it lacks enough soil to grow in. Western society has so many unhelpful elders because we're indifferent to and lack responsibility for our environment. It comes from the illusion that because you fulfilled the terms of your social contract, your work is done. Many of us are following a path that will come to a halt at the end of our lives as we wait for our reward.

Support or Isolation

Your personality is a set of unconscious habits and thoughtful intentions. A fungus grows out from a central point, creating a starburst of tendrils in all directions as it looks for nutrition. This is how your thoughts develop from a central idea or condition, searching outward for recollections and encouragement. You're attracted to some ideas and repelled by others. These triggers, once set off, dominate your attention until you put them out of your mind or turn your attention to something else. They create a set of focus points that act like bits of food for thought.

When you encounter something toxic, your thoughts will try to disarm it. We work to avoid, divert, neutralize, or forget toxic areas. To hide or turn them off. The pervasive myth of the hidden monster emerges from our efforts to hide our monsters.

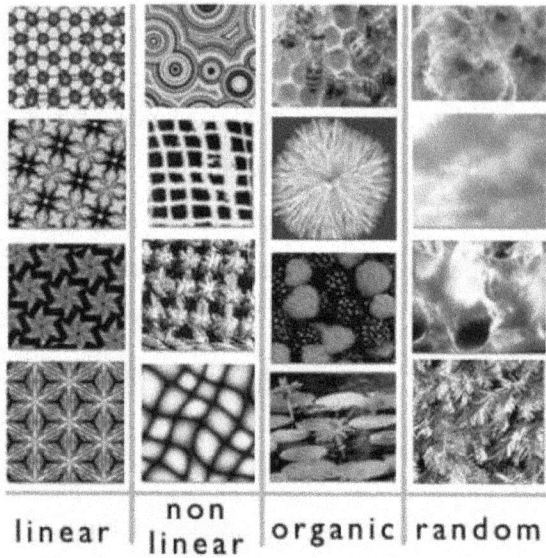

Figure 13: Structures that offer metaphors for different ways of thinking.

You won't notice what you choose to avoid, as that would bring it to your attention. This could include trauma you've experienced or inflicted on others. Just as we justify what we prefer to think, we unconsciously distort our memories.

Our two greatest fears are isolation and rejection. We're always assessing ourselves in social terms, and social support is as necessary as breathing. To be rejected for achieving our goal is seen as a defeat. It takes a strong character to be indifferent.

Flexibility

Few of us are even aware of our style of thinking and rarely suit our style to our problems. We blame elements of the world, the problem, or ourselves for our lack of solutions when the real problem is how we're thinking. We would do well to be more flexible.

Many of my clients struggle with the unhelpful issues and attitudes of others. They feel external events cause their problems when the actual source is their lack of boundaries. There is chaos in the world and it will drag you in if you let it. Chaos is a natural consequence of destruction and creation. If you need to be part of it, that's your issue.

There are reasons for our inflexibility. We're rewarded for being skilled at one thing more than we're rewarded for being skilled at many. I have found the truth is different: deeper rewards always come from broader skills and deeper thinking.

One gains skill in the usual way: by practice. You learn what you practice, but practice will not make you skilled unless you do it correctly.

Practice often embeds poor performance. Repetition does not lead to improvement, it leads to more of the same. Improvement changes what's being repeated, and it can happen even if you're not aware of how you're improving.

Even good performance doesn't assure you of skillful thinking. You don't learn skillful thinking when you learn a skill. Feedback is essential, which is why most teachers, whose skills are marginal at the start, never improve.

You learn what you practice; repetition strengthens existing patterns. Memorizing a perfect performance doesn't assure you of an improvement.

A student who succeeds at rote learning has learned nothing. Learning to perform a musical passage perfectly only indicates skill when you can reapply this performance in other contexts. Skillful thinking is a step beyond performance.

Because novel thinking is unknown territory, you must go into unknown territory to develop your thinking. Thinking is inherently creative, and there is no one measure of creativity. No one can test you on thinking because your creative potential is unique to you. Creativity cannot be measured according to someone else's goals.

A reasonable approach to any field is to get good at one thing first and then broaden your skills. This works in sports, music, art, science, relationships, and thinking. There is one big difference between these and thinking: no one teaches thinking.

It's possible to teach thinking, but I question the wisdom of it. One learns to think in actual situations; without actual situations, one doesn't really learn to think. The best way to learn to think is to perfect yourself in a variety of circumstances.

You want the ability to navigate a variety of seas. The worst way to learn is to do nothing, to avoid the water entirely.

The second worst way to learn is to get no feedback and consider nothing. A rudder doesn't work unless there is something passing over it. You drift with no control.

The third worst way to learn is to become a specialist so that you see everything from a single perspective. You are a tool with a single setting. In each of these circumstances, you are not developing the skills to compare, decide, or react. You learn by reacting to what you don't expect.

Styles

Most of our conclusions can be predicted given our style of thinking, regardless of the details of the problem. A lack of thinking skills is a fundamental problem. If you explore what people say about having the right attitude, you'll be encouraged to be positive, solution-focused, collegial, and realistic. However, for a person who is depressed, oppressed, overpowered, or defeated, such encouragement has no traction.

Positive

> "Don't waste your time in anger, regrets, worries, and grudges. Life is too short to be unhappy."
> — **Roy T. Bennett**, author

"The power of positive thinking" is a thinking style. For most people, this means seeing things in a positive light. This weak interpretation imposes a bias that's indifferent to reality. Positive feeling is a strength; positive thinking is a coping strategy.

Seeing things in a positive light can help you see the positive potential in situations, but it will not clarify what is holding you back. The overly optimistic thinker develops a strategy that presumes rather than protects the desired outcome. They will fail because of circumstances they did not see or control.

Negative

> "You can always turn no into yes, and usually make people happy, but it's a lot

harder—sometimes too late—to change yes to no."
— **Bob Knight** (2013), basketball coach

Thinking of all threats to a positive outcome is seen by many as negative thinking. Such a negative thinker is always seeing dangers, threats, and problems, but that does not mean that these obstruct their goals.

In order to judge a strategy's chance for success, see beyond the method to the goal. Our goals are often unclear because we presume them rather than explain them. We may see our near-term goals and be blind to where they're leading.

Negativity or positivity should be a property of reality, not perspective. Recognize whether you're talking about goals or means. Negative means will lead toward positive goals if you aim to avoid the negative. Recognize the means you employ toward the positive goals you want to achieve. The means and goals are separate parts of the process, but in some situations, the journey is the destination.

We are often unsatisfied with our goals once we achieve them. Your attitude along the path may be more of a reward than what you accomplish. Beware of climbing other people's ladders.

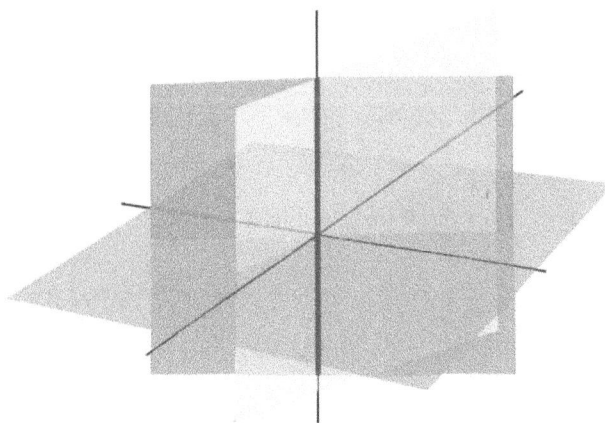

Figure 14: Planes that intersect offer different perspectives with a line in common.

A positive perspective will not assure a positive goal, nor will a negative perspective assure a negative outcome. If you aim for success and secure a job that makes you miserable, is that positive or negative? Can you balance the emotional with the intellectual? See paths and goals from both perspectives.

Duality and Dichotomy

"In order to eat, you have to be hungry. In order to learn, you have to be ignorant. Ignorance is a condition of learning."
— **Robert Anton Wilson**, author, from *Leviathan*

Some spiritualists espouse a non-dualist philosophy and condemn dualistic thinking. But non-duality is a nonstarter because if you are really avoiding duality, then it does not exist for you to avoid. Thinking is dualist. It requires a separation between what you think and who you are. Non-dualist thinking is an oxymoron.

We are duality machines. All analytical thought is built on contrasts. Rhythms are built on alternation. Duality is fundamental to the currents, frequencies, and resonances that are the building blocks of existence. Without duality, you cannot have the phenomena of time.

Dual thinking is fundamental, but dichotomous thinking is not. Dichotomy is the existence of conflict and dichotomous thinking is thinking that creates conflict. This is a mode of thinking in which strife is a source of illumination such that without conflict, situations fade from view. A dichotomous person is one who exists for conflict and feels a lack of existence without it. I suspect that non-dichotomy is what most non-dualists are looking for. Until they use their language correctly, I don't think they'll find it.

Here is a dichotomy disguised as a duality: "Seeing the mud around a lotus is pessimism, seeing a lotus in the mud is optimism." The duality lies in seeing contrast. The dichotomy lies in assigning opposite values to each.

The non-dualist doesn't distinguish mud from solid ground, nor flowers from brambles. They don't notice or appreciate the differences. It's all the same to them. We need duality.

A non-dichotomist sees the benefits and drawbacks of both the ground and the plants. Mud and earth are both good and necessary. Flowers are as good as brambles, and neither are of greater value. All the many roles that duality reveals require your support.

Reduction and Its Opposites

"He that breaks a thing to find out what it is, has left the path of wisdom."
— **J.R.R. Tolkien**, author, from *The Fellowship of the Ring*

We reduce in order to analyze. Our brains seem to be hard-wired to prefer simplicity. We think we have to reduce in order to understand things. This is an odd mistake.

The world isn't reductive. It doesn't need to understand anything, and it has no trouble operating. The difference for us is that we're trying to predict things so that we can pick our future.

You don't need to be reductive to figure things out, but you do if you want to think linearly. If you think linearly, you reduce complexity to single events in order to understand them. There are several situations where this does not describe what's happening, and where being reductive does not work.

Think of the future as if it were a maze. At every intersection, you would like to know which way to go. You want a formula. The formula is only useful if it's simple, which means the maze needs to be simple. Most of our games and entertainments center on maze-like situations where the choices are simple.

We like reductive pictures because they let us focus on the steps of a path. This is reassuring. We focus on chains of events. We identify these with paths to our destinations.

This search is for formulas that we can use. We train specialists to positions of authority and follow their directions. We assume this kind of thinking will always work, but it's a faulty assumption.

The more complex the situation, the less likely it will be reducible. In order to protect ourselves and assure success in thinking linearly, we build for ourselves limited and linear worlds. You can see this in our lifestyles, our economy, culture, and politics. It all starts with how we think.

There are several alternatives to being reductive. They are not opposites, as there are more than two alternatives. Here are a few.

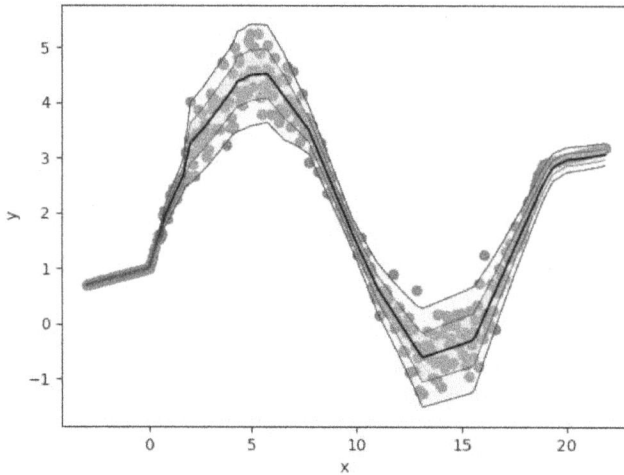

Figure 15: Nonlinear processes generate patterns not easily described.

Nonlinear

"My core philosophy is that I might be wrong."
— **Asaad Almohammad**, author, from *An Ishmael of Syria*

Nonlinear things don't go in a straight line. Nonlinear thinking advances in ways that are difficult to predict. Creativity is a version of limited nonlinearity.

To think non-linearly, stop following your path when you get to a point where you need to decide. Now, consider a different rationale, consider a new direction, make a new decision, and then proceed in your usual, linear manner.

Nonlinear thinking applies new tools, or existing tools in novel ways. If you drove a car and now you ride a bicycle, then there will be some changes in your thinking that are nonlinear. If you had a childless marriage and now you have children, your life will no longer move in a straight line.

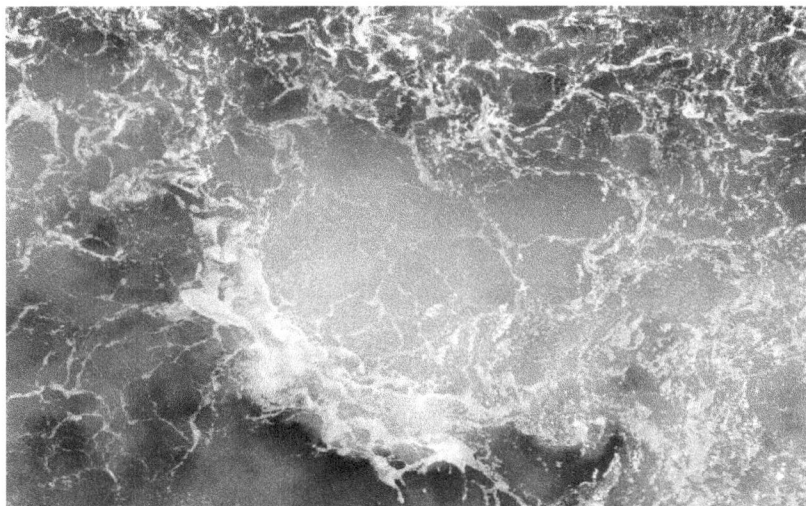

Figure 16: Patterns in randomness can describe the object, event, situation, or point of view. (photo Aaron Ulsh)

Random

"If complete and utter chaos was lightning, then he'd be the sort to stand on a hilltop in a thunderstorm wearing wet copper armor and shouting 'All gods are bastards!' "
— **Terry Pratchett**, author, from *The Color of Magic*

Taking a random direction is not being creative, and it's not acting mindlessly, it's accepting a loss of control. Random changes, and the thoughts that accompany them, need to be controlled to prevent them from being destructive.

You can't expect a random change to solve anything, but it will introduce novelty. The more novelty you want, the more accepting or nondiscriminating you want to be. To accept a random change, defer judgment, realign yourself, and step into a new situation.

Judgment is useful in novel situations, but which judgment and when to judge are uncertain. Your judgment may be linear, some extension of what you thought before, but it should be different. If you apply the same linear thinking as usual, this may return you to your previous situation.

Random changes are nonlinear, but nonlinear changes need not be random. The weather changes non-linearly, but it appears to change randomly. Usually, we try to undo the changes in

265

the weather by rearranging our environment. This allows us to continue our routine without interruption. In other cases, we might return to some previous routine, such as when the power fails or some plans get canceled unexpectedly.

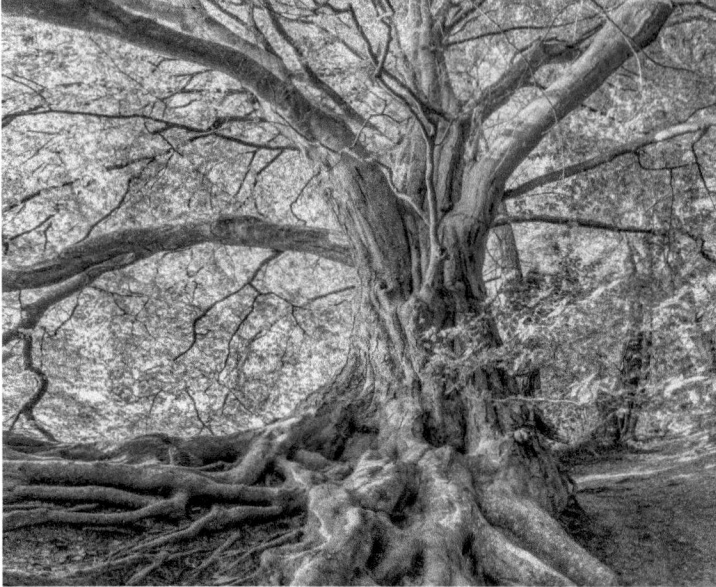

Figure 17: Organic structures reflect both the environment and the structure's interaction with it. (photo Felix Mittermeier)

Organic

Organic thinking involves constantly reevaluating the situation and making choices. You are keeping your perspective but making new choices. New ideas come from the environment and you must be open to them. The organic thinker holds few presumptions or preconceptions. They are attentive to needs and opportunities, perhaps unreliable but not irresponsible.

Resilience is key. A metal bar bends but regains its shape when released. Pushed beyond its elastic limit, the metal loses its original form.

Organic thinking has its limits too. Below this limit, your thoughts adapt to stress but return to their original form when relaxed. Pressured beyond this limit, your thinking may change permanently. There is no one limit that applies to all situations.

The organic thinker holds adequate structure for the present situation but responds to small pressures. When change is large, the organic thinker is an opportunist. Changing both balance and direction, an organic thinker can be mercurial.

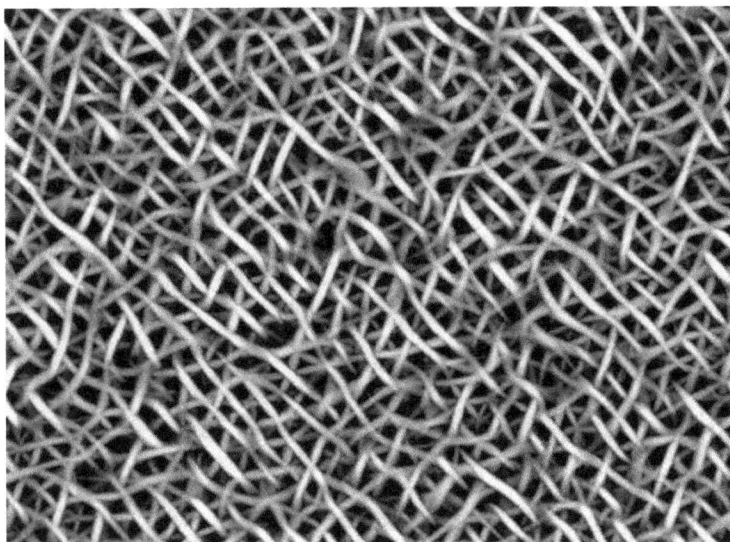

Figure 18: Chaotic structures are only chaotic from some scale or perspective. Defining chaos requires some reference.

Chaotic

"He had just about enough intelligence to open his mouth when he wanted to eat, but certainly no more."
— **P. G. Wodehouse**, author

To think chaotically is to think without structure. We mistake a lot of extreme behavior as being chaotic, such as psychotic or manic behavior. These are not chaotic, they are radically different. Even hysterical and uncontrolled emotional behavior need not be chaotic.

Chaotic thinking lacks structure. It can include anything and have any outcome. Because this could be dangerous, it is a limited part of any strategy.

Where organic thinking draws inspiration from the environment, chaotic thinking adds noise. Because it's influenced by elements you cannot perceive, chaotic thinking can seem preternatural, either loaded with insight or absent of any.

Chaotic thinking is fertile, but difficult to follow. It can conflict with everything and generate ideas that fit nowhere. Dreams exhibit chaotic thinking.

Sudden Savant Syndrome is a chaotic change. In these rare situations, an unlikely event causes the appearance of an unprecedented skill. Restoring a person's sight or hearing would be a chaotic change. It would be a logical process for the surgeon, but a chaotic experience for the patient.

I am always trying to trigger chaotic thinking with my clients. I use trance and daydreams. Past life regression is, at its best, a chaotic experience, as can be a psychedelic experience.

Chaotic does not mean uncontrollable, it means unpredictable. You can throttle it back, but when you release it, you won't know where it will take you.

Your Thinking Potential

I'm seen as a therapist, but I'm not comfortable with that description. I work with people to explore alternative modes of thinking in a search for new discoveries. If you think of yourself as disabled, then this might be called therapy, but I encourage people to see themselves as enabled.

This work is just as important for a person who considers themselves free of difficulty. If you're engaged in change, it doesn't matter what you think you are. You can develop any ability you lack and expand the abilities you have. It's not true that you only use 5% of your brain, but that you only use 5% of your ability.

Lacking challenges, you have no needs. When you're challenged, it's not what you lack that limits you, it's what you're unable to become. Authentic change creates something that does not exist.

References

Knight, B. (2013). *The Power of Negative Thinking: An Unconventional Approach to Achieving Positive Results.* New Harvest.

T19 – Reality of Craziness

October 20, 2021

Get to know all the other people who you think you are not.

"One person's craziness is another person's reality."
— **Tim Burton**, film director

Thoughts Aren't Reality

You are a musical instrument with a mind of its own, a resonator that can take action. Some primary actions are built into you. These are the urges that arise in you in the normal course of doing things. For simplicity, they are of four kinds: survival, maintenance, attraction, and indulgence. This is an abbreviated list—like Maslow's hierarchy of needs—but I will build on them.

Survival is ever-present. Sometimes it dominates, but mostly it just colors our perception. Maintenance compels us with click-like regularity: eating, sleeping, and busying ourselves. Attraction is our response to opportunity. Attractions are triggered by associations. Indulgence is what we want most of the time: relaxation, contentment, comfort, and happiness. Indulgence provides the lines on the roads we travel.

Within this context, we have thoughts. Our thoughts resonate with our preferred actions. Our thoughts keep us in the neighborhood of what we would like to control, acquire, or secure, although this can extend quite far. Some of us experience the world widely and others narrowly. We may speak the same language, but we don't share the same world. Our thoughts are not real, they are strategies.

What Isn't There

Many of our problems arise from a lack of clarity or conclusion. When things are clear and conclusive, we don't have many thoughts, and that's the way we like it. We reward ourselves with relaxation when all is going well, and we indulge.

269

Humans like to think in the way hamsters like exercise wheels; repetition is calming. People are most comfortable with inconsequential thoughts. This puts us in a state of mental idling and, in this state, the world is a haze of recreational good feeling. In this state, we are least engaged with reality. It is the state of comfortable illusion.

We also need stimulation. Your brain has different rhythms of attention, and they all like to be kept busy. That way, we feel we are fully alert and aware. But we are not really alert or aware, we only feel as if we are. In the hamster wheel metaphor, we have several hamster wheels that spin at different rates, and we feel most comfortable when they're all spinning.

Your average Hollywood movie provides a constant mix of stimulating sounds, images, actions, characters, themes, and issues. Nothing goes on for long and nothing requires much thought or attention. The scenes are short, the cuts are quick, and all topics are glossed over. It's all an unthreatening, amusing, distracting blur, and this makes people feel their needs are being met.

Reality is what's happening outside of your conceptual bubble. It is incomprehensibly complex. Reality is the changing, interconnected world, not the static world of separate events. This is the basic source of human confusion: we want a static state that has no threats, but we languish in stasis. We are enervated by curiosity, but threatened by novelty. As long as this prevails, we can never be satisfied.

What you ultimately want is a sense of emergence with a sense of safety and eternal youth, and you cannot have it. It's not that you have not found it. It cannot exist.

What you can achieve is something that may not attract you: the threat of change, or the boredom of sameness. The spectrum from change to sameness is something you can measure. We measure our prospects and predict. The spectrum from threat to boredom is subjective. It exists in the realm of feeling and these feelings are inside you. To change what you feel, change what you think. This is called reframing.

Beyond What You Think

Reframing is the foundation of changing one's mind. All stuckness requires a frame or boundary, a mindset. Opening, changing, or breaking out requires new thinking. Novelty can come as new ideas, emotions, sensations, or rhythms.

You may think you know these territories, but I assure you that you do not. There is always a boundary to what's familiar. What's outside that boundary is shrouded in fog and is infinite.

Some limitations are a matter of deduction, as new deduction requires a new insight. Our greater limitations are matters of induction, situations where generalizing has gone wrong. These are situations where we're limited not so much by what we do think, but by what we can think. We are limited by what we think is possible.

Consider your thinking as having two parts: what you know or think you know, and what you don't know and don't think about. An easy way to see this boundary is to consider what you believe in versus what you don't, or what's reasonable versus what's outrageous. Contentment versus horror, or what's for dinner versus extra-terrestrials. The boundary may be vague, but what lies on either side is clearly of a different nature.

Thinking consists either of connected thoughts: causes and effects or reasons and understandings, or disconnected thoughts: wonders, confusions, and unknowns. Connected thinking creates boxes, limitations, and constraints. Disconnected thoughts are shattered containers, their limitation is also their opportunity. Some of our greatest times of personal growth result from disasters because they cause us to change our thinking.

Our thoughts must disconnect in order for us to have a new idea. They might reconnect afterwards, but it's better if your thoughts remain disconnected. Let connections develop organically, free from pressure and interference.

Imagine that every one of your problems has some kind of resolution outside of any thinking that you know. Imagine that none of your problems will be solved using your current approach. This is almost certainly true of any problem that has been long-standing. If your understanding of any problem has not led or is not leading to a resolution, then it most likely won't, no matter how much time you give it.

Einstein's Special and General theories of relativity came in a flash. They were some of his first papers and had no precedent. He spent the rest of his life trying to apply this same thinking to other field theories and got nowhere.

Give Rhythm a Try

One of the easiest forms of novelty comes from rhythm. It is also one of the most elusive. Most of us are unaware of our rhythms and how our rhythms determine our awareness. Consider whether it is what you think that alters your heart rate, or whether your heart rate alters your thoughts. Does one come first?

Being in synchrony with your daily rhythms will have a greater effect on your moods than your moods will have on your daily rhythms. We operate on frequencies that range from fast radio frequencies to slow solar cycles. We try to control our daily rhythms and moods, but make little effort to control the effects other cycles have on us, or our response to them, if we're aware of them at all.

The main purpose of meditation is not to control your thoughts, but to control your rhythms. You become aware of your rhythms by first disengaging from your thoughts. You cannot stop feeling present, but you can separate being from presence. You can be aware of your being without supporting it with your presence. In this disengaged state, you can appreciate your different rhythms and the feelings, emotions, thoughts, and sensations associated with them.

Try this simple exercise. Seclude yourself for five or ten minutes. Find a quiet place where nothing is happening, nothing is changing, and there is no disturbance. Close your eyes, relax as much as possible, and imagine yourself experiencing regular waves of thoughts, sensations, or images.

You might picture or recall yourself experiencing some rhythm in the past. Focus on a rhythm and recreate it in your imagination. Experience one rhythm for 30 seconds and then move on to another.

After 10 minutes, open your eyes and spend one more minute letting thoughts and sensations appear and disappear without attachment. Pay attention to the various rhythms without attempting to constrain or control them. Notice the mood that each frequency brings. Then, find a sense of calm and return to your normal affairs.

Obligations of Learning

There are parallels between developments in the current time and those of the Dark Ages and the Medieval periods of European history. With hindsight and using modern language, we can identify how this age now differs from those ages then. What stands out most is the limited transfers of power and knowledge that predominated in the Dark Ages and started to break in the Medieval period.

The Dark Ages—and it's argued that this period was not as dark as it seems to us now—was dominated by the feudal system. It was half a millennium of relative stability—between the years 500 and 1000 CE—not for lack of need, but for lack of opportunity. Wars were frequent but small, interests were local, transportation was nonexistent, and literacy was nil. The structure was horizontal, composed of local lords who purchased armies and alliances. They were weakly allied to a sovereign, and they were all constrained by the regressive Roman Catholic Church.

Throughout this period, and well into the 19th century, state-sponsored terror and repression were the norm. Justice was nonexistent. Law, such as it was, was defined as whatever kept things in place at a low, functional level. Authority was preserved at all costs. As their authority started to fail, the Church began 700 years of inquisitions, starting in the 12th and continuing until the 19th century.

Although communication was limited, the structure was something like our internet. The structure common to both is that the governing nodes were independent. You could take down one baron, duke, or lord, but this did not weaken the feudal system. The lack of any opportunities within the system and the rewards of keeping things small resulted in five centuries of stability, stasis, and suffering.

In the Medieval era, literacy was still rare. Nation-states built industries. Alliances between states became more consequential, as did the rewards of conquest. Then, as now, there were great information wars.

With the invention of the printing press, the continent became literate and, with that, ideas spread. Without writing, spreading ideas is a sort of telephone game that's only as effective as the weakest link. Writing fostered change, it coordinated propaganda. Through written propaganda, Martin Luther—an otherwise unconvincing man—loosened the stranglehold of the Church of Rome.

What we call progress is really a system of feedback combined with instability. This has brought rapid improvement, but it has also brought insanity, chaos, and suffering.

We cannot talk about individual enlightenment outside of the context of cultural enlightenment. Today we recognize people like Dante Alighieri and Leonardo da Vinci as agents of change, but in their time, they fought a losing battle. The opportunities for change in the Modern Era, which started with Europe's expansion, resulted from new ideas. Your change will also succeed or fail because of your new ideas.

> "The thoughts that you hold most dear and are least willing to bring into question are often the most delusional thoughts of all."
> — **Charlie Ambler**, Founder of @dailyzen

T20 - To Be Confused I - Physics

May 4, 2022

Considering closed loops in space-time.

"Truth is ever to be found in simplicity, and not in the multiplicity and confusion of things." — **Isaac Newton**, physicist, alchemist, and theologian

Confusion

In his book *Reaching Down the Rabbit Hole* (2014), Allan Ropper says confusion "is not, technically, a disease, but a syndrome, a collection of problems." Confusion exists on an interesting spectrum. We have a rough idea of what it means to have no confusion and what it means to be entirely confused. But on closer inspection, a complete absence of confusion has much in common with being completely confused. The difference between the two extremes is subjective. It's what you decide to be.

A completely certain person is not sane or else they're not living in the real, uncertain world, and we can say the same about a completely confused person. In either case, the person involved may claim themselves to be at either extreme; what determines whether they are or are not confused depends more on our judgment, not theirs.

"Be confused. Confusion is where inspiration comes from."
— **Robyn Mundell**, author

In this series, I'd like to contrast different confusions in order to clarify that we all are confused all the time. Insanity can bring confusion, but there is nothing insane about being confused.

I'd like to contrast the confusion we experience in our well-balanced minds with the confusion that exists when we feel unbalanced. I'd like to show that we never really know where we are on the spectrum. Not only can confusion not be operationally defined, but the best we can do is to define it relatively. It's relative to what's needed at the movement, and it's relative to what other people expect.

I want to begin with a confusing concept in physics. At least I hope it will confuse you. In this way, I would like you to experience the intellectual confusion of a sane and well-balanced person, namely yourself. I would like to show that our minds have a particular way of isolating confusion so that we can cope with it.

In the next chapter, I want to consider the emotional confusion of a sane and well-balanced person, again yourself. I want to explore how we deal with what we don't know. How we resolve our confusion and how we make excuses for it.

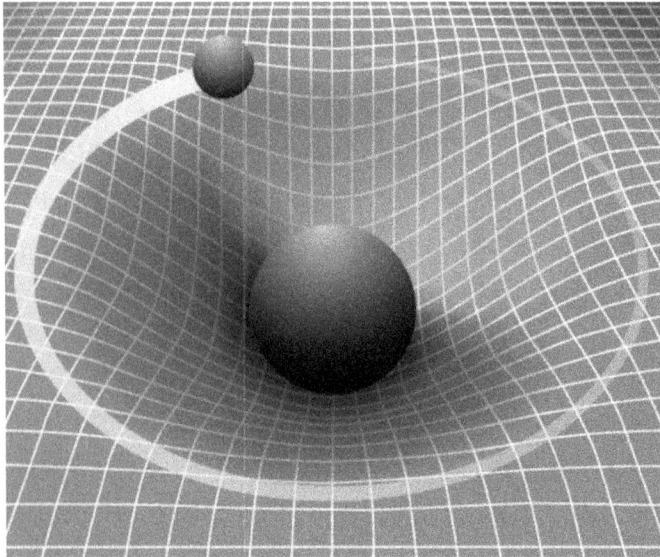

Figure 19: The geometrical picture of a gravitational orbit as a ball rolling around the perimeter of a cup. The gravity of the central object creates the cup-like distortion of space-time.

Gravity

To fully appreciate Albert Einstein's General Theory of Relativity, you must really see the mathematics. That's because most ideas develop from the specific to the general. You begin by understanding core things and then you generalize them. The thing about General Relativity is that there is no specific core idea that explains it. That's why it's a general theory.

There are some core formulas, but they depend on each other and upset each other. Space-time everywhere depends both on the mass of objects everywhere and the energy of everything in between. To get any "general idea" of what General Relativity says, you must specify everything in the universe. It's a brilliant theory if you want to generate confusion.

A good place to start is with the fundamental mathematical object of General Relativity: the metric tensor. Watch the YouTube video, "Demystifying the Metric Tensor in General Relativity," at https://youtu.be/Hf-BxbtCg_A

In 1949, Einstein's estimable and tragic friend Kurt Gödel—tragic because after Einstein died and for lack of friends, Kurt starved himself to death—found an exact solution to Albert's equations. Gödel found a description of the entire universe at all times in the past and future. Remember, these are equations for the coordinate system of the universe itself, not for anything in the universe. These are equations for space-time, the firmament of existence.

That Gödel found any solution at all was notable, but what the solution said of the firmament was untenable then, and is still untenable today. However, there's little doubt that everything he found would be true if the conditions he assumed prevailed. That these conditions are not the conditions of our universe offers little consolation. That's because regardless of Gödel's assumptions, the properties true of the firmament in his model universe remain true in our real one.

Dust

> "All are from the dust, and to dust all return."
> — **Ecclesiastes** 3:20

Gödel took dust as his starting point, but he added one thing: the dust was uniformly rotating. His universe was uniformly filled with rotating dust. Gödel found the space-time curvature of this universe could be described exactly. With the right density of dust rotating at the right velocity, his universe had several odd properties. Of these, the property I want to describe is that of closed loops.

You've heard that space-time is curved, and you may have heard that the trajectories of light rays bend as they pass near stars. That is spatial curvature. There is time curvature as well, but time doesn't curve. It stretches or compresses, so it's called time dilation. As light rays pass stars, time first compresses and the light's frequency increases as it approaches a star. Then time stretches and the frequency decreases as the light moves away.

If you moved in or against the direction of the rotation in Gödel's model of the universe, the spatial curvature would bring you back to where you started. This is roughly the 3-dimensional analog to moving fully around the equator on a globe. You feel no force, you always feel that you're moving in a straight line, but you eventually return to where you started.

We can swallow this. The globe provides a familiar example. And while this circularity limits the extent of the universe, just as the globe limits the extent of the earth, it doesn't mess with our future. There may be a limited amount of space on the Earth, but there isn't a limited amount of time.

The funny thing about Gödel's special model is that it has a limited amount of time, too. Starting at any point in this dusty model, as time goes forward, it eventually comes back to where it started. We have no analog for that, and that is the puzzler.

To get a grip on this, we have to be careful what we assume is happening. These are statements about space and time, not the behavior of things in space or time. From the point of view of any local region of dust, life is normal, life is good. Everything seems normal and there's no human way to reach the edge of the universe or the beginning of time.

Also, this is not our universe. In our universe, so far as we know, space may be finite or not. We don't know. Space might wrap around itself, but time does not.

This is a small consolation because it's the same dynamic in both cases. The rotating dust universe highlights what appears to be the truth, which is that time is just a measure of change. It's not some kind of eternally changing beingness.

Time may not wrap around on itself in our universe, but it is still, according to Einstein's theory—which has never been shown wrong—a thing that "does not pass." It does not pass and nothing "happens" in it. Time is just another degree within which we describe the configuration of things.

Time

Look at time more carefully in Gödel's universe. What does it mean for time to wrap around? Consider a simple model, different from Gödel's, that has only one dimension of space and one dimension of time. This is called the 1+1 dimensional model.

It's not a 2-dimensional model that you would picture on a flat plane because you can't rotate from space to time just by turning a corner. It's not the two-dimensional surface of a globe because space exists along a single line at any one point in time, and time exists along a single line at any one point in space.

> "Space by itself, and time by itself, are doomed to fade away into mere shadows,
> and only a kind of union of the two will preserve an independent reality."
> — **Hermann Minkowski**, physicist

In the 1+1 model, you can only travel left or right and you move in one future direction around the time loop. You may start at any point in space or time, but there are only two aspects of your motion. You can move in either space direction, but only one future direction in time. You can't "turn" a time corner.

Drawing space and time on the surface of a torus gives us a picture of what it means to be "closed" for this 1+1 dimensional model. This torus, or donut, is shown in Figure 20. Here, lines of spatial extension circle the hole parallel to each other. Each of these encircling lines represents the different points in space at one point in time. Lines of temporal progression encircle the torus in the other direction, each describing a full round-trip through time at a single position in space.

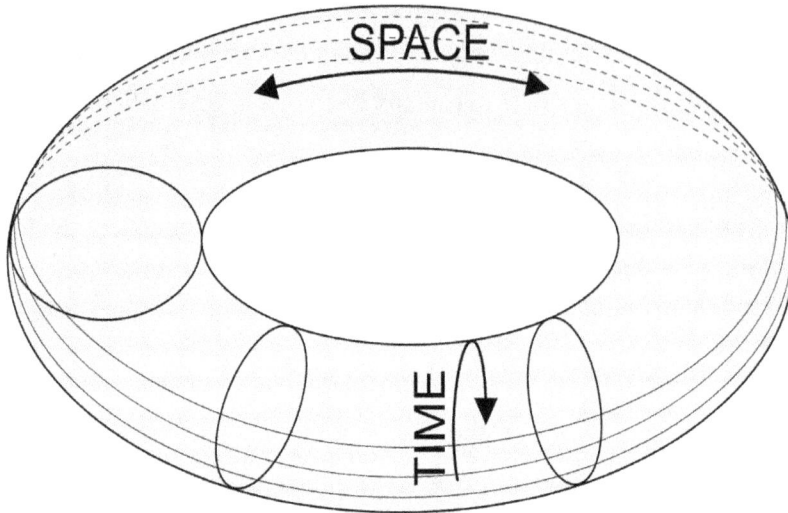

Figure 20: The 1+1 geometry of a looping space and looping time universe maps onto the surface of a torus.

Within any small area on this surface, things are relatively normal. We can always choose our direction and time would seem, for those of us living there, to always move forward. Were we to move left or right far enough, we would come back to where we started, but we'd never know we'd completed a circle unless we left something behind to remind us.

The same is be true of the time circles. Time would always seem to move forward and we'd never know we'd come back to the start unless there was something there to make that starting time special.

Being

What we call time is not time, it's being. It's being that moves forward as the clock ticks, not time. Time is just the fabric across which we move. As time passes, our being changes, not time.

This is true of all things. At least that's how we see it. Rocks "be" and stars "be" and all the cars, pets, and people "be." And they all "be" at the same rate because they're all made of stuff that changes at the same rate. That is the case as long as time is not distorted.

In fact, space-time is distorted, but the effect is infinitesimally small in our neighborhood

(Siegel 2016). To see a discrepancy in the "being" of things, things must travel through extensive regions of warped space-time. We see this happen constantly on subatomic timescales, but it evens out on average. We suspect this happens in the neighborhood of supermassive objects, but they're too far away to affect us. What might happen if changes didn't cancel out on average? What would this do to our sense of being?

Space Looping

After we complete a circuit of our closed-space universe, we come back around and encounter things that have not moved as they were and still are. If time was not "closed," then new events would continue to unfold. This is similar to our current 2-dimensional lives on the surface of Earth.

Completing this circuit would lead to either consonance or dissonance. Dissonance means the starting and finishing situations don't "fit" and there is some kind of reckoning. If you raced a car around a loop to the starting line and encountered your car idling on the starting line, then you'd crash into it. This would feel dissonant.

But if you completed the loop and found your car racing away from you at a speed equal to your own, then you would follow this car without conflict. This would be consonant. At a microscopic level, we expect things to be consonant because there is nothing distinctive about any point on a space loop.

For things to repeat, as we might expect in a closed loop that offers no other point of view, all points must be consonant. This means that the end of the cycle must "fit" the beginning of the cycle.

We can visualize the world of one closed dimension of space and one open dimension of time as an infinite cylinder. We circle the outside while time progresses along the cylinder's infinite length. If we move constantly around the cylinder, then our spacetime path would spiral upwards.

Imagine racing around the equator to return to your starting point. If there is nothing at the starting point upon your return, then you simply continue around and around, corkscrewing into the future. If there is something at the starting line, then it had better be moving forward at the same speed as you, or it must be off to the side so that you can get around it.

But in a world of one spatial dimension, there is no "off to the side" to provide the room to get around. In one spatial dimension, all cars must go around at coordinated speeds if they are to move in perpetual circles. This doesn't mean that speeds can't change, it only means their changes must be coordinated to allow continuity. All kinds of patterns are allowed as long as no car slams into another.

In this world, a space loop involves one person remaining stationary while another person continues forward, adding milage, executing the circuit, and coming back to meet the person who never moved. One person has clocked some miles while the other hasn't moved at all, and they're both back where they started.

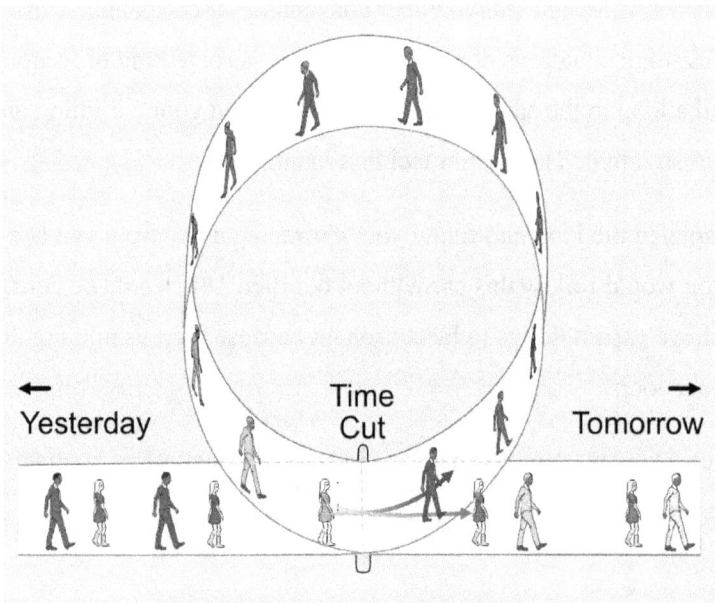

Figure 21: Visualizing a time-loop ruptures our notion of time as continuous and progressive.

Time Looping

In our 1+1 dimensional universe, we have to limit ourselves to travel one way or the other around the cylinder in the open-time universe, or around the donut in the closed-time universe. Time goes up the cylinder or through the hole in the donut, and the flow of time carries us in those directions with no effort on our part.

In this world, a future time loop involves one person remaining stationary in space and time, while another person continues forward in time only, adding hours, continuing through the hole in the donut, and coming back to meet the person whose time never moved. One person has clocked some hours without moving in space, while the other hasn't moved at all. Then, they're both back where they started.

However, remaining stationary in time is to stop time, and this makes no more sense in this universe than in ours. It's equally nonsensical for a time traveler to execute an instantaneous time loop through the future and back to the present before a second person has a chance to move at all forward in time. This is what's shown using a "time cut," in the time loop of Figure 21.

The simplest thing we can do in this universe is nothing. Just sit in the car on the starting line at time zero and wait for time to come forward enough to return to zero. What happens then? We're still sitting on the starting line. Do we feel any change in being? Not if we don't remember anything. If we do remember something, then it's because we've left something behind, namely the memory of what was and the measure of time passing.

A memory is not nothing, and time only "passes" if you record it. To record it, you need a device to measure it, and this device is much like the car that travels through space. It measures your passage along your temporal "road." Call this your clock. You don't actually need some mechanical device if your memory is good enough.

Memory

Memory is a time structure, and the longer the period over which you remember, the larger the time structure it represents. If the memory is large enough, then it would extend from the start to the end of your universe. What happens then?

When you return to time zero, you must meet yourself in consonance or dissonance. But a finite-time universe offers no alternative future in which dissonance can occur. The physical laws, whatever these laws are, require consonance upon returning to time zero in a time-looping universe.

You cannot return to time zero and say, "Ah, here we are again!" because that would mean

283

that mean you uttered a new expression and time was not looping. You could only say "Ah, here we are again!" if you had said that at the start of the last time loop.

The Sci-Fi series *Atropa* (STUDIO+ 2018)—coincidentally released on a channel called Dust—is a Sci-Fi story in which time loops. But, as is usual for time-looping plots, it's not a real time loop because no one would know it if it was. Instead, it's the "going back in time to change things" theme, which does not work, makes no sense, and is not supported by any physics. Yet this is what people keep imagining when they think of time travel.

Note that in a closed-time universe, time is a circle, not a spiral. There is no breaking of the circle's symmetry, every subsequent cycle must match the previous cycles. If they didn't, then one cycle would mark a different cycle and a different time. But there is no "different time," so there can't be any different cycle.

What does this mean for your being? It means that you cannot say to yourself, "Oh, I've made the circuit and now I'm on my second time around." That would count the cycles and there is nowhere to "put" that "number two." If the universe was flat or if it spiraled forward to infinity, we could keep counting. Here, in a model with closed circles, everything must match and each cycle must be the same.

What would this feel like? There are endless ways to match up, but in every case, subsequent time loops feel exactly like the first. And, because this universe is also spatially closed, the locations of things also repeat themselves. The configurations of all things repeat themselves. Nothing can be added and nothing can be taken away or even moved on subsequent cycles.

Everything works out. We can draw little pictures representing the state of everything at every point on the surface of our 1+1 dimensional universe. There is no "time" outside of these pictures, the surface is "inside time." Whatever way you turn the torus, wherever you point your finger, there is a "state of being." Your being feels normal at every point.

You could even imagine there being a car crash at some point. Such an event could still be part of a consonant picture as long as all the pieces are reassembled to be consonant with the past when it comes back around.

One final note: in a nondeterministic universe, time loops need not be identical. But that's another story.

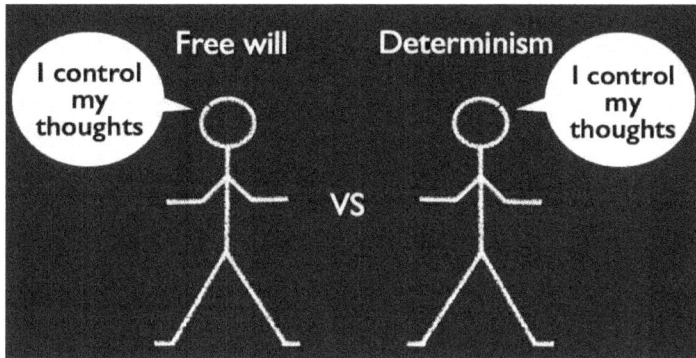

Figure 22: Our experience of having free will says nothing about our role in causing anything to happen.

Free Will

"Confusion of goals and perfection of means seems, in my opinion, to characterize our age."
— **Albert Einstein**, physicist

Does the Gödel universe have free will? Well, everything feels just the same as our universe at every point. It only reveals itself as different to those inhabitants who have a memory that persists longer than the duration of the time loop… but there can't be any such thing. There is no "duration" longer than the time loop.

By clocking the light from old stars, it appears our universe is over 13 billion years old, is expanding, and is continuing to expand. A Big Bang is proposed at the start, it is something that wipes out all memory. We don't seem to live on closed time loops, but if we did, then the Big Bang would assure us we'd never know it.

There are other models. They are intellectual curiosities. The structure of space-time does not seem to impinge on our notion of free will, even if we live on time loops and ultimately don't have free will.

We have another definition of free will which pertains to the choices we make at each moment. In a mechanical universe in which every state of things is predetermined, there is no room for free will because there are no choices. There are several alternatives to a mechanical universe. Quantum mechanics offers one choice and multi-dimensional models of the world offer others.

The free will of being is not a consequence of time. We can discard time as some fundamental change in being. Time is just the board on which our pieces move. If our universe was closed and consisted of time loops, then we know free will would not exist because there would be no room for any other choice the second time around.

Assuming that we don't live in a closed universe, there is a chance for free will. This depends on what makes choices happen. This might be subatomic or it might be divine. There is still room for new theories of being. Physics is always wrong as long as there are new realms to be described.

I hope I have confused you. It took me a week to come to these conclusions and I doubt you've thought of these situations before. The point of this monologue has been to illustrate how we isolate confusion. As long as we agree among ourselves that a confusing issue won't affects us, it won't. As long as we agree among ourselves that a confusing issue won't affect our behavior, it won't. It won't until it intrudes. At that point, there is dissonance.

The recent movie *Don't Look Up* tells the story of a pair of astronomers who realize the Earth is about to be destroyed by a comet. This is a confusing situation that citizens find too uncomfortable to entertain. Because the need for consonance is too great, the dissonance is ignored, and the world refuses to listen to these astronomers.

Free will engenders choice, and choice can lead to confusion. Our discomfort with confusion feeds back and limits our free will.

References

Grave, F. (2008 Nov). "Visiting the Gödel Universe." *IEEE Transactions on Visualization and Computer Graphics, 14* (6):1563-70. https://doi.org/10.1109/TVCG.2008.177

Momin, A. (2002 Mar 24). "The Gödel Solution to the Einstein Field Equations." Al Momin. http://www.math.toronto.edu/~colliand/426/Papers/A_Monin.pdf

Siegel, E. (2016, Sep 30). "How Do Photons Experience Time?" *Forbes.* https://www.forbes.com/sites/startswithabang/2016/09/30/how-do-photons-experience-time/?

sh=285d2f07278d

STUDIO+ (2018). "Atropa." https://movies.how/show/atropa

T21 - To Be Confused II - Awareness

May 11, 2022

How we play with, be in, and create in our awareness.

"An understanding of confusion has yet to be operationalized... (it's) a syndrome, a collection of problems." — **Allan Ropper**, MD (2014), neurologist

Confusion

Compare the confusion in our heads to the stock market. The stock market is a marketplace where everything is sold at auction. Shares of ownership in thousands of public companies are sold and nothing has a fixed price.

Despite periods of fluctuation and uncertainty, stocks always have a "last price." They don't have a "next price," only a last price. They don't even have a current price, only a variety of bid prices offered by those willing to buy and a variety of offers made by those willing to sell. There is no price on anything and no advertised value. Bargaining is everything.

Imagine you went shopping and nothing had a price on it, only a "last price." If you want something, then you are invited to make a bid. Of course, that would not be enough. You would need to know the price at which your item was being offered. You might also like to know who else was bidding and what they were last willing to pay for it. The only price at which you could be certain to get what you want is the price the store is offering.

One can say a lot about auction markets. If you thought items should have prices, an auction market would confuse you. An auction market is like a fencing match in which contestants advance and retreat along a single line. The last price is the point on that line where the last point was scored. It's a game.

Offense by one player and defense by the other will lead the aggressive player forward for the moment. Defense by both results in stability: no action and no change. Offense by both generates a frenetic clashing of their foils. Your decision-making process is like this: a conflict of parties, usually a conflict between two main opinions. Often more than two.

Stability

We say we like stability, but in those areas where we're subject to confusion, we are not satisfied with it. If you're happy with stability and you're not confused, then there's no more to say at the moment. Chances are you'll remain stable until support runs out or pressing novelty appears.

Confusion comes from an imbalance that could lead to change or could lead to being locked in struggle. We often mistake confusion for imbalance, but lack of balance is a situation, confusion is our reaction to it.

There are three kinds of imbalance: leading confusion, trailing confusion, and uncertain confusion. In leading confusion, you're considering an action that's proactive. You think you know where things are going and you're almost ready to commit. You're ahead of the pack. If "the pack" is your range of opinions, then you're taking the lead in forming an opinion.

In trailing confusion, the action you're considering is reactive. You're joining the followers. You're feeling pressed to catch up, desiring to avoid further losses or avail yourself of a waning opportunity. In this case, you're committing to the idea that things will continue getting worse or stop getting better.

There's an odd asymmetry between leading and trailing uncertainty. The confusions feel similar, but the calls to action are different. Leading uncertainty requires courage, aggression, or inspiration; trailing uncertainty is driven by fear, need, or obligation. Each camp is a group of odd bedfellows, and each camp is at odds with the other.

The third challenge to stability is struggle or contest, where both sides are demanding a response or urging immediate action. Some of us are proactive, others are reactive, and still others need conflict in order to take any action at all.

What happened to stability? Stability went out the window.

When I think of stability, I think of Buddhism, a religion that espouses stability and works to mitigate confusion. The interplay between stability and confusion has been a dominant meme in culture and religion. Remember this point: change does not require confusion.

"The world, harmoniously confused, where order in variety we see, and where, tho' all things differ, all agree."
— **Alexander Pope** (1688–1744), poet

Change

The reason we want to see into the future is to change without confusion. This enables us to remain in consonance with our environment. If we can discern the rules governing events of the moment, then we can navigate change with understanding and stability.

We're always looking for these rules. They could be physical laws, moral prescriptions, or market forces. The first thing we try to determine is which of these is operating. What are the forces leading to change, and can we change with them?

If you're considering ketchup, then you'll weigh the cost of the ingredients, the integrity of the market, and your desire for a hot dog. If you're considering suicide, then you'll weigh the value of your life, whether the world will treat you justly, and your longing for relief. Which will make you the happiest, the hot dog or death?

"A single (hot) dog could chop 36 minutes off your life."
— **Sarah Wells** (2022), journalist

Buddhists will say, "Six of one, half a dozen of the other. Only stability will bring you peace." You will respond, "But I must choose. No action is not an option." Buddhists will say, "No action is the only option because there is no genuine change. Conflict remains in conflict. There is no winner; it's just a game."

Awareness

The first rule in obtaining clarity is figuring out what you're confused about. If you know what you're confused about and you see the conflict, then you're playing a game that you cannot win. You do not resolve confusion by seeing in it, but by seeing beyond it.

Confusion is the nature of games. They place you in confusion and expect you to resolve it. In a society that throws Christians to the lions, the only ones who win are those who don't play. Even the spectators are players and they lose too. You're led to believe that clarity leads to the winning choice. Don't believe it. In a society that asks you what you want to be when you grow up, the only successful answer is, "Whatever I want to be."

The right choice in the hot dog contest is a salad. The right choice in the suicide contest is to go out and find the world. The right choice in the stock market is to ponder the chaos. In each case, the right choice is the one that makes you the designer of the game, not an avatar in it. We rarely realize that the player is also a piece.

The fallacy lies in the dichotomy of winning versus losing. A reward is like money. You can trade it, but you can't eat it, and trading money just puts you in another game. Greater awareness in playing the game won't reveal the ultimate solution because that lies outside the game.

The game is a fallacy of clarity. Real clarity lies in discarding the rules and becoming comfortable with the ensuing confusion. Confusion is reality. There is no reality to the game. It's a simulacrum. You do not win it; you navigate it. The reward is in playing ever more inclusive games that are images of how you see yourself.

I had a dream in which I was trying to find my way out of a horrible, maze-like house. I woke up in distress before it was time to arise and resolved to return to the dream on my own terms. I fell back to sleep, found the house, and destroyed it with a bulldozer.

> "If you use your mind to study reality, you won't understand either your mind or reality. If you study reality without using your mind, you'll understand both."
> — **Bodhidharma**, 5th or 6th century Buddhist monk

Games

Just as there are better or worse actions, there are better or worse Buddhists. The better Buddhist, in keeping with their tenet of stability, considers your situation and flows with it. Stability does not mean stasis and games have consequences.

Choices that end in death and choices that end in hot dogs both require consideration. The rewards may be relative, but there are always consequences. The Buddhist is right: the game is not over until you choose to stop.

Life offers many games: hot dogs, suicide, the stock market. The mistake people make—the mistake we're encouraged to make—is that we can only choose the game, but not the rules. That is the first and the last error because the only one who benefits in any game is that character that exists only in the game. None of us exists only in the game. Not in any game that has clear and separate boundaries from real life. All real people must take their game results and make something of them.

Games are simulations of limited realities. Unreal players exist within the game only. For real people, the game is just an exercise. The benefit is in the playing, not the winning. No one knows this better than the game designer for whom winning and losing are two sides of the same coin and neither can exist without the other.

If the playing of the game you're in is not intrinsically rewarding, then you're not a mature player or a Buddhist. You are an expendable resource consumed in the game's playing; a resource that is fodder for the game itself.

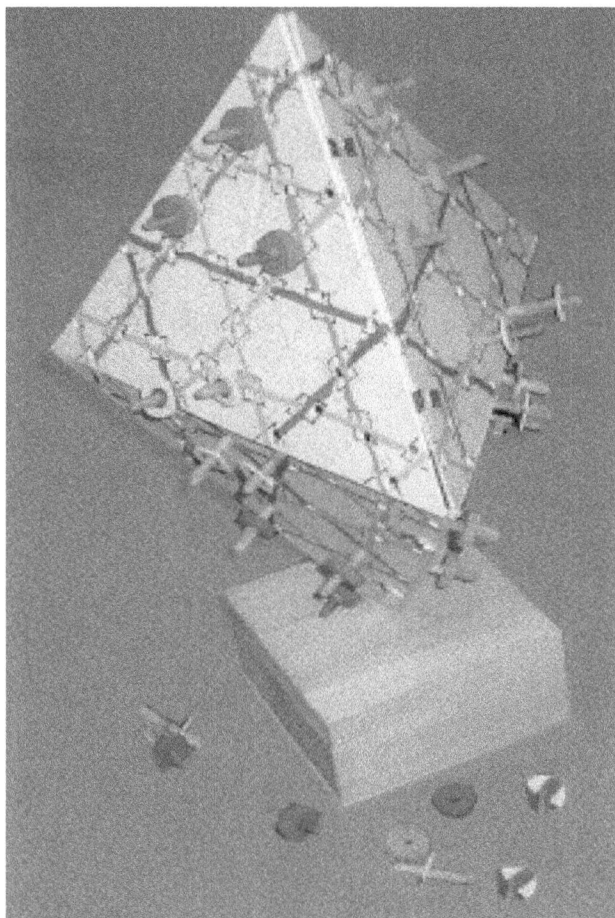

*Figure 23: Ugluk: a 3-Dimensional board game
whose puzzle lies in its confusing geometry*

I design games. In these games, the object is not to win or lose. The object is to finish, discard, and start again. Here are some of the board games I've built:

Ugluk: A fast-playing shooting game played on a 3-dimensional globe-like board where players' moves overlap, and no one can seem to get away from anyone else.

The player's arrows continue to travel around the octahedron's encircling trajectories as players try to fire new arrows at their opponents while dodging the old arrows still flying around the board.

https://www.mindstrengthbalance.com/alternative-education/games-abstract/#ugluk

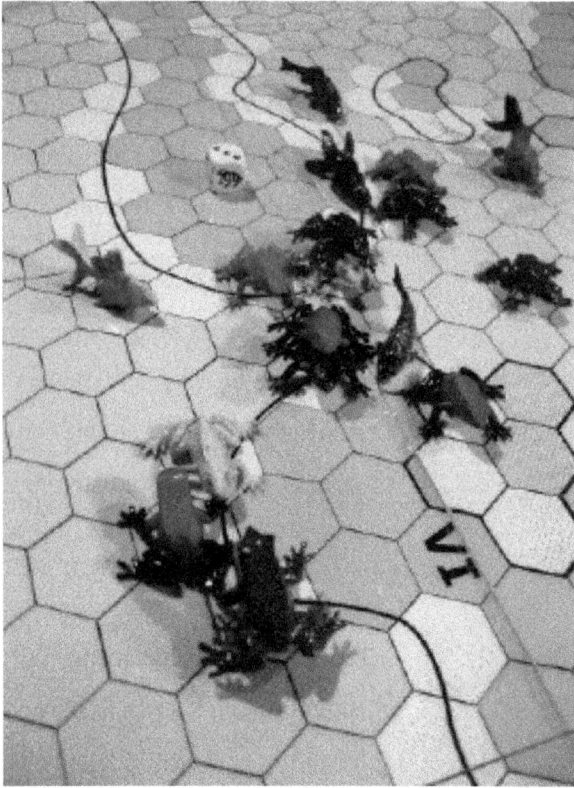

Figure 24: The Mating Game: to win a game of many players, the leading player exploits the trailing player.

The Mating Game: Each player is one of up to five populations of frogs striving to reproduce only with the frogs of other players in order to dominate the pond while avoiding the fish and birds.

Frogs travel over land and water to mate, but they're only safe in the shallows. In the deep water they can be eaten by pike. When crossing land, they can be eaten by heron.

Starting with small colonies of frogs, birds, and fish, as mating progresses, the number of pieces on the board can grow dramatically.

https://www.mindstrengthbalance.com/alternative-education/games-system/#matinggame

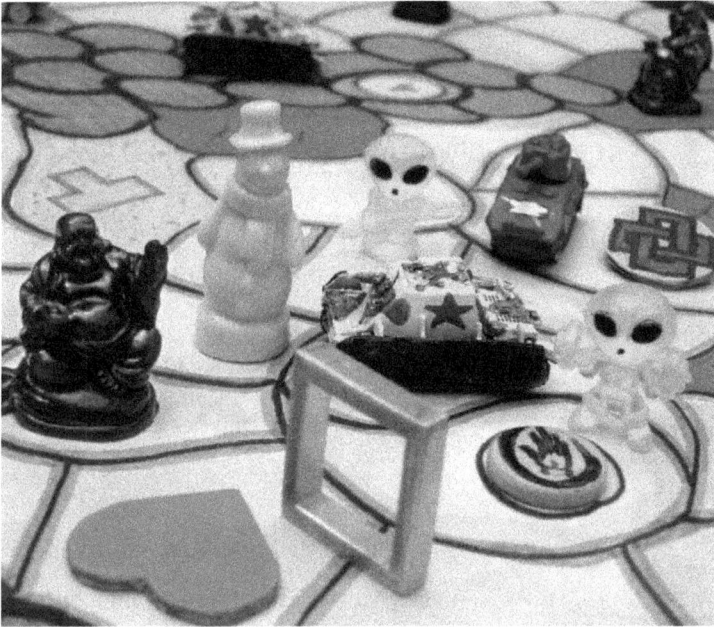

Figure 25: In Chinese, Buddhists & Aliens: three players with entirely different pieces and powers move in different ways to achieve different goals.

Chinese, Buddhists & Aliens: A three player game in which the Chinese want to destroy the Buddhists, the Buddhists want to return to their homeland, and the Extra-Terrestrials want to abduct humans.

Each player plays a different group with unique powers and an entirely different objective.

The Chinese have tanks, the Aliens teleport, and the Buddhists travel slowly on foot to collect the sacred relics. They're aided by their solitary, powerful friend the Abominable Snowman.

https://www.mindstrengthbalance.com/alternative-education/games-system/
#chinesebuddhistsaliens

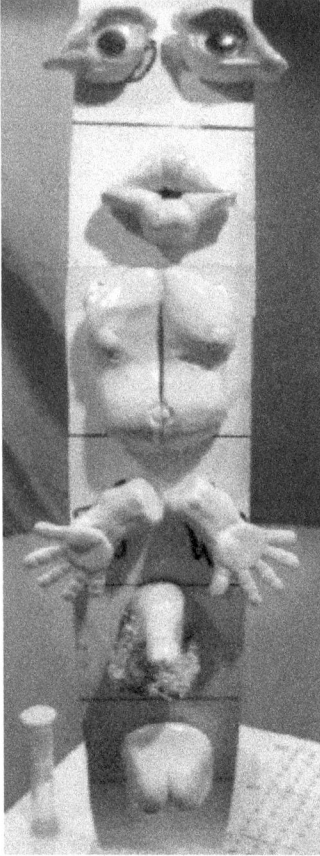

Figure 26: Orgy of Moderation tests your ability to separate strategy from morality.

Orgy of Moderation: four naked people of four races—two males and two females—move their unattached, magnetized body parts around a flat metal Möbius strip, striving to have sexual encounters.

As the body parts scatter on this one-dimensional, one-sided world, the encounters of certain body parts with those of opposing players generate points.

You gain points for voyeurism. Even masturbation offers a few points, but comes at the risk of losing an eye.

Each of these games is ridiculous, and each is designed to put you into a position you'd never find in real life.

https://www.mindstrengthbalance.com/alternative-education/games-social/#orgy

References

Ropper A. H., & Burrell, B. D. (2014). *Reaching Down the Rabbit Hole, A Renowned Neurologist Explains the Mystery and Drama of Brain Disease.* St. Martin's Press.

Wells, S. (2022). "Are Hot Dogs Bad For You?" *Inverse.com.* https://www.inverse.com/science/do-hot-dogs-shorten-your-life

T22 – To Be Confused III – Music

May 25, 2022

Music, as structure in time, is the opposite of confusion.

"Music's exclusive function is to structure the flow of time and keep order in it."
— **Igor Stravinsky**, Composer

I observe music as having similarities to brainwave training, and these similarities offer insights important to your understanding of confusion.

Cycle

Why should my observations be important to your understanding? The difference between my understanding and your understanding is what each of us does about it: I speak and you listen. In order to complete this cycle and create understanding, you must speak and I must listen. With the completion of that cycle, a new structure can take form. Without that completion, these ideas fall on fallow ground.

Music makes cycles manifest. It makes the cyclic nature of our being evident to us. It also manifests in cycles, but that is different. To say that music manifests in cycles only means that you'll find music within repeating structures, which is trivial.

Experimental music that violates cycles serves to show their necessity. Without cycles, sound can claim to be music only by reputation, or else it is noise.

Cycles have dimensions. Patterns can be cyclic in some aspects and not others. Animal songs only sound musical once their repeating pattern emerges. Until that happens, they may be harmonic, but they're not musical.

What makes sound music is its entrainment of human beingness. It is the effect music has on the working of our brains that makes music important. Of all the things that define our humanness, it is amazing that we overlook music as part of our definition. We are virtually the only animal that is musical.

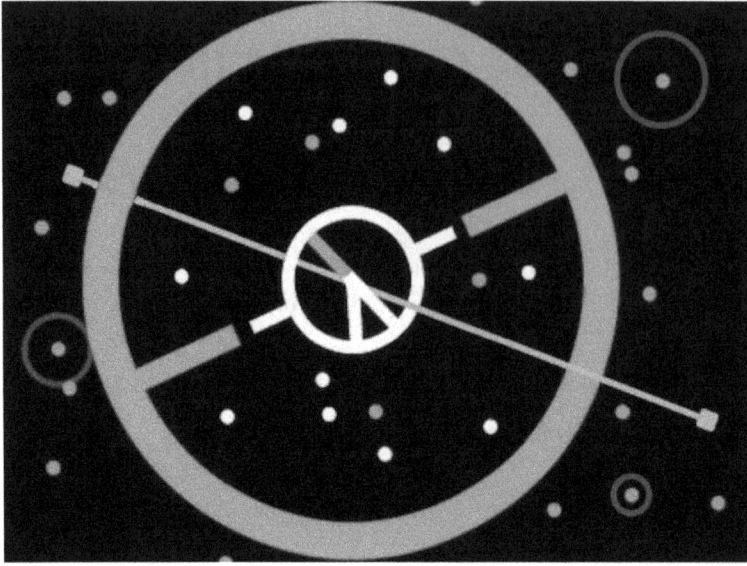

Figure 27: Tempo is a regular and constant pattern that contains synchronized but irregular structures inside it.

Tempo

"Drums are to be felt and not heard."
— **Max Roach**, jazz drummer

Music and language share common elements, tempo being one. Language with tempo is said to be poetic, but tempo is an important part of all language.

Tempo is a form that encapsulates a structure. A drum beats a tempo, but the tempo is not the beat. It acts as a musical foundation.

The ideas in our language can be measured in the musical sense: they emerge with the beats. The lack of tempo in speech is a sign of imperfectly organized thought. Tempo is a container of organization that says nothing of the structure it contains but can make its impact greater. The statements of a mellifluous speaker have a far greater impact.

When you read a text, your mind tries to recreate the tempo that was in the author's mind. Texts that lack tempo lack an organized structure and are increasingly difficult not only to read but to comprehend. Tempo is an essential ingredient in what we call thought.

Readers of Western music think of tempo in terms of meter and measure, but that is little more than sentence structure. The greater detail of tempo is in the repeating sound patterns which can exist outside or inside the measure. The thoughts themselves can be melodic.

Tempo exists in your thoughts too, but I doubt you're aware of it. While we are acutely aware of the absence of tempo in speech and writing, we have little awareness of it in our thought processes. This observation can play an important role in your self-understanding: your comprehension stands or falls with tempo.

Tempo is so important to humans that we confuse it with being sentient. A speech pattern that lacks clear cadence and meter is heard as being disorganized and undirected. The speech of a person who is drunk or half asleep has a particular half-conscious form. The natural disorganization in our thinking forces us to rely on tempo in holding our thoughts together. Animals whose thoughts are constrained to a rigid dictionary of signs don't rely on tempo. At least, we're not aware of the appreciation of tempo in most animals. The exceptions are those animals that can keep a beat, which include parrots (Ceurstemont 2009) and sea lions (Mullis 2013) and a few others.

> "Making sense of sound is profoundly governed by how we feel, think, see, and move."
> — **Nina Kraus** (2021), neurobiologist

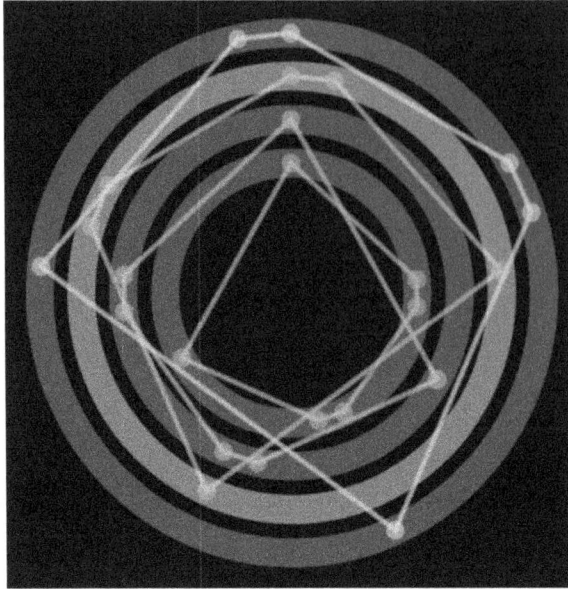

Figure 28: Rhythm is the repetitive and irregular structure of emphasis layered on top of the regular structure of tempo.

Rhythm

"Music creates order out of chaos: for rhythm imposes unanimity upon the divergent, melody imposes continuity upon the disjointed, and harmony imposes compatibility upon the incongruous."
— **Yehudi Menuhin**, conductor

Recognizing a tempo in a situation is the first step in its organization; the first step in lifting oneself out of confusion. Finding rhythm is the next step.

Rhythm is the pattern that follows the tempo. It is a pattern, not a structure. While tempo is infinitely repeatable, rhythm is a pattern within the tempo, something particulate that's built out of waves. Rhythm is what you hear, tempo is what you feel.

The feeling of being confused gradually remits as we add more structure. It is a mistake to isolate particular confusing elements when there is no overall pattern. Rhythm is the first localized pattern one can create within the tempo.

Finding a rhythm to your thoughts enables an incipient sense of meaning to emerge. While both tempo and rhythm are patterns, rhythm is the pattern that reflects ideas. Signals coming from outer space are full of tempo, but rhythm is rare. A rhythmic signal implies that it has been created by a structure that's localized somewhere in space or time. This is a requirement of thought.

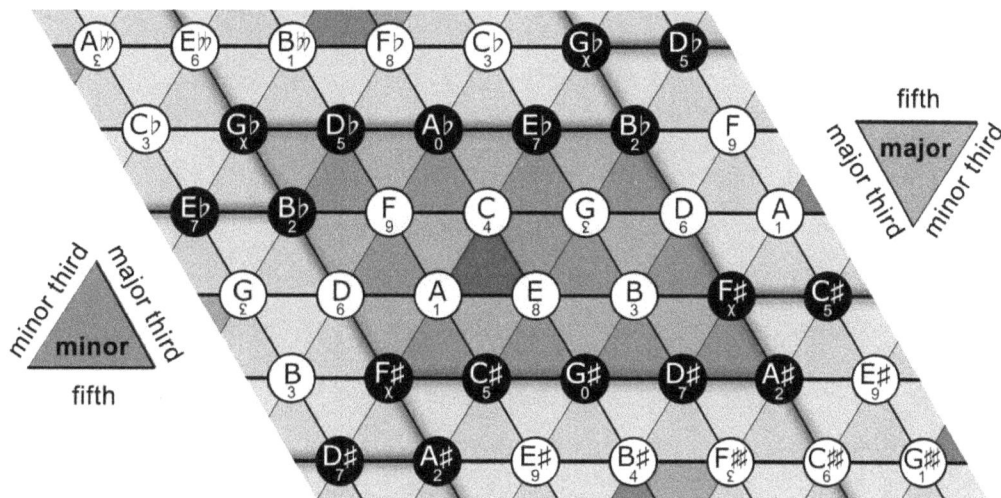

Figure 29: The geometry of musical key signatures generates definable emotional tones.

Rhythm is not enough, however. You must find rhythm in your confusion if you're going to achieve clarity. If you find nothing beyond rhythm, at least you have something to work with. Depending on your level of confusion, finding rhythm may be enough to settle you. I can calm my most distressed clients by speaking in a gently rhythmic pattern. These are people who are otherwise overwhelmed with anxiety and try to shut out the chaos in their heads. To speak with calm, musical reassurance is a basic form of hypnotic patter. I am hypnotizing these patients out of a state of panic and into a state of comfort. If you understand hypnotic means focused, then you'll appreciate all states are hypnotic states.

Pattern

"I often think in music. I live my daydreams in music."
— **Albert Einstein**

Animals use sound as songs that sign, but they don't modulate their song patterns into unique thoughts.

We don't know if this is really true as there are some animals that make up unique song patterns that they use like we use words. The "whup" pattern in the song of the humpback whale is not uttered in exactly the same way by each whale. The sound is spoken differently by each whale because it appears to refer to each whale or pod by name. What we hear as a single "whup" is actually an infinity of possible different names, none of which our ears can distinguish (Science Friday 2021).

For an animal to revise their song into words that convey new thoughts, would be like a human making up words to express themself. An animal's song is one thought in the way the word is one thought. For an animal to make up their song would be like a human making up their words. It would be gibberish to other animals in the way your invented words would sound like gibberish to us.

For us to distinguish confusion from understanding means we can distinguish chaos from structure. Chaotic thoughts are confusing, while structured thoughts may be understandable. Chaotic sounds are noise, while structured sounds can be musical. Structure alone does not make meaning or music, but it is necessary.

Structure

"A new language requires a new technique. If what you're saying doesn't require a new language, then what you're saying probably isn't new."
— **Philip Glass**, composer

Structure is the final form of thought and music. It is the statement that has meaning. Most of our confusion will not generate structure, as that is not its nature. Like panning for gold, we impose structures on what we hear to filter out confusion. We create a kind of sluice to help us find what's valuable in the communications we receive.

Paul Dirac was an unusual physicist, who some claim was on the autism spectrum. In his public presentations, he responded to questions but not to statements. If someone contested his results using reasoning that was not his, he did not respond. Some inferred from this his great confidence, but I suspect he simply did not see the statements of others as things that applied to him. His work was creative, unique, and complete. The means he employed were justified by the ends he achieved, and he was creative in both. He thought up the concept of antimatter. He was uninterested in why other people could not understand his ideas.

There has to be confusion in order for there to be novelty. The confusion itself is not the problem. Our problem is our need for order in a situation that lacks order. This is like staying afloat when you don't know how to swim. Swimming is the structure of movement and buoyancy that one needs when immersed. You need some structure in order to keep your head above water.

As a counselor, therapist, or coach—all versions of the same—my task is to find rhythm in confusion, but not to find structure. Structure is the individual stuff of intentional thought. We use words to give our thoughts structure. I work to help contain my clients' thoughts while encouraging them to add structure.

A person's authentic structure can't be expressed in words any more than an animal's feelings can be expressed in song. You may cry with true feeling, but that communicates few details. Our typical response to a crying person is to say, "What's wrong?" My task is not to create structure. I also do not presume that I'll be able to understand your structure. I'll look for indications of your meaning, such as tempo, rhythm, and association, but I'm guessing in the end.

Psychotherapeutic modalities that aim to coral behavior do just that: they create fences. They take the wild animal of your greater perception and train you to stay in your stall. This feels better than chaos in the sense that being in a lithium-induced stupor is better than suicide. And it is better, but it's animal training, not understanding.

Think about music, don't just listen to it. Listening to music entrains you, like reading someone else's story. Thinking about music creates it, like writing your own story, and that's what you want to do.

Musicians are better thinkers if they both think and make music (Ying et al. 2018; Kraus 2021). That doesn't mean you'll be good at either if you do both, but you'll think better if you do. In particular, your ability to appreciate emotion will be enhanced. That being said, I know at least one musical person who is emotionally disabled, so music can be a crutch. Music is just a way of finding structures, not a guaranteed way of creating good ones.

Try this experiment. When you are next in touch with your confusion, try making music. Forget that dumb idea that only musicians make music. That's a despicable idea. Go to this website, https://tonematrix.audiotool.com, and play with the interface for a few minutes. Then, return to your confusion and see what you can make of it.

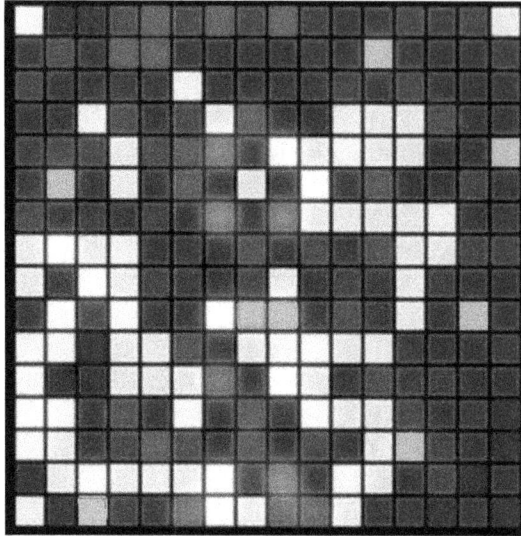

Figure 30: The graphical interface of the Tonematrix audio software.

Cherish your confusion. It's the realm of your wilding. Consider the structures it may contain.

References

Ceurstemont, S. (2009 May 1). "Dancing Parrots Could Help Explain Evolution of Rhythm." *New Scientist*. https://www.newscientist.com/article/dn17065-dancing-parrots-could-help-explain-evolution-of-rhythm/

Kraus, N. (2021). *Of Sound Mind: How Our Brain Constructs a Meaningful Sonic World.* MIT Press.

Mullis, S., (2013 Apr 2). "In the Name of Science: Head-bobbing Sea Lion Keeps the Beat." *NPR*. https://www.npr.org/sections/thetwo-way/2013/04/02/176047593/in-the-name-of-science-head-bobbing-sea-lion-keeps-the-beat

Science Friday (2021, Jul 23). "How the Humpback Says Hello." *Science Friday*. https://www.sciencefriday.com/segments/humpback-documentary-fathom/

Ying, L., Guangyuan, L., Dongtao, W., Qiang, L., Guangjie, Y., Shifu, W., Gaoyuan, W., & Xingcong, Z. (2018 Nov 13). "Effects of Musical Tempo on Musicians' and Non-musicians' Emotional Experience When Listening to Music." *Frontiers of Psychology, 9*. https://doi.org/10.3389/fpsyg.2018.02118

T23 – To Be Confused IV – Facts and Feelings

March 2, 2022

Confusion is its own kind of order; accept it and understand it.

"It may sound trite to say that confusion is the most confusing syndrome in medicine, but it is. A confused person behaves in a way so foreign to common experience that it can be unnerving, even for professionals. It is an alternate state of being. Portrayals of confusion in popular culture—the town drunk, for example —may look funny, but in the case of a truly confused person, the sight of someone who can't find his own mind can be overwhelming."
— **Allan Ropper**, MD (2014), neurologist

Our goal here is to be less confused. In order to get there, we want to know what confusion is. While confusion is a confusing syndrome, the experience is clear even as its roots are obscure.

Confusion can be:

- Situational: too many plausible choices, or no plausible choices.

- Cognitive: emotional or intellectual uncertainty.

- Neurological: the inability to find or make sense.

Clarity Comes with Obscurity

In physics, a greater understanding of chaos came when people stopped trying to find order in chaos and started looking for the order of chaos: chaos as a thing in itself. It's profitable to do the same with personal chaos.

Intellectual chaos generates confusion, and when narrowness and certainty are wanted, confusion is not helpful. But are narrowness and certainty always appropriate? In situations where change is needed, and where that change is significant or broad, narrowness and certainty will not get you there. To embrace significant change means moving away from what's narrow and certain.

Change leads toward confusion from the old vantage point. What seems like confusion from the old vantage point could offer clarity from a new vantage point. Do we need to know what

306

we're aiming toward before we start to change?

To insist that new thoughts and theories be more orderly and inclusive than what has come before is classic, reductive thinking. It is typical of naïve science and facile problem-solving. It happens sometimes that old thinking can resolve new problems, and we're encouraged to believe this is the right approach.

Most of the physicists I've known believe this, and some of them are successful in applying this belief, but most are not. The application of old thinking makes incremental progress and yields diminishing returns. Those who are expert at applying old thinking lack foresight and creativity. But to have foresight and be creative takes a certain amount of competence, but less than you think, and less than is assumed.

Many breakthroughs are made by accident, and most pioneers are more creative than expert. The skills required are not expertise and authority; they are determination and focus. The greater obstacle to new insight is not technical difficulty, it's chaos.

We resist moving into confusion because it seems there are more wrong ways than right ways. If there's some reason to change, some pain or push that's motivating us, we want clarity before we invest. We want something delivered, usually comfort or security, and confusion is neither comfortable nor secure.

In the leading quote, Allan Ropper was thinking about confusion as a neurologist. This is the 3rd point on my list of sources of confusion. He was talking about diagnostic confusion, which is structural rather than situational. One is diagnostically confused when the situation is within the range of normal, but our ability to navigate what's normal is disabled.

I'm focusing on points 1 and 2 on my list, having more to do with knowing facts and feeling centered, and having less to do with neurological ability.

We think facts are intellectual and feeling centered is emotional. This is part of the problem: facts are often relative and not absolute. We believe facts that support what we feel rather than accept what might be facts that cause us confusion. We have a hand in recognizing confusion. What appears as confusion can more reflect the error in our thinking than the complexity of the situation.

307

Our most common confusions are conflicts in our preconception, not a lack or excess of choices. As long as we are not neurologically impaired, our confusion is mostly of type 2: emotional or intellectual. Our situation is signaling us to think differently, and our confusion reflects our resistance to doing so. The ideas we are attached to are causing conflict and confusion.

The Action Bias

We are biologically inclined to act on issues, and we all behave this way. This works to our advantage, especially in emergencies where time is critical and doing nothing is not an option. The action bias is our tendency to see things as urgent. The result is rarely the best, but often better than nothing.

From an urgent mindset, confusion is an obstacle. We'd like to act, and for that, we want to know. But consider this from another point of view. Most cases are not emergencies; careful thinking that incorporates more information generates better outcomes.

If you want to know what to do, do you need to know more facts or more feelings? How might confusion help you in these situations? Confusion is the feeling that there is more to know. If you can become comfortable with that feeling, then you'll be more open to learning and change.

Confusion can be seen as informative in both respects. Finding information is an outward search for connection, while getting more in touch with your feelings is an inward search. You will feel confused if you cannot resolve your facts and feelings. But you'll have a deeper understanding when you accept you cannot understand all that you see or feel. Accepting what you cannot yet know is a significant insight.

In the formal, mathematical sense, information is what cannot be condensed. The more succinctly and definitively something can be stated, the less information it contains. From that point of view, your aversion to confusion is an aversion to learning more. This comes from your compulsion to act.

If you can re-conceive of taking no action as an act, then you're more likely to see confusion as a source of direction to take the action of not acting. This will feel counterproductive if you feel pressed to ACT NOW, but then that is an underlying bias.

The New Paradigm

When you're pressed to grow, or after you have experienced growth, you are moving into new territory. Expect things to make less sense when seen from the old paradigm. You'll have to find the new sense present in the new paradigm. The problem with the action bias is not the desire to act, but the urge to act now.

Sometimes everything works normally, and new information fits in the old paradigm. When this happens, we have little trouble waiting to act. We can see the path, we know what's adequate, and we're comfortable with the result. We accept the facts.

But when the facts lead us along a path that ends in dissatisfaction, then we can either resign ourselves to the inevitable or embrace confusion in a search for change. Most people who are troubled with their confusion have taken the second approach.

One of the most fertile goals in counseling or coaching is to relax into what appears to be confusing. If I can find calm in not knowing, and become sensitive to what previously made little sense, then I can begin to appreciate another person's situation in their own terms.

To reach this point, one must get beyond expectation. Cognitively, this means accepting contradiction. Emotionally, it means releasing need. Spiritually, it means accepting a deeper sense of meaning. The source of confusion is the differences in these three directions. You must sort through facts, feelings, and needs in a new way in order to realign them. The picture that results may be incomplete, but it will be more spiritually valuable.

Confusion

"Clinically, confusion is defined as a loss of the usual clarity, coherence, and speed of thinking, but this description, while accurate as far as it goes, captures only a snapshot of confused behavior."
— **Allan Ropper**, neurologist

Confusion is often a good thing. It's a sign of fecundity. It's one of the two things that stand just outside any structure, the other being the sterility of absence. Too often, we are more comfortable with what's sterile than what's fertile. We learn to be fearful and this becomes a bias. As a result, we're more comfortable with what's static than with what's dynamic, being more attracted to what's certain.

Think about this from a learning point of view: you will not learn with certainty. Certainty will not lead you to change and growth. Perhaps you are at a point in your life where you want certainty, but will that benefit you in the long run?

This confusion between stasis and change is fundamental. As long as there is life, there is change, and with change comes confusion. It's natural. The question is, how do you approach it? If the origin of your uncertainty is organic—a natural outgrowth of the situation—then the more you resist, the further you'll be from understanding. Seen from the old paradigm, there is contradiction. Seen from the new paradigm, the problem is confusion.

This is the essence of counseling and coaching. It's the essence of learning and change. To be a good scientist, you must welcome confusion. To be a good teacher, you must incite confusion. To be a grounded person, you must accept confusion, too.

References

Ropper, A. H., & Burrell, B. D. (2014). *Reaching Down the Rabbit Hole, A Renowned Neurologist Explains the Mystery and Drama of Brain Disease.* St. Martin's Press.

T24 – News, Memory, and Truth

July 20, 2022

We must do more than remember.

"Life can only be understood backwards, but it can only be lived forwards."
— **Søren Kierkegaard**, theologian, philosopher, and poet

News, memory, and truth have little to do with each other. None of them stand up to scrutiny.

Our language does not distinguish between the two radically different meanings of memory. We equate the meaning of these two phrases that mean entirely different things: "Can you describe your feelings?" and "Can you recall how you felt?"

Requesting a description asks for a summary in terms of signs and signifiers. In contrast, asking you to recall how you felt could mean asking you to re-experience a past feeling, or to create in us what you felt. A description bears no more resemblance to a feeling than a label can be equated with a sensation.

A description is a communication made of things and actions. A sensation is a phenomenon that is experienced. It's understandable that we should ask for a description, but this doesn't recreate the sensation. We allow the feelings that other people create in us to define the terms we apply to them. For example, we might equate feeling proud with nationalism or feeling angry with being disadvantaged.

When you say that something was red, we accept that because red is a relatively constant thing. But when you say you feel angry, no one attempts to quantify your feeling accurately. Aside from distinguishing between being slightly angry and being furious, we have little means of measuring anger. Without measuring, how can we know what another person means?

There has been a rash of random public shootings recently. If those shooters said they were "very angry," would we understand what they were talking about? We would not.

News

There has lately been a fuss about the quality of the news. Low-quality information frustrates everyone who is trying to understand things. We like to think that if the information is correct, then we can arrive at the truth and navigate the future. People like to think that if they were better informed, they'd be able to figure everything out.

We want to know the facts in order to record events properly. The facts are the events that caused things to happen and which, in a similar context, will cause the same things to happen again. I wonder if people would be as upset with their memories if they understood how poorly we remember things.

In the article "The Influences of Emotion on Learning and Memory," Chai Meei Tyng (2017) and colleagues report, "Emotional experiences/stimuli appear to be remembered vividly and accurately, with great resilience over time."

I understand what it means to have a vivid and resilient memory, but what does it mean to have an accurate memory? It does not mean what you might suspect. It does not mean factually accurate; it means recollectively accurate. That is, you can better recall thoughts that triggered emotions than you can thoughts that did not. That does not imply these thoughts were accurate at the time or ever.

Memory

In the BBC Viewpoint piece titled "His Dark Charisma," Laurence Rees (2012) quotes Emil Klein, who heard Hitler speak in the 1920s, as saying, "The man gave off such a charisma that people believed whatever he said."

In the article "Emotion and Memory Research: A Grumpy Overview," Linda Levine and David Pizarro (2004) note that, "The vividness and detail that often characterize memories for emotional events do not necessarily imply accuracy." They conclude:

"The types of situations that evoke emotions such as fear, anger, and sadness vary dramatically with respect to the responses required of the individual. Once evoked, these emotions appear to trigger selective processing, encoding, and retrieval of information that is important for responding to these differing emotion-eliciting situations. The selective encoding and retrieval of motivationally relevant information would typically be adaptive, but depression and anxiety disorders remind us that this is not always the case."

We don't remember the truth and we don't remember the facts because neither exist. Like the cat who jumps on a hot stove, we remember what appears to be useful based on what we want. We don't have to think about this, and it's not reasonable. Remembering what's reasonable is little more than programming for comfort.

I drag my son through mathematics. He's 11, and he thinks mathematical reasoning is pointless. I don't think he'll remember much of what I've told him. I drag him through modern history, and I tell him why certain events were important, but they're not important to him. He has no "reason" to remember them. His reasoning is not based on argument, it's based on usefulness.

When I say, "Time is not really a fourth dimension because it does not behave like the other three," my audience falls asleep. When Hitler said, "The doom of a nation can be averted only by a storm of flowing passion. Only those who are passionate themselves can arouse passion in others," his audience woke up.

Levine and Pizarro note that, "Fearful individuals display enhanced memory for threat-related information and poorer memory for threat-irrelevant details." As with Hitler's audience, so also did Donald Trump's audience hear redemption when he said:

> "From this day forward, a new vision will govern our land. From this day forward, it's going to be only America first, America first."
> — **Donald Trump**

You don't remember the truth; you remember what emotionally rewards you. A leader is not someone who clarifies what's true as much as a person who confuses everyone into conformity.

> "My definition of a leader in a free country is a man who can persuade people to do what they don't want to do and like it... The truth is all I want for history."
> — **Harry S. Truman**

Truth

In a 2001 paper, Levine and Prohaska report, "Memory for past emotions changes over time and... the changes are systematically related to current appraisals of the emotion-eliciting event." That is, your memory of past feelings is influenced by your current feelings.

Unless you question how you feel, your feelings will bias and exaggerate what you now remember, and distort what you learned from the past. If you're currently afraid, you'll exaggerate your fearful memories. If you're currently in love, you'll exaggerate your loving memories.

I went to relationship counseling with my last partner after she expressed no further interest in being part of our family. The counselor asked her to recall how she originally felt about me when our relationship began. She responded, "I never had any positive feelings for him."

This would have been offensive if it were not pathological. It was an extreme case of distorting reality, which furthered the new direction she was taking. This demonic reconstruction highlights a tendency that we accept as normal, and where our language fails. We do not recognize the difference between labels and the feelings that are labeled.

We don't recognize the role of bias in memory. More simply, we don't recognize our bias. This twisting of truth supports the persistence of grudges, feuds, and prejudice. Errors of the past are made worse by your attachment to them, and to your continued investment in going forward with them. How can we "learn from the past" if we can't remember it?

This is the crux of the issue: what is true in memory? If it is true, as has been observed, that "memories for the emotional significance of events are stored permanently [in] and mediated by different brain circuits, than memories for events themselves" (LeDoux 1992, 269–88), and these memories don't agree, what then?

If we're going to get our heads straight, then we must do more than remember, because recollections are not accurate. Our recollections do not recall how we felt in the past, even when they retrieve the labels we attached to those feelings. Our memories inaccurately reflect the important aspects of the past. They recreate aspects of the past pertinent to how we feel today, and along the lines we're thinking today.

Clear thinking—if there can be such a thing—requires recalling multiple memories: what we thought, what we saw, and how we felt, and our circumstances in the past. Most importantly, clear thinking depends on being aware of the connections between the present and the past. If this burden seems unwieldy in forging future decisions, then reflect on the German experience from the 1920s: what are you really trying to achieve?

> "When awareness is brought to an emotion, power is brought to your life."
> — **Tara Meyer Robson**

> "All learning has an emotional base."
> — **Plato**

References

LeDoux, J. E. (1992). "Emotion as Memory: Anatomical Systems Underlying Indelible Neural Traces." In *The Handbook of Emotion and Memory: Research and Theory*, edited by S. Christianson. Erlbaum. https://books.google.ca/books?hl=en&lr=&id=dXMs_dloSEcC&oi=fnd&pg=PA269&dq=Emotion+as+memory:+Anatomical+systems+underlying+indelible+neural+traces

Levine, L., Pizarro, D. A. (2004 Oct). "Emotion and Memory Research: A Grumpy Overview." *Social Cognition, 22* (5): 530-54. https://www.researchgate.net/profile/Linda-Levine-5/publication/240611983_Emotion_and_Memory_Research_A_Grumpy_Overview

Rees, L. (2012 Nov 12). "Viewpoint: His Dark Charisma." *BBC News*. https://www.bbc.com/news/magazine-20237437

Tyng, C. M., Amin, H. U., Saad, M. N. M., & Malik, A. S. (2017, Aug 24). "The Influences of Emotion on Learning and Memory." *Frontiers in Psychology, 8*: 1454. https://www.ncbi.nlm.nih.gov/pmc/articles/PMC5573739/

Emotions

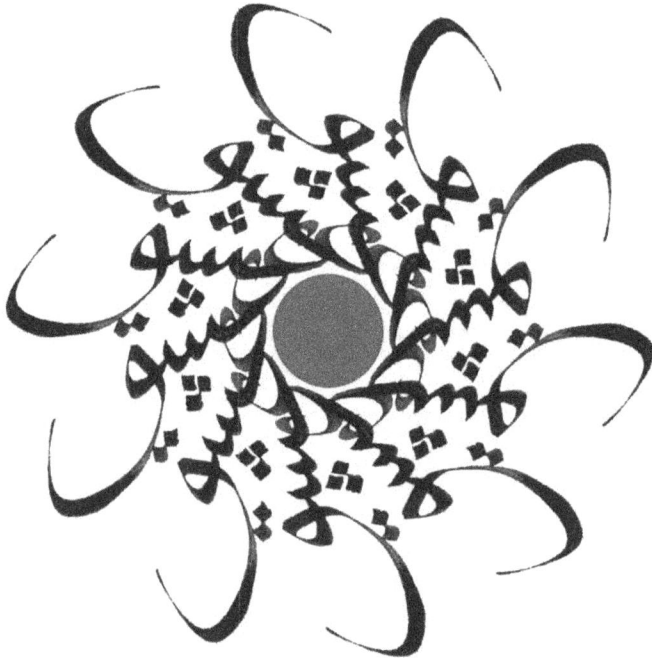

E1 – Emotion

Emotions are signs, not things. Don't be them, read them.

"The emotionally intelligent person is skilled in four areas: identifying emotions, using emotions, understanding emotions, and regulating emotions."
— **John Mayer** and **Peter Salovey** (1990)

These writings on emotion compile thoughts I feel my therapy clients need to hear. They are thoughts most people need to hear because most people have little understanding of emotion and think nothing of it.

As I survey the perspectives I explored, I want to provide a holistic structure for understanding emotion. I've not found such an approach in what I've read.

Exposing the shortcomings of small ideas is like raking the rocks out of the earth in the garden. It's necessary, but it's not the same as creating fertile soil. This piece is an attempt at fertilizing the garden.

Forget What You Know About Emotion

Emotion is not unintelligent, undirected, disconnected, or extreme. We think of emotion in these limited ways because we encounter emotion in these dysregulated forms. But just as blood is not a red liquid that flows on the ground after a murder, emotion is not an expression of inner meaning that pervades a relationship after a crisis.

Emotion is also not one thing. Our emotions serve different functions in different ways. Blood serves many functions, and we have other liquids: saliva, sperm, lymph, plasma, bile, stomach acid, mucus, and milk. Some of these are functionally specific and others are vehicles for nutrients, hormones, and chemical signals. Like bodily liquids, emotions are like mental liquids.

We once equated the body's liquids with emotions. We called them humors: sanguine, choleric, melancholic, and phlegmatic. It was a poor system, and it didn't work, but I laud the attempt at seeing emotions as fundamental.

Today, we deride the old theory of humors, but we forget it was a great step forward from the theory of evil spirits that preceded it (Hendrie 2021). As frightening as the theory was, it introduced the concepts of balance, nutrition, and hygiene that are the foundations of today's medicine.

Emotions in General

Emotions are not structurally fundamental, as the theory of the four humors suggested. They do not control the body's functions, and they are not carried in separate substances. But they are fundamental to one's attitude.

Reinterpreting the medieval theory of humors on a purely cognitive level gives us something better than modern psychotherapy. Today's psychotherapy seems to overlook emotions entirely. To flesh out the territory, start with functional emotions, such as feelings that are positive, negative, detached, or controlling. Add to these the interpretive emotions of anger, fear, love, and comfort. You need to have some map of the landscape of emotions before you can understand how emotions provide a map of your decisions in the world.

Today's theory of emotions has led to attempts to find where emotions are localized in the brain. This is increasingly seen as unsupportable. The localization of emotions is a reasonable conjecture only if you overlook what they're made of. They're made of too many disparate things to have a single origin.

Few people examine what emotions are made of; psychologists who research emotions don't seem to. Given the subjective nature of emotions and the objective bias of researchers, researchers may be the least qualified to understand emotions. We learn more about our emotions by watching a skilled actor.

Many people assume emotions have no components and see them as primary things. On that basis, it's plausible that they are the product of some organ within the brain.

Emotions are complex signals. They are collections of associations that differ more in how they direct us and less in what they are composed of. They're all composed of associations, inclinations, urges, and ideas. Most are not singular things.

They serve the purpose of sculpting the landscape on which we build our thoughts. If that landscape provides a poor foundation, then you'll have a difficult time organizing your thoughts. As hormones regulate our biochemistry, emotions regulate our thinking.

Some Emotions in Particular

Comfort, as an emotion, is a combination of physical and mental relaxation. This means both a lack of tension and attention. To be comfortable is to have a detached view of the past, a placid view of the present, and a relaxed view of the future. This kind of comfort is a cosmology that supports a happy conclusion.

Love is more complex than comfort, as it adds a feeling of satisfied attachment, support, trust, and intimacy. These general terms mean different things to each of us. It is embarrassing to recognize that the Greeks of 2,000 years ago had a better understanding of love than we do. Their eight words for love are hardly used in our language. We can explain them, but we confound them.

The eight words for love in ancient Greek are erōs for passion, philia for affection, agape for selfless love, storgē for family love, mania for obsession, ludus for playfulness, pragma for enduring love, and philautia for self-love. These words were not used equally, and even though these distinctions were made, they were not consistent or clear (Hurt 2013).

> "In Plato's *Symposium* the most common word for love was erōs, and it denoted a kind of enlightened pederasty. One of the earlier speakers said there could be a good erōs and a bad erōs; the bad version was typical of a 'Popular Aphrodite' who merely loved having sex with a good body. Eventually, when Socrates spoke in the dialogue, he defined true erōs as the love of virtue in which no physical intimacy was ultimately necessary."
> — **Carla Hurt**, philologist (2013)

Our culture would gain much by studying what love means to us. C. S. Lewis wrote an influential book called *The Four Loves* (Lewis 1960), but that was sixty years ago and I just found it. Our fascination with love combined with our lack of interest in better understanding it, suggests that either our brains or our cultures are not developed enough to appreciate the differences.

Love and comfort play a relaxing role in our parasympathetic nervous system. Their components differ with each person and we do not have, and never will have, a consensus definition of them. This works against gaining control over our emotions. It also undermines our ability to understand ourselves and communicate with others.

Other emotions, like fear and anger, are more biochemical and neurological. These emotions are more a part of our sympathetic nervous system, the system in charge of activating us. They don't tell us how to think or act, they just tell us we need to think and act. They often lead to what we later consider poor thoughts and actions, but that's a misunderstanding of their purpose. Fear and anger motivate actions and responses. They are filters that focus our thoughts. If we focus incorrectly, that's because we understand them poorly and have failed to refine them.

I have a client who complains that she and her 30-year-old daughter always fight. She does not want to fight; she says she wants the anger to stop and get her "baby back." However, the issues that arise trigger my client and she says she cannot control herself. My client's driving emotion is fear, and she admits this. She says she sees her daughter "stepping into the fire."

I tell my client that she is in an emotionally violent situation. As in all violent situations, the first thing one must do is stop the violence. I point out that while she says she wants to regain a loving relationship, her actions are destroying it.

It's likely that we can understand the fear this person is experiencing. We don't need to know what she's afraid of because we have a consensus understanding of how we're motivated by fear.

We can't say the same thing about the love my client wants to foster. I have pointed out her notion of love includes a great deal of control and righteous authority. One might exercise such control over a 10-year-old, but this kind of mothering is inappropriate for an adult. It is no wonder her daughter rejects her.

Her daughter wants her mother's love, but not the love her mother is offering. The mother is stuck in demanding a love her daughter sees as immature, unjustified, and unsupportive.

I find myself educating my clients about the emotions they feel. I ask them, "What does your anger mean?" "Do you want control or do you want alliance?" "Which part of you is yelling and which part of you is crying?"

A person should have some control over their feelings before they enter a conflict, especially if that conflict is with someone who is close to them. Not only do many have no emotional control, but they have not even considered it. We erroneously think that our emotions are justified and true. We often examine our thoughts at least superficially, but we rarely examine our emotions. We are led by them, and this creates most of the problems that my clients encounter.

Another client is analytical. They have arranged their plans and resources. They say they feel change is happening too slowly. After concluding that they would benefit from better management of their time and resources, I asked them if they felt they might also be burdened by some personal problems they have not disclosed. To my surprise, they said, "Yes." I asked if they wanted to explore this further, and they said, "No."

In contrast with the mother, who was possessed by her anger, this client could not act on their feelings. I reassured the mother that by recognizing her need to control her emotions, she would make progress. The client who could not recognize their feelings may not return. They need a crisis to force their recognition.

Reading the Signs

Emotions are not something you have, they are something you read. When we are emotional, we are enacting the sign rather than understanding it. My angry client is getting the message to be angry and acting it out. Instead, she needs to see why she's getting this message and make adjustments to it.

My evasive client is not even getting the message. Like a person with a stone in their shoe, this person is not removing the stone. Instead, they're walking in an unbalanced fashion in order to avoid feeling what their emotions are trying to tell them. In both cases, it's not the control of the emotion that's needed, it's the understanding of why these feelings arise.

Similar situations occur with depression, heartbreak, and confusion. In each case, we mislead ourselves by thinking we must act as the emotional signals direct us. When the result of the emotion is distress, accepting its direction is probably the wrong thing to do. The right thing to do is to explore the emotion, to understand why an emotional warning light is flashing red.

Exploring Emotional Change

Emotions are famously immune to argument. Simple analysis is the wrong tool, but analysis can be used to understand emotions if the analysis is deep enough. Most of our analysis is too shallow to affect our emotions, but we can learn to do better.

One way to use analysis to understand emotions is to regress into the past or conjure feelings into the present. In either case, you are recreating scenarios that support your feelings. These don't need to be true stories. In fact, they will never be any more factual than stories can be. The stories you create from regression or conjuration are symbolic. Their symbols are the triggers of your feelings. It is these triggers that you want to manage.

Part of one's success in managing emotions lies in how you approach them. If you are confrontational and combative, then that's the relationship your emotions will bring you. My angry mother client cannot escape violence because she is taking violence as her starting point. If you start from the wrong frame of mind, which is not the frame of mind which you want to build, then you won't reach the right frame of mind by following those feelings that contradict it.

Your engagement with your emotions is the next step. You are not your emotions, you can only allow yourself to become them. If you can separate yourself from your emotions without suppressing them, then you can communicate with them without becoming them. My evasive client cannot yet do this.

The final step is integration: the bringing together of what you feel with how you would like to feel. Here, the conflict is in yourself. At this step, you stop projecting onto others and external situations. The integration step shows you a bigger picture of what is not working.

Something new needs to happen if you're to form a new emotion. This may be part of the integration process, or it may be something beyond. Here, we're entering unfamiliar territory both personally and therapeutically.

References

Hendrie, A. (2021). "The Four Humours: Understandings of the Body in Medieval Medicine." *Retrospect Journal*. https://retrospectjournal.com/2021/05/02/the-four-humours-understandings-of-the-body-in-medieval-medicine/

Mayer, J., & Salovey, P. (1990 March). "Emotional Intelligence." *Imagination, Cognition and Personality, 9* (3): 185-211. http://gruberpeplab.com/3131/SaloveyMayer_1989_EmotionalIntelligence.pdf

Hurt, C. (2013 Aug 17). "Greek Words for Love, in Context." *Found in Antiquity blog*. https://foundinantiquity.com/2013/08/17/greek-words-for-love-in-context/

Lewis, C. S. (1960). *The Four Loves*. Geoffrey Bles. https://gutenberg.ca/ebooks/lewiscs-fourloves/lewiscs-fourloves-00-h.html

Moore, C. (2022 Aug 15). "If You Can't Always Find the Right Words, These 8 Greek Words for Love Will Help You Better Define Your Closest Relationships." *Parade*. https://parade.com/1274015/charli-moore/greek-words-for-love

E2 – Emotional Thinking

February 23, 2022

Emotions process information without thinking, and you do too.

"Everybody gets so much information all day long that they lose their common sense." — **Gertrude Stein**, novelist and poet

Intellect

We're under the illusion that thinking is putting ideas together to reach conclusions. Even those of us who are artistic fall into this trap and see the creation of good art as a conclusion of our thoughts. For Homo sapiens, thought is good when it produces a result. Thinking is a prison of misery, and most of us are locked in.

The obsession with executive function explains why few of us can communicate with animals. It also explains why few of us can express our authentic nature. We believe we are thinking beings, but we are not; we are feeling beings. It's our pursuit of an independent identity that forces us into our thoughts and away from our feelings. The idea of our independent being-ness is a sterile construction.

> "We have for so long defined ourselves as separate personalities that we have fallen into the hypnotic spell of believing that separation, not unity, is the underlying reality."
> — **Larry Dossey**, (2006, 72), in *The Extraordinary Healing Power of Ordinary Things*

When we talk about intelligence, we're talking about the properties of our intellect. The idea of emotional intelligence is an oxymoron because emotions do not act intelligently. They don't plan, formulate, strategize, solve, or construct. Intellect is our tool for navigating our separateness within a landscape of meaningful events. Emotion makes our landscape meaningful; emotion is the geography of the meaningful.

By "thinking" emotionally, we assign meaning to what's within us and around us. This is not thinking in the intentional sense. You can no more "think emotionally" than you can think yourself to sleep. There is no process or output, but it is not static either. Let's reserve thinking for intellect and use feeling for emotions. The two feedback into each other, but they operate using different processes.

Our reality is our emotional landscape. It is a living system that grows of its own accord. You do not think your emotional world into existence any more than you think how to walk. You can think and you can walk, and you can think about how you walk, and you can focus on walking and become more aware of it.

You can think yourself to focus and become more deeply aware, but being is not focus, and focus is not thinking. Thinking is structural and computational. Thinking can trigger feeling, but it's the feeling that is the being.

Most of us cannot stop thinking, and some of us cannot start feeling. We've grown up in a world that so obscures feeling and so denigrates our having feelings that many of us don't even know how traumatized we've become. Given the chance to feel, many of us behave psychotically, believing in our delusions of the past. We create dichotomies, projections, and conflicts in the present that we never learned how to resolve in our childhood. Our behavior appears repetitive, but it's not without reason. We recreate situations we want to resolve. It's too bad that we rarely can without help, but we keep trying nonetheless.

Much of psychotherapy patches up this container and convinces us that our disembodied minds will make it to the nonexistent finish line. Unfortunately, therapy is not as much a "helping profession" as therapists would like to think. Psychology has more to do with coping than healing. Commodity therapy aims to keep your eyes on the road and your mind on our shared social obligations.

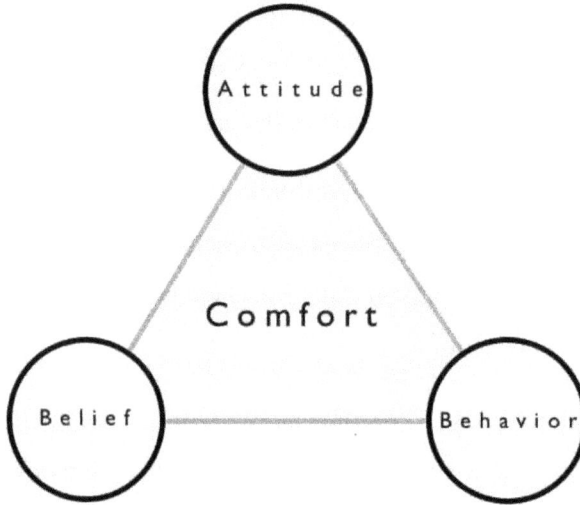

*Figure 31: Comfort as the combination of
attitudes, beliefs, and behaviors.*

Emotion

We have not found our personal, social, or ecological balance because our intellectual world has none. It is not intelligence we lack, a flame that disintegrates everything it touches, it's emotion. We lack a secure emotional identity. We won't have a secure emotional identity if we're immobilized by scarcity and fears of encroaching destruction. Lacking an intact pyramid of family, community, and culture, our world is threatening. It borders on being our enemy. If we know nothing but struggle, then we manifest a state of war around us.

To be emotionally able does not require emotional intelligence, as intelligence presupposes decisions that require intellect. Emotional ability consists of identifying, understanding, using, and regulating emotions.

The intellect rests on beliefs, attitudes, and behaviors. Emotions also rest on beliefs and attitudes, and lead to behaviors. The intellect operates by connecting ideas in sequences. Emotions operate through recognitions, associations, and impulses. The six steps pictured in Figure 32 proceed from appreciation to definition, ideation, orientation, testing, and, finally, implementation. These describe intellectual or emotional understanding but mean something different in each case.

Emotional ability requires no intellect. If you had an accurate map of how everything behaved, even given the uncertainties of nature, then you would have no fear in being and in expressing yourself. You would eat, live, hunt, and mate with whatever gave satisfaction and didn't bite you.

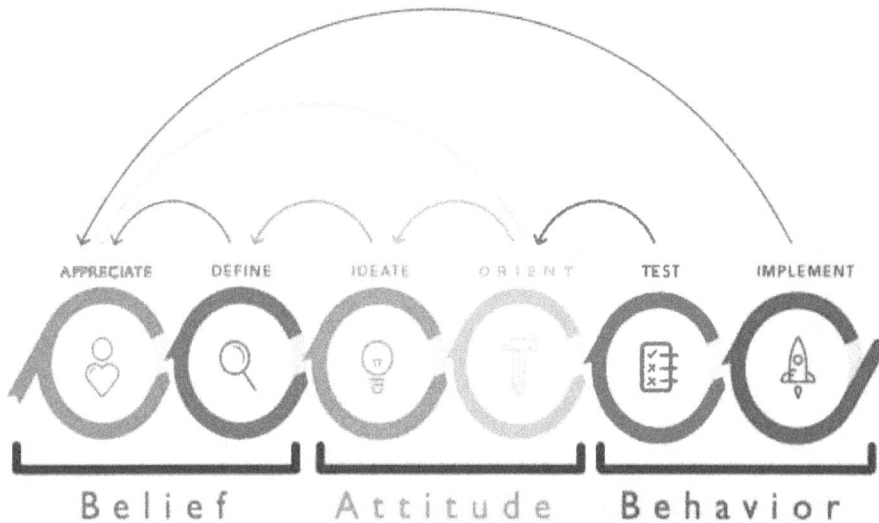

Figure 32: The progression from beliefs to attitudes to behaviors, and how each feeds back to strengthen or weaken the others.

Think Biologically

Animals are emotionally able, and they have intellect. They configure their reality, but they don't introduce unnatural constructions. They don't pollute their environment by making abstract conflicts real. They don't project their frustrations onto their families and warp their children's minds. They might eat their children, but that's a survival instinct, not a pathological behavior.

Modern human societies behave pathologically. We live in an emotionally unbalanced world in which we are always on the defensive. Obstinance and aggression are never far from the front burner. We attempt to achieve balance on a material level while building on an emotional swamp. An emotionally able solution would be to drain our swamp, quench our conflagrations, and find solid ground.

Instead, modern culture encourages emotional myopia in order to overlook our disabilities.

327

Modern culture wants us to think alike. Members of a balanced culture depend on and collaborate with each other. By thinking differently, diverse points of view create a more accurate and resilient perspective. Where people depend on and support each other, we find healthier communities. But when people exploit each other individually and institutionally, we find sick communities.

Intelligence operates in both healthy and unhealthy minds, but only those who are emotionally able are healthy. These people build balanced and resilient bonds both outside and inside of their circle of dependents. In contrast, unhealthy cultures prevail by enslaving and exploiting. They fail when they run out of resources.

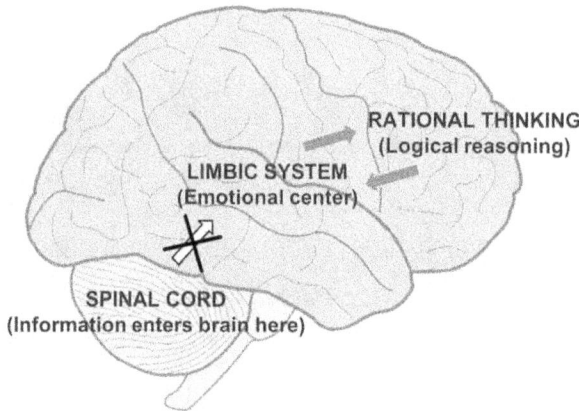

Figure 33: Feedback between the lower limbic and upper cerebral system

Despite the tyranny of our intellects, we all enter emotional states when we dream. These non-executive functioning states of mind return us to a non-Homo sapiens level of awareness. A dog's waking reality would be like a dream to us.

Dreams build the emotional landscape, the landscape on which we build our waking life. Here, we build our intuition and instinctual awareness. Our dreams are the artwork of animals drawn with dirt, tooth, claw, and feces.

Each night, we take our life's worth of jigsaw puzzle pieces, including the day's new pieces, and explore the expanding picture. In this hodgepodge, nothing fits, but everything of importance is included.

Dreams are your attempt to terraform your emotional landscape. Notice that although dreams explore many odd combinations, they do not violate your essential feelings. For example, I doubt you dream of having sex with your parents. If you go to sleep weighted down by particular situations, they will appear in your dreams in some form.

Hypnosis Is Emotional Thinking

Any freely associating state is a hypnotic state. The signature of hypnosis is being fully invested in the moment, in the way you're fully invested in a dream. The difference between dreams and hypnosis is that in hypnosis, you have the option to take a greater or lesser part.

If you enter a dissociated, emotional state without the guiding, filtering, and interpreting effect of the intellect, you are in a hypnotic state. When awake, your intellectual filters ensure that your intellectual perspective dominates for your protection.

An emotionally able person, like a hypnotically able person, can suspend the intellect. They can fully embrace the reality of their feelings without forcing their feelings to conform to preexisting beliefs and attitudes. However, as they become more deeply emotionally enmeshed they lose a degree of control.

We define non-hypnotizable people as "analytic resisters." These are people who are too cautious, vigilant, controlling, insecure, or frightened to set aside their intellectual identities. Many intelligent people suffer from this condition. It's not the intellect that's a disability, it's being unable to do without it. You are at a creative disadvantage if you cannot hear your feelings or appreciate the feelings of others.

Some persistently intellectual people create separate environments in which they explore their emotions. They will relax their intellect only under controlled and protected circumstances. They take off their intellectual garb and skinny dip in the shallow end of their pool of emotions.

With help from a hypnotherapist, people feel comfortable going into the deep end. As a hypnotherapist, I act as an ally or lifeguard. I come from an emotionally curious place that is both nonjudgmental and unfiltered. I discard my intellectual knowledge, assumptions, and interpretations. It's not that I don't care, it's that I don't presume to know the truth. You don't know the truth, either. Emotions open us to feeling, not knowing.

Wisdom

Let's get away from the word therapy and use the word wisdom instead. What you want—and I'm pretty sure I can speak for you as the reader—is the wisdom to handle your emotions. You want to feel safe in the exploration of your emotional extremes.

They say, at the end of their lives, people rarely regret what they've done. Instead, they regret what they did not do. But, of course, acts of doing mean nothing in and of themselves. It's the feelings we're after. What people regret is never fully engaging with their emotions.

Everyone needs a safe environment in order to explore what we need to do, learn, and feel. This is why we must stop abusing ourselves, and stop abusing others in our families and communities. Living in emotionally unsafe environments—a defining pathology of our culture of scarcity—prevents us from learning how to become emotionally able. We all need safety. We can create safety by recognizing what safety feels like.

Create a safe boundary within which you can explore. Even if you are alone inside that boundary, that is better than tolerating the company of those who are hostile or would exploit you. You have allies that will emerge in the solitude of your retreat. If you're like most people, being entirely alone with your feelings is a lonely and disheartening experience.

Emotional support is valuable, and few therapists or counselors can provide it. Wise people provide support, and these people appear in healthy cultures as elders. In our culture, few of our elders are wise because their growth was stunted.

Wisdom can be found in non-directive colleagues and advisors. Such people are emotionally able coaches, partners, and mentors. Some religious, contemplative, physical, and athletic pursuits foster non-directive wisdom. Wise people don't project their pathologies onto others. They don't attempt to "fix" anything.

Don't wait until you become sick to grow yourself. Sickness begins with a system out of balance. If you don't recognize what it is to be in balance, then you will surely move out of balance before you recognize something is wrong. If you require injury to attend to your growth, then you're creating the situation for this injury. Be proactive.

You're not seeking help—that's the therapy model—you're seeking growth. Modern life is a maze of empty streets. All healthy cultures rely on wisdom keepers, but our culture has driven most of them away; consider the injured or imperious characters presented in the media. Find the wisdom that will help you. We need to support each other in regaining health and balance as individuals and as a culture.

E3 - Emotional Ignorance

March 16, 2022

Maybe humans aren't so smart after all.

"We are dangerous when we are not conscious of our responsibility for how we behave, think, and feel." — **Marshall Rosenberg**, psychologist

We are biased against the negative and biased against confronting the negative. What is negative is considered bad, and talked about in hushed tones. This has been going on ever since people noticed that thinking about things has a way of making them happen.

Extolling the positive and condemning the negative distinguished Christianity from its tribal competitors, according to Peter Kingsley (1999). Appropriating the good and projecting evil elsewhere—a universal component of nationalism—has become so ingrained as to be considered a virtue rather than a misdirection. The good and the bad jostle for time in our minds, no matter what culture you're from.

Endorsing the good has become culture's "high road" and none of us are immune. This might be fine as a guide to intentions, aspirations, and morality, but it's not fine when it comes to repairing psychological damage. To reshape yourself, you must address those forces that continue to distort you. Various agents who we believe protect us—such as teachers, politicians, the police, and other public servants—commonly cause anxiety, fear, and deprivation. We are obliged to accept their behavior, which they see as their right. An aspect of our damaged self-worth is our acceptance of authority. The role of all these authorities, even those who are competent, is to constrain thought and limit change.

As a therapist, if you can't help your clients integrate their dark sides, then your future impact will go down the bleak road of cognitive-behavioral therapy. This is the psychological correlate to law enforcement which follows the much-flogged dictum of, "Nothing to see here. Move along." Those who can't see the negative are easily misled by promises and attractions. Enduring change must build on a firm moral foundation and a fearless awareness. An effective counselor is one who stops you from moving along and draws out from you what more there is to see here. Moving to a new state of mind requires an intermediate state of chaos.

Amoral behavior is not the problem, nor is illegal behavior. The Seven Deadly Sins are symptoms, not causes. Thinking is not the solution, because thinking can be manipulated. It's your emotions that lie at the root of your thoughts and actions. If something feels bad, then it probably is, regardless of who tells you otherwise. The thing about emotions, and what makes emotions so important, is that they grow slowly and can't be ignored. Thoughts are like the leaves on a tree, constantly growing wherever there is light. Emotions are the trunk and branches whose structure represents a commitment or, often, an injury. Ideas guide our mouths, but our hands and feet follow our emotions.

Short-sighted thinking is also a symptom, not a problem. The problem is a lack of empathy, altruism, and awareness of the whole. We might call this a lack of "emotional intelligence," but since that doesn't tell us how to do it, it's not clear this is intelligence at all. Just because psychologists have tests for emotional intelligence doesn't make it real. Just because there are tests for psychologists does not make them real either. In fact, they are unreal.

Psychology is a fictitious profession. Compare therapy to driving. Driving is both a skill and a set of rules. We need rules to limit the situations we might encounter. We're not agile, attentive, or responsive enough to drive without rules, but those are not the skills of driving. They just constrain the situations. Psychologists are trained in the rules of behavior, but those are not what drives a person, they are what constrains them. Skill as a therapist, for yourself or others, lies in your ability to attend, understand, and respond. In every case, when I am working with my clients, I am mentoring them to become their own therapists.

Problems arise because emotions are difficult to measure. Emotional forces may be primary, but the evidence of emotion is elusive. Emotions don't leave fingerprints while actions do. Actions always seem to be justified intellectually. A therapist is a detective looking for the insanity that underlies everyone's reasonable emotions.

Tyranny

Successful tyrants are intellectual geniuses and emotional idiots. I suspect this describes Vladimir Putin and Xi Jinping. Western politicians also qualify on these criteria, but let's focus on these two. There are less powerful tyrants in corporate leadership, three percent of whom are also estimated to be sociopaths.

Pundits and politicians speculate on the goals of leadership. There is talk about tyrants as autocrats, but little talk about them as regular people. We're concerned with predicting their effects on our investments, as that's where we feel them. If you're more sensitive, then you'll also feel them in your heart.

The tensions ongoing in Europe and Asia are centuries old. If there is any silver lining to these clouds, it is the golden opportunity to learn world history. This would be a small consolation, even if people could learn. Maybe there's something you can do?

Most of us avoid focusing on what we don't want to see; it just doesn't seem to help. And while we don't want to wear the boots of tyrants, we'd like to have that kind of power. Their dark side is our dark side, and it remains dark because we—like tyrants—are more attached to our emotional needs than our evolution. We need to evolve.

Cultures have emotions. Just as a person can lose control and commit crimes, cultures can too: the Vikings, Romans, Huns, Colonial White America, Germany, and Rwanda. Remember the Alamo but forget Wounded Knee. Cultural crimes make people especially uncomfortable. When confronted with class accusations, we're quick to shout "Prejudice!" We exonerate ourselves in victimhood, and so the underlying emotions stay dark.

Ukraine has its own culture, territory, and language. Its people have suffered the ravages of Russian imperialism since well before the dawn of the 20th century. One of Stalin's lesser-known initiatives was the mass murder of Ukrainian poets.

> "Kobzars were a unique class of musicians in Ukraine, who traveled between towns and sang dumas, a meditative poem-song. Kobzars were usually blind, and required the completion of a three-year apprenticeship in specialized Kobzar guilds, in order to be officially recognized as such. In 1932, on the order of Stalin, the Soviet authorities called on all Ukrainian Kobzars to attend a congress in Kharkiv. Those that arrived were taken outside the city and were all put to death."
> — **Wikipedia**

Let me put in a plug for my friend Julian Kytasty and his album, *Black Sea Winds: The*

Kobzari from Ukraine. (https://youtu.be/3x79AI63ZYY)

Their enmity toward the Russians led the Ukrainians to ally with the Nazis. Twenty-five percent of the Jews murdered in the holocaust—one million people—were Ukrainian Jews from the Ukraine. Ukraine then suffered the brunt of the ground and air war. Five to seven million Ukrainians, 25 percent of the country's population, died in World War II.

Brutality, depravity, psychopathology, and carnage are nothing new. Putin's invasion cannot be seen as new opportunism. It is a combination of 19th Century monarchism, irredentism—the recovery of lost territory—and revanchism, otherwise known as pure revenge. It won't be resolved by victory or compromise. Real resolution lies in an integration of the dark side.

Putin's moves can be ascribed to certain intellectual arguments: it worked before; his time is running out; he's sitting on an otherwise unprofitable war chest; Russia's control of almost half of Eastern Europe's energy and a tradition of entitlement. Donald Trump called Putin's invasion "genius" (Gedeon 2022), but Trump's problems are more than emotional ignorance.

These factors are mirrored in the situation between the People's Republic of China (PRC) and Taiwan. Putin's strategy may not bear fruit, but members of the PRC need to foresee the world's otherwise inscrutable behavior (Matthews 2022).

Democracy

Democracy has been compared to two wolves and a sheep deciding on what's for dinner. Democracy easily slips into populism, as we have repeatedly seen (Michener 2023). It was for this purpose that republics are created, where representatives are empowered to govern. Representatives, responsive to broader pressure and being more informed, are better able to see all sides, including the dark side.

It is republics, not democracies, that are implemented in what we call "the free world." The concept has its roots in the indigenous society of the pre-colonial Iroquois Nation. There, social control was woven into a more psychologically integrated culture. Today, this is forgotten.

Russian and Chinese territories have been ruled autocratically for over a millennium. Russia's experiment with democracy in the 1990s was without precedent, and it failed.

China's army of 8,000 life-sized terracotta soldiers protects the burial mound of Qin Shi Huang, the first emperor. It is 40 years since its rediscovery, yet only 1% of the burial mound has been excavated. Qin Shi Huang's mountain-sized mausoleum was erected to ensure his immortality, but the horror of his rule led to his subjects erasing him from history. China's legacy of tyranny has yet to be broken.

These states have a history of autocratic power and monarchic governance. They have no cultural model for autonomy. Their rapid ascent to power in the 20th century is a combination of forced organization and the stimulation of foreign trade. In the equation of globalism, greater trade is supposed to foster greater alliance and less imperialism. Do you see it?

As outsiders who live in what we call a free world, our response to the expansion of autocracy has been appeasement, opportunism, and gamesmanship. Those living under tyranny have little choice. Maintaining complacency is the autocrats' aim. The conservative Cato Institute has an interesting appraisal of people's attitudes toward aggression at the start of WWII (Powell 2014). Regardless of your political persuasion, this is a good time to review history.

Monarchs, emperors, tsars, and kings take credit for improved conditions. They never take blame and need not tolerate it being assigned to them. It reminds us of abusive parents who subjugate their children to subjugate and profit from the family. When there is no one to object, what else can we expect?

The Dark Ages was a European period of roughly 800 years, presided over by tyrannical governments. The period was marked by economic, intellectual, and cultural decline. Land was the major resource and states fought wars to steal land and labor from their neighbors. Laws were capricious, resources were wasted, and justice didn't exist. A suit of armor cost five oxen. Which was more productive? What did we gain? The invention of the horseshoe.

Mentality

What are the roots of a tyrant's mentality? What are the roots of the craving for power? Are these social aberrations or the dark side of ourselves that we deny? Just as winning athletes are not people with normal psychologies, neither are leading politicians. These are not personalities that develop without a social context. We create them.

Wars are a cultural event. It makes no more sense to blame one individual for causing a war than it does to credit an acorn with causing an oak tree. Pontius Pilate may have condemned Jesus Christ, but Christ's execution was the will of Rome. To understand wars and other inhumanities, we have to understand the collective action of people to install and obey sociopaths.

> "The most essential fact to bear in mind is that the key to Western European society in the Central Middle Ages was land, or, more specifically, the ownership of land. As a result, the interests of landowners often shaped warfare."
> — from **Warfare in Western Europe in the Central Middle Ages**,
> https://www.swansea.ac.uk/history/history-study-guides/warfare-in-western-europe-in-the-central-middle-ages/

Many of us contribute to efforts we don't believe in, averting our eyes from the ill uses of our labor. This comes so naturally that we don't think twice. I knew a gentle grandfather who worked on missile launching systems and an enthusiastic colleague whose theories modeled uranium projectiles passing through steel. "Just like a bullet passing through water!" he said enthusiastically. Einstein, the pacifist, triggered the atomic arms race.

Vladimir Putin ordered the invasion of Ukraine. Major General "Buck Turgidson", the anti-hero in the apocalyptic movie *Dr. Strangelove or: How I Learned to Stop Worrying and Love the Bomb* (Kubrick 1964), was modeled after General Curtis LeMay, the real-life commander of the US Pacific Fleet. LeMay ordered the firebombing of Tokyo, the most destructive act of war in history, most of whose casualties were civilians.

Acts of war are defensive in theory, but offensive in practice. By the time war is conducted, there is no room for discretion. The intellect is driven to prevail and emotions are driven by fear. We not only support this but support situations that lead to it. This includes leaders who accept it, cultures that condone it, and economies that prosper from it.

It should be clear to us all that as long as we're paying for the armies to fight wars, we are responsible for them. We will say, "Yes, but we only fight just wars!" This is exactly the point: the people we install will justify anything, and we think that's okay.

It's not really the tyrant's mentality that's the problem. There will always be sociopaths and there will always be nice people making destructive machines. The problem lies with those of us who either support building the machines, give sociopaths the power to use them, or are indifferent to the consequences.

Change

I see three causes of this problem:

1. the power to wage war, which is a power that we create;

2. the authority to wage war, which we fail to control; and

3. a collective feeling of responsibility, which we don't have.

These all relate to our individual failure to integrate our darker nature. This is closely related to our resistance, fear, and sorrow. We are afraid to develop a full emotional awareness of our effects on others, our environment, and ourselves. This stems from our emotional sorrow in fully remembering and empathizing with our past and our low self-esteem.

Just as we build weapons to protect our territories, we build armor to protect our egos. The seeds of indifference grow into culture-wide attitudes of entitlement. Some of us try to improve ourselves more than others. But many of us feel no obligation, and there is no social imperative for self-improvement. Social and personal isolation is a pervasive social attitude to which we've grown indifferent. This is hidden by choreographed behavior, useless social interaction, and ineffectual involvement.

To go down another layer, emotional disconnection is considered good professional practice. As managers, we watch the bottom line leaving morality to religion. As therapists, we're told, "Don't make friends with your clients." Have unconditional positive regard, but have no personal investment in it. Much of what the therapy profession does maintains the status quo. I don't toe this line.

Nations go to war because their citizens are maladjusted. People are reluctant to heal themselves or their families. Healing isn't always happy, it can also mean setting boundaries, starting over, or opening up to one's own disquiet. It means entering the dark side. This is not simply transference and counter-transference, but matters of incidental reflex and projection. There is always a dark side. Real therapy takes risks.

Major dysfunctions at the top of Maslow's pyramid of needs have their roots in thousands of smaller dysfunctions at the base. The top of the pyramid is the area of spiritual discretion, while the base is the realm of necessity. The base is also the foundation of personality and unexamined needs. Intellect holds this pyramid together. We use thinking to get what's necessary. This is thought's main purpose. But comfort requires more than thinking. Intellect is the boat we sail, but emotions are the currents of the ocean. As Homer wrote in *The Iliad & the Odyssey*, take any boat you like, but the ocean will determine your fate.

Greater empathy starts with each of us. We all can become more sensitive. We don't have to know why, gain more power from it, or notice a change in those around us. Small changes won't make big differences, and even big differences may change nothing. The pace of change is set by the currents that distribute it.

The change required today, from global war-mongering to global stewardship, is at least as great as our path out of the Dark Ages. That took 600 years, but change happens faster today. I guess meeting today's challenges will take us 300 years. We can be subversive, and we can cause change, but we have to stick our necks out. As a hypnotherapist, I'm told to avoid giving unrequested suggestions. That is unacceptable. I'll drop the seed of greater empathy into my client's unawareness without waiting to be asked. I'll plant seeds in an effort at reforesting empathy.

Healing has many levels, and there are many perspectives to any story. As a therapist, I've learned that the presenting problem is a symptom. The real problem lies deeper down. The problems of culture lie further down still, in our personal darkness, but you can see them if you know where to look.

In his book *LSD and the Mind of the Universe*, Christopher Bache (2019a), a morally well-grounded and otherwise innocent professor of religious studies, arranged over 70 carefully planned and supported LSD excursions into the depths of his psyche. These gradually deepening excursions took him to the depths of humanity's hell. They left asking himself,

"Where is this place and why am I here?" He concluded it was really there. Current events remind us that hell is alive and well.

> "We have to face our shadow in order to get to the gold on the other side of the shadow... how many of our children and grandchildren are going to have to die before we will be willing to make the changes that we are not willing to make today?"
> — **Chris Bache** (2019b), religious scholar

We can ask ourselves, "How would your situation change if you had greater feelings for others, and they for you?" We can suggest a growing concern for the safety of others and that others have greater concern for us. In a more empathic world, you see others differently, you understand them more deeply, and they will react with a deeper understanding toward you.

We are never healing just one person. Every person who comes to us represents part of our whole species' thought form. Big healing works to heal what is big, but it also heals us as individuals.

> "Most of us Westerners are afraid of spiritual phenomena. They are strange to us. We need some conceptual context to help us make sense of these phenomena so that we can be more at peace with our own and more supportive of others' spiritual awakening."
> — **Emma Bragdon**, psychotherapist (2006)

References

Bache, C. M. (2019a). *LSD and the Mind of the Universe, Diamonds from Heaven.* Park Street Press.

Bache, C. M. (2019b Jan 1). "Conversation with Christopher Bache." *Journal for the Study of Radicalism 13* (1): 155–178. https://doi.org/10.14321/jstudradi.13.1.0155

Bragdon, E. (2006). *A Sourcebook for Helping People with Spiritual Problems, 2nd Edition.* Lightening Up Press.

Gedeon, J. (2022, Feb. 23). "Trump Calls Putin 'Genius' and 'Savvy' for Ukraine Invasion." *Politico.com.* https://www.politico.com/news/2022/02/23/trump-putin-ukraine-invasion-00010923

Kingsley, P. (1999). *In the Dark Places of Wisdom,* Golden Sufi Center.

Kubrick, S. (1964). *Dr. Strangelove or: How I Learned to Stop Worrying and Love the Bomb.*

https://youtu.be/LNC0YwuGLqg

Matthews, C. (2022 Mar. 8). "'Xi Is Using Putin as a Test Tube.' Here's How China Is Assessing the U.S.'s Russia Sanctions as It Eyes Conflict with Taiwan." *MarketWatch.com.* https://www.marketwatch.com/story/xi-is-using-putin-as-a-test-tube-heres-how-china-is-assessing-the-u-s-s-russia-sanctions-as-it-eyes-conflict-with-taiwan-11646766286

Powell, J. (2014 May/Jun). *Woodrow Wilson's Great Mistake.* Cato Institute. https://www.cato.org/policy-report/may/june-2014/woodrow-wilsons-great-mistake

E4 – An Unusual Awareness

Sept. 11, 2019

In your hypnopompic state, you may be able to clarify issues otherwise inaccessible to you.

"I know how much a dream can be worth, but, alas… 'Hello.'"
— **Richard Brautigan**, from his short story *The Library*.

Lucidity

In my book about lucidity (Stoller 2019), I emphasize that lucidity is becoming more aware. And depending on what state you're in, becoming more aware can mean different things. There is not one state of greater awareness. There is not one state of enlightenment. There are many states of awareness, and you can become more enlightened in any of them.

I'm involved with hypnotherapy and for me, that means leading people into states of greater self-awareness. Hypnosis itself is not a state of greater awareness, though it's not a state of lesser awareness, either, as it's sometimes misunderstood to be. Hypnosis is more like a dream state, and dream states are states of great potential.

My research in dreams and hypnosis has led me to an article by David Kahn and Allan Hobson (2003) called "Dreaming and Hypnosis as Altered States of the Brain-Mind." This article talks about the discernible differences in brain states between hypnosis and sleep. In one experiment, it's observed that people just waking up are more able to make creative associations than when they're fully awake.

This connection between dreams and hypnosis was also brought to my attention by a client who deals with inner conflict only when they wake up. We overlook these brief states of being between asleep and awake. The parallels between my client's experience and these laboratory observations show something interesting is going on.

The state of transitioning to wakefulness is called the hypnopompic state. The definition should be more specific because it's an important state that can play a useful role in your waking life. I'll focus on the hypnopompic state when awakening from a dream.

The Hypnopompic State

Hypnosis is said to be a state in which you're vulnerable to suggestion. Hypnosis is a way to change inclinations or plant suggestions, leading to a better state of mind. There is a fair amount of discussion over the meaning of better and worse, and whether bad ideas can be implanted.

It's said that ideas cannot be implanted if they go against your will, but this doesn't make much sense. Most people exhibit a great variety of wills, and most of us are full of tendencies that are not only negative but self-destructive. I tread carefully when someone gives me access to their inner feelings, not just because I don't want to offend them, but because I don't want to mislead them. A person in hypnosis accepts the spin that's put on any idea. As in a dream, a hypnotized person seems to take things at face value. What is accepted in hypnosis sticks at an emotional level, and what you accept in a dream may stick as well.

Our brain's analytical functions largely limit the way we experience things. Our mind works to give us a smaller view of what's going on outside us. This must be so, because any analytical picture of reality is just one version of several. The more you can focus, the more you can attend to the details, and the fewer details there are to attend to. By analyzing what we see, we attempt to make sense of what's going on; and we usually think we succeed, but we never really do. We limit ourselves to what we think we see.

Out of Thin Air

We contrive the agreement between what we think and what we perceive. Our ability to fabricate reason is the foundation of hypnotic suggestion. This changes our fabricated memory, leaving our sense of free will intact. Reason floats over emotion like a spectator explaining a magic trick. Hypnosis speaks to your inner viewer; your inner viewer controls the actions that you think are of your free will. But your inner viewer is not your identity. Your inner viewer does not speak directly to your conscious mind. What you think of as free will is an explanation you concoct after the fact.

You are convinced free will precedes your decision to act, but it does not. Even as you're forming your decisions to act, you're making up your reasons for the way you feel. Stage hypnotists make use of this by inciting ridiculous actions in fully awake people who then fabricate ludicrous explanations of their behavior. The lesson is clear: your conscious mind is making everything up as you go along. It's not really controlling anything that you do—it's your subconscious that's deciding. Your conscious mind is just reading the press release.

There are limits to this, and you might regain conscious control. Some people don't fall for suggestion. We can't identify the factions of mind that vie for control. We've noticed certain aspects of more hypnotizable people, but there's no simple test of who is suggestible, or how suggestible they might be. In order to get you to act on a hypnotic suggestion, there must be some part of you that will go along with it. Under normal circumstances, you can't manipulate a person to violate fundamental aspects of themselves.

Here, again, dreams are an interesting counterpoint. We don't have dreams that are completely unrecognizable; there is always some level of reality in them. That does not mean our dreams are always understandable; in fact, they usually are not understandable. Our dreams are our inner viewer talking to us. The confusing nature of dreams is a measure of the vastly different mode of thinking between your inner viewer and you.

In the movie *Arrival*, the protagonist, a linguist, is tasked with communicating with a highly developed alien intelligence. She eventually figures out that the aliens do not experience time and space the way we do. They experience many simultaneous realities over many periods of time. When the movie ends, we're left to wonder what kind of awareness this could be. It's like the holistic awareness of our inner viewer. It's that alien.

Dreaming takes advantage of our free time to rearrange, reconsider, and consolidate what was or might have been. That is also why we forget our dreams. Most of our dreams are a sense-making process, they are not the final version of anything. To remember all our dreams would produce a result more confusing than a plot built from all the ideas the author discarded. A lot of it would just appear as confusing garbage to our analytical prefrontal cortex. Dreams are multi-dimensional cubist paintings. Our ego has the mind of a child. It can be no other way. Order is built from disorder, and it's disorder that's presented to us.

Cat and Mouse

Last night I had a strange dream. I am where I grew up and I have a dog. I am close to dogs, but I cannot see this dog. A large orange cat appears, and it is teasing the dog. We never had a cat when I was growing up. The cat has brought in a mouse and released it. Someone has picked up the cat as the mouse runs down the hall. I shout, "Let the cat go!" The cat pounces on the mouse, bites it on its back, and releases it again. The mouse twists around as I pick it up by the tail. It's terrified, but it's not a mouse—it's a gerbil, and I had pet gerbils. This wasn't a wild animal; it was my pet.

I'm not completely awake, but I'm waking up. I'm in the hypnopompic state where I can still create images. I resolve to take the mouse outside. The action is now in my mind, the mouse in my hand, and I am heading outside. I'm feeling resolved, but without a conclusion, and it seems I've run out of time. I feel the state slipping away as if I'm being sucked out of direct experience and into the normal waking sense of being lost in the world.

I'm entering the latter part of the hypnopompic state in which one is relaxed, mostly awake, and mentally fluid. It's as if I'm in contact with two conversations at once—one is considering the dream, and the other is starting to think. I want to be in contact with all of what's happening, which I do by sitting with the whole feeling. Then I take the situation into my body.

I identify four entities in the dream: the dog, the cat, the mouse, and my stress. I get in touch with sensations in my body: my heart, my gut, my genitals, and my feet, and I associate one of these entities with each of those body sensations. The dog goes into my heart, the cat into my gut, the mouse into my genitals, and I let the stress settle into my feet. Then I just let myself marinate as I rise into wakefulness.

Nothing happens. My mind is unclear, but my anxiety settles. I become grounded. This is not a logical process; I did not rationalize these connections. I simply let things arrange themselves in ways that seemed right, and this is something that one can more easily do in the hypnopompic state. I can still feel those places now. The entities are no longer ideas; they're feelings, and my body will process them.

My initial feelings were a reflex. A deeper connection comes from realizing these feelings don't pertain to an event but are an ongoing sense of being. I initially felt I needed resolution, but it's not resolution I need—it's introspection. This might take hours or days, but now that I have embodied the dream, it will happen.

Thinking from an Altered State

We think we wake up from dreams but, rather, we contract into a reduced state. It's not that we're lost in a dream—it's that we no longer exist as who we consider ourselves to be. While we are dreaming, we are a larger, more self-aware person.

Waking up is a state few of us take advantage of, but we can. According to Kahn and Hobson, you are more creative in this state. In *Becoming Lucid* (Stoller 2019), I offer a guided visualization to further explore this state. In it, I lead you to new ideas and help you watch them as you wake up.

That brief state of waking up is a time when you can be receptive to insights that might otherwise evade you. But you may also encounter conflicts that you otherwise overlook. This creative state is available to all of us.

Becoming Lucid explores what you can become lucid of in your waking state, your sleeping state, and the two states that separate them, the hypnopompic and the hypnagogic (falling asleep) states. Each of these states offers different doors to lucidity, and to different kinds of lucidity.

Read the book for more details. It's available in digital, print, or audiobook formats.

References

Kahn, D, & Hobson, A. (2003). "Dreaming and Hypnosis as Altered States of the Brain-Mind." *Sleep and Hypnosis* 5(2): 58-71. https://www.sleepandhypnosis.org/ing/Pdf/8365c49769944e359320fab7a052d933.pdf

Stoller, L. (2019). *Becoming Lucid; Self-Awareness in Sleeping and Waking States*. Mind Strength Books. https://www.mindstrengthbalance.com/becominglucidbook/

E5 – Thinking, Time, and Identity

March 3, 2023

How nonlinearity can help you understand your mind, your thoughts, and your future.

"Intelligence is something we are born with. Thinking is a skill that must be learned." — **Edward de Bono**, MD, psychologist, author, and inventor

"Being able to 'think out of the box' presupposes you were able to think in it." — **Bob Lutz**, Vice President of Ford, General Motors, and Chrysler.

Linear Thinking: Sequential, Causal

Many things come naturally to us, but thinking is not one of them. Many things are taught to us; thinking is not one of them. Some forms of thinking are taught, such as logic, but there are many forms. We primarily employ two forms of thinking: linear and emotional. We develop these by mirroring the behavior of others.

Linear thinking is sequential and causal, and it forms a template for our perception. We learn to see in terms of sequence and we learn to think in terms of causes. Our constantly rationalizing minds attach the notions of sequence and cause to all we see in the world. And if we don't see it—and, in fact, most of the time we don't see it—we make it up. We make it up so much that not only won't we see what doesn't fit this model, but we can't.

You cannot "see" something for what it is if you don't understand it. You can see something you misunderstand, but you cannot see something you don't understand: it does not compute. As a result, our sense of self is limited to our perception of time and thought. These are mental constructions.

Nothing exists as we measure it. Measurements are just an imprint; they are containers we force objects into. No actual object can be reduced to a measurement. We measure the imprint, not the thing.

Consider your foot. You measure its length from heel to toe, approximate its width, and then try on a shoe. The best shoes are built to fit our feet, but those are expensive and take time to construct. Instead, we try to find a close fit and hope the shoes will mold to our feet. No foot is the measurement of it, but if we take enough of the right measurements, we hope to get close.

Time does not exist as we measure it. What does a second have to do with anything? To us, time is a sequence of events scarcely measured, fleetingly recalled, and not understood. That's enough to get by as long as things remain ordered. The problem is that we think that is all there is and, as with any habit, that becomes all we perceive and imagine. With effort, you can perceive and imagine more. If you cannot, then you will not understand most of the workings of the world, which are not linear.

Linear thinking proceeds in steps and, just as in walking, these steps only touch the ground at isolated points. These are the points of experience, and between them, there is only the assumption of continuity. When "A causes B" we're asked to accept the reality of A and B, and to take on faith the notion of cause. In physics, cause is based on an abstract notion of invariance, but just about everywhere else, cause is metaphysical. Linear thinking is a metaphysical chain of perceptions.

Circular Thinking: Deluded, Deceptive

Circular thinking is a flawed approach to nonlinear thinking, though many people are drawn to it. Circular thinking attempts to solve a problem by connecting dots that follow a linear path that concludes at the point where it started. All arguments for the existence of God or gods are circular because they start and end with what cannot be explained. A concluding argument that follows a hidden path back to its starting point can appear logical, consistent, and substantive. And it is all of these things, but it's also wrong. Like all tautologies, a circular argument is just a restatement of its premise.

We are asked to accept the point to which the circular thinking brings us as embodying a greater understanding, but it is the definition of false thinking. Circular thinking is alive and well in the higher realms of argument, rhetoric, and discourse, where it appears as sophistry. It also pervades the lower realms of gossip, hearsay, and spectacle, where it appears as prejudice. We feel compelled to present a reasoned defense for our beliefs, but we lack the skills or interest to create one. Most of what we hear in politics and conversation is circular thinking.

I was recently privileged to meet an intelligent person who believes the Earth is flat. I much appreciated his showing me some of the evidence for this, which consists mostly of puzzling photographs and conundrums. This was wonderful stuff for the breadth and scope of the ideas it encompassed. The arguments were careful and logical and I could not find the errors in many of them, though I could in some. They were wonderful examples of clear, reasoned, linear thinking assembled to justify their assumptions.

The arguments were frightening for their blindness. They lacked far more than they contained, and in this, they are a brilliant example of thought being used to represent a feeling. They were disguised as reasonable feelings that were entirely emotional. The emotion supporting the flat Earth hypothesis is fear—fear of social control, political exploitation, and organized deception. These are all valid fears. Circular thinking does not resolve these fears, is powerless, and lacks understanding. It can lead to paranoia, but it can also create a community of cult-like believers.

Nonlinear Thinking: Chaotic, Non-rational, Creative

Nonlinear thinking departs from being sequential and risks losing its logical bearing. At the same time, nonlinear thinking allows you to see the multiplicity of the world. Structures emerge from the multiplicity of the world. The greater the multiplicity you can see—which is to say, the connections between many things—the greater the structures you will comprehend. And by "greater" I mean larger in scope, size, time, duration, or effect. A galaxy is a gigantic structure, but so is a chromosome.

The ignorance of most specialists follows from the limits of their thinking. These boundaries constrain their thinking to a circumscribed domain. We are all guilty of this ourselves because we need to quickly predict sequential events. Nonlinear thinking makes it harder to put ideas together effectively.

Understanding is not the same as performing or reacting, and our understanding is often tested by situations that require us to predict where things are headed. Nonlinear thinking does not lend itself to rapid predictions. But whatever it does, it is equal to or more insightful than linear thinking. Charting the path for a rocket to travel to the moon requires linear thinking. Understanding climate change requires nonlinear thinking.

To think non-linearly requires giving up the title of being an expert. I know many smart people who cannot think non-linearly because their sense of self is attached to their authority. To think non-linearly, you must admit your ignorance. Only the most able people do this. This is a serious political problem because politics fosters order, not insight, and in some conditions, these cannot be combined (Hitchen 2022).

The paradox is that by thinking non-linearly, you become smarter, but few people can do it and most people are not allowed to. In most situations, control is more important than understanding. The first step to becoming smarter, in this sense, is recognizing your attachment to authority and control.

Emotional Thinking: Insightful, Intuitive, Experiential

I am working to better understand emotion. It's a hot topic. I have some useful things to say, but I cannot yet distill them. I will only say that I feel emotion, as a general thing, is a form of collective intelligence. Emotion embodies entire blocks of experience. Different emotions represent different experiences.

Emotion does not lend itself to thinking, as we know thinking to mean. It is closer to a form of interpreted perception. We experience emotion; we don't construct it. Emotion informs us; we don't assemble it. In this, emotion, or the totality of our emotions, provides direction for us. People who are emotionally disturbed, dis-regulated, or dysfunctional have an impaired sense of direction or, as I prefer to say, they cannot understand the truth.

We don't learn to think emotionally, but think using emotional perception. The processes and conclusions of this kind of thinking, which I'm calling emotional thinking, differ from reasoned thinking. It's still the same "us" that's thinking. We feel ourselves into existence more than we think ourselves into existence.

To some extent, we learn to think emotionally; but to a larger extent, we are born with the ability to perceive emotionally. What we learn is how to assemble, apply, and react using emotions. Some of us are much better than others at this. There is a wide spectrum of emotions and a wide spectrum of skills.

I believe emotional thinking is a key to thinking non-linearly because emotional thinking is neither logical nor sequential. It is reasonable in its own way, and those emotional reasons enable us to use emotions as a foundation for how we feel about the world. Unfortunately, there is little agreement on or training in emotional reasoning. This is the focus of my work.

Time: Nonlocal, Non-sequential, Multi-threaded

The perception of sequential time is a cognitive trap. Time appears to proceed from the past to the future. We see this between both the longest and the shortest events we can discern. But this does not mean that time proceeds at the same pace, or in the same small steps over larger spans of time as over smaller ones. The non-linearity of things, the chaos that prevails at small scales, and the unpredictability of things, means that we don't really know how things proceed.

The environment in which things occur, be that ecological, atomic, social, or astronomical, is shaped by things that happen slowly, quickly, near, and far. A layering of different things, sporadically connected, supports or creates other structures which themselves emerge, interact, and disappear, only to have an effect at distant times and places. We try to make sense of this, but there are forces we cannot make sense of because, like asteroids, they appear so rarely or not at all. Yet, when they do appear, they can change everything.

It is not that time is a fiction, though it might be—it's that our sense of all things being well-ordered, recognized, and recorded at every instant is a fiction. There is much in our universe that simply does not exist now as we know it, did not exist in the past, and will not exist as we presume in the future. These "things," or events out of which we assemble our time-ordered reality, are metaphysical. They are concepts grounded in indirect observations and erroneous theories. To be clear: all observations are indirect, and all theories are erroneous.

Identity: Self-awareness, Focus, Meaning

None of this would be a problem were it not for our habit of building our behavior based on predictions of the future. If we were less cerebral, we would simply form habitual patterns that did not extrapolate into the future. We might call these "zero order theories" in that they predict no change in any pattern: the days repeat, as do the seasons, and other phenomena. But we don't do this. Instead, we predict change based on our thinking, and we position ourselves for it. Rather than waiting for consequences, we endeavor to make them.

We ask if animals think and feel. I assume they do, and most would agree. I wonder, instead, who they think they are? I don't mean whether they think they are, as I assume they do, but who?

We, as humans, are what we create ourselves to be. We have an identity, and that seems partly to be our ego, or our ability to make statements about ourselves. A few weeks ago, I asked this question of who we think we are. I was told our sense of self was just our mind's attempt to envision itself. "You have a soul!" I was told, to which I said, "Thank you!" But that was not really the question.

I was not asking whether I could conceive myself as something, but what that "thing" amounted to. To say, "It is your soul" is flat-earth thinking. It is linear, as it requires no new thinking, and circular, as it leaves you just where you started. It's certainly metaphysical, which also misses the point. The question is: of all the nonlinear things in the universe that I comprise, how much of them do I appreciate?

I believe this is a valid question, but I also believe it does not admit an answer in the system from which it's asked. There are other ways of thinking that are more expansive and inclusive than linear thinking—ways that do not presuppose that time scans existence like a moving spotlight. Ways that are not based on perception and prediction. Maybe we can't know them, but that's our problem.

References

Hitchens, T. (2022 Aug 11). "The Nuclear 3-Body Problem: STRATCOM 'Furiously' Rewriting Deterrence Theory in a Tripolar World." *Breaking Defense*. https://breakingdefense.com/2022/08/the-nuclear-3-body-problem-stratcom-furiously-rewriting-deterrence-theory-in-tri-polar-world/

E6 – Consilience: Reason and Emotion

June 20, 2020

Consilience: the linking together of principles from different disciplines to form a comprehensive theory.

"Salvation is not a reward for the righteous, it is a gift for the guilty."
— **Steve Lawson**, author and pastor

Learning

Learning is change. We use the term "learning" to mean something conscious or intentional, but even if we're unmotivated or the change is unintentional, learning still changes us. We also talk about machine learning, and we can think of species learning, or environmental learning.

When we think about learning, we think about teaching, as the two seem to go together. But who teaches a machine, species, or environment? Learning describes something that happens, teaching is a concept we've invented. What we call teaching is an act of changing the environment so that learning, which happens anyway, happens differently. The best learning is accomplished without teaching.

Teaching is interference to bring things to the learner's attention. There has long been a confused discussion whether better learning requires better teachers or better learners. We observe that better performance, happiness, security, and control follows from better learning. We presume it comes from better teaching.

We focus on the credentials of teachers but not on the quality of teaching—if teaching even exists as a quality. Certainly, some situations are more conducive to learning than others. Some of those more conducive situations involve people designated as teachers, but, as most people would agree, the most important learning doesn't involve people who see their role as teachers.

I've studied under teachers ranging from abysmal to award-winning. They were all teachers in the sense that they were not emotionally invested in my learning. The best were perfectionists, but not passionate about me. And from the best of these, I was given reams of details in the subjects that interested me. Little was useful because it was not exciting, and they did not inspire me.

I have learned from passionate people. They were mentors who were personally and specifically involved with me and the subject. Some of these people were not smart or insightful, but they were involved and sincere. The details I learned from them required the heat of emotion and personal meaning.

For example, a college student learns many things, but most of what he or she learns doesn't happen in classes taught by teachers. Similarly, most of what parents and warriors learn is not learned in school but on the battlefront. What we learn is embedded in our character. Who teaches this?

Evolution is a learning process. Evolution can be variously described, and natural selection —the old Darwinian idea—is the accepted description. Natural selection does not arise from basic physical laws, but it's easy to understand and simulate in a lab or using a machine.

Natural selection is anthropomorphic. We make selections, so we presume nature does too. Even when combined with random mutation, natural selection is insufficient to explain the incrementally positive changes in form and function (Gurova 2010; Laland et al. 2014). Molecular genetics has found a host of nonrandom evolutionary mechanisms (Shapiro 2023).

Structures change in order to explore the consequences of the as-yet unattainable. In thought, we call this dreaming; in atomic and particle physics, we call it tunneling. In psychology, it has been called "the collective unconscious."

In evolution, we don't recognize it at all. That is because evolutionary biologists do not recognize what Rupert Sheldrake calls "the morphic field" (Sheldrake 2006). I don't recognize it either, but I accept that some additional thing is going on.

It is worth digressing to clarify that the notion of physical laws is based on the assertion that things follow patterns. Suggestions that there are unexplained patterns, such as the idea of morphic resonance, are invitations to observe new things in need of explanation. Asserting that statements of the unexplained constitute a theory is itself a kind of morphic field, which Sheldrake maintains with a plethora of unreferenced claims. They are not theories or hypotheses, and cannot be approached in this form.

> "But no one knows what these fields are or how they work."
> — **Rupert Sheldrake** (2006, 32)

Presenting invitations to new thinking as conjectures of new theories invites confusion. As invitations, these suggestions of incompleteness lack any demonstrable or even conceivable mechanism. The empiricist cannot measure them. Since they assert that our knowledge is inadequate, the theorist is threatened by them. They require a creative scientist to appreciate them, or a self-confident person, at least.

There are few such scientists, and the science culture works to exclude and devalue such people. As a result, the people who have explored the perimeters of what we believe we understand are denigrated as outsiders or nonconformists. This disrespect has been experienced by every creative scientist. Creative thinkers are only accepted when their ideas generate money and power.

This cultural behavior is itself evolutionary. It rewards the short-term gain of power, not the long-term gain of progress. When we think logically, we recognize and test the choices, accepting some and rejecting others.

The natural world does not operate this way. Natural processes do not evolve through thought, consideration, argument, conjecture, testing, and application. Humans display this in the evolution of consensus, but ecologies operate by some other means.

This is quite important. If evolution—or learning—followed logic, doing only what yielded the greatest advantage, then exceptions would not occur. For this reason, random mutations, otherwise known as mistakes, must be added for ecological selection to work.

Ecological selection, or "natural selection," is a process of exclusion. It is a destructive, not a creative process. It works to exclude options that offer fewer rewards. It does not create more rewarding options.

Creating something better remains a process we cannot explain. We have a theory of how this happens in quantum mechanics. It's called the theory of least action. It works because it is forward-looking in time. Quantum mechanical systems "see" the future and "remember" the past.

We have a mystical theory of how this happens in consciousness. It's called insight or inspiration. Darwinian evolution plays this role in biology, but what it involves is unclear, and what it predicts does not adequately explain many things, such as morphogenesis, which is the evolution of new forms.

Ecological systems learn through nonlogical means. We might call them statistical, many-threaded, or holographic. Most learning in nature occurs in a chaotic fashion in which old structures collapse and new ones emerge. Much of our learning is done by nonlogical means. There's more to our learning process than what's rational because there is so much more to us than our rational awareness.

I suggest using the word rational instead of logical because we rarely use logic. Logic rests on certainty while reason only requires the plausible, and that's usually all we have. We develop strategies based on what's plausible.

This happens at a superficial level. Making strategies is how we test things, but it's not how we learn things. Most of our learning is done by association, metaphor, and emotion. This allows for creativity.

Covid-19 is a learning situation. The chaos the virus has fomented—disorganized as it might be—is a learning environment. The "solution" to the Covid-19 "problem" is not a rational strategy because none of the rational strategies available are big enough. Covid-19 is here because we've been thinking too small for too long.

The virus has exposed aspects of our social structure that we have ignored. Not the reasoned personal and national identities we believe define us, but the way individuals and groups find direction. And how have we been deceived into making flawed decisions? We designed our parents, teachers, and leaders to teach them to us. Our parents, teachers, and leaders are our "morphic field."

Reason

I offer you three related points of view: physics, neuroscience, and behavior. As you move from the first to the second to the third, the rules governing behavior degenerate toward chaos.

Part of this is historical. It's certainly easier to learn, teach, and navigate systems that are well-ordered. It's easier to write history according to the fiction that causes and events made sense. One version of events provides a rationale for the narrative. But as one's awareness broadens, the reality that chaos is a dominant force becomes clear.

When you study any historical event, you "go down the rabbit hole." This means that what's going on under the surface is unlike what we see on the surface. It also refers to rabbit holes as full of passageways, rooms, twists, turns, and alternative destinations. The rabbit hole metaphor is a more accurate description of history and a better model for learning.

Things are organized and logical in isolation. The number of choices can be limited. As systems get larger and more components interact, we're quickly overwhelmed with choices, forces, and outcomes. Chaos is just a label for a situation we no longer understand.

We can't understand big, complicated systems because we cannot contain them in our awareness. The human brain may be the most complicated system in the universe, but it can barely cope with the reality it confronts. You can barely remember a string of over seven digits, and you can only hold one thought in your head at one time. We're underpowered given the problems we face.

Our minds can operate holistically, and most of our learning happens this way. This is what dreams are, and this is what we spend all of our sleeping time doing, though we remember next to none of it. We are probably also dreaming while we are awake without being aware of it. We actually have many mental processes going on at once, with the conscious, logical process being the only one we're aware of.

Understanding our experience of Covid-19—our understanding of anything, really— depends on our incorporating multiple perspectives. No one perspective is complete and no one story is complete.

Looking for a "complete description" is a dead end. There is none because the virus lies at the intersection of many systems. Many of these systems were not designed, or did not evolve, to respond to this infection. The virus has disrupted medicine, politics, economics, science, genetics, and ecology, not to mention your physiology and metabolism. No story written from any of these points of view will be complete.

Awareness

We think of attention as an action, as "to pay attention," but it's also a state, as "to be attentive." We identify attention with awareness and apply the binary quality of awareness—of either being aware or unaware—with a binary quality of attention, either paying attention or not.

> "My experience is what I agree to attend to."
> — **William James**, psychologist

Watching brain states reveals that attention lies on a spectrum. One can only pay attention to what one can discern, and discernment requires change. Our minds need change in order to maintain focus, which is why we use rosaries, mantras, dialog, legends, and spectacle to hold our attention. It's next to impossible to meditate on nothing; you can do it only by going into an intermittent state of thoughtless awareness, a kind of listening state with distant boundaries.

As your brainwaves become faster, you become more attuned to rapid changes and memories of shorter duration. I also believe slower brainwaves enable you to be more aware of slower changes and memories of longer duration.

More extensive memories support a more integrated understanding, while narrower memories collect greater detail. Childhood is dominated by more extensive memories, which is one reason we lose touch with those memories as we age and our focus turns to memories of shorter duration.

The character of your brainwaves changes with your situation, your age, your energy level, and the time of day. You can also train your brainwaves. With practice, you can voluntarily control what you're aware of. This hyper-focus supports higher-level performance (Thomas

2018).

The character of your thoughts and speech follow the nature of your focus. The range of your brainwaves—which is your focus—defines your personality, your responses to your environment, the ideas you hold, and the friends you make.

To one extent, this is obvious: when your brainwaves stop, you're dead. But to another extent, it's profound: you can change your awareness. We don't know how much control you can gain, or the full range of characteristics controlled by it, but controlling your brainwaves controls your ability to attend. You can voluntarily become more aware, engaged, and insightful.

Identity

You are what you're aware of. This is quite different from your personality.

Your personality determines your success in your interactions with other people, but not your control over your environment. Patience, temperateness, and good humor will help you solve problems, but intelligence, insight, and artistry exist in a different realm.

Our personality is shaped by school, work, and society, and is a measure of our maturity. With our personality, we navigate social situations. The major focus of modern schooling—nonsectarian schooling of the last 200 years—is in the shaping of personality.

Our awareness—which includes intelligence, insight, and artistry—is not considered to be a learned skill. Yet, our awareness determines our ability to navigate our environment. My experience training people's brains, and the entire field of neurofeedback therapy, is all about enabling people to become more aware.

You learn through feedback. You stretch your awareness by encountering elements outside your full awareness, but partially within reach. You typically have, or can be directed to have, a small awareness of larger phenomena. Understanding complex music, for example, can be achieved by learning to hear its distinct parts. One experiences a kind of cognitive fine-tuning.

There are limits to how much you can change—you can't become a musician overnight. You can only learn to do later what you can almost do now. New skills build on existing skills. Growth occurs at the boundaries of your awareness.

Before schools were invented, we learned through apprenticeship and play. These forms share a multiplicity of scales, time-frames, and points of view. In its largest sense, nature contains all scales—many more than we're aware of. Nature offers learning situations that cross many boundaries.

The virus is a crash course in environmental education. It has stretched or broken the personality-based structures—like politics and culture—that we build around the idea of control. The virus resulted from a global experiment in production that made humans vulnerable at many levels. From the virus's point of view, globalism has made humans a resource.

Interconnection

People connect with each other through personality, and modern culture is largely personality-based: it's based on our needs, wants, and vulnerabilities. We've become increasingly less aware of our environment as we've become less concerned with it.

We have little control over what we're unaware of, and we're not aware of how vulnerable we've made ourselves to viral transmission and infection. We need to quickly gain more awareness. We need to understand what we've done to enable this virus to appear, infect, and exploit us.

These questions span the gamut from our impact on our environment to how our cells defend themselves. They are not answered by knowing which pharmaceuticals benefit ill patients, which vaccines will protect us, or which policies will restore our economy.

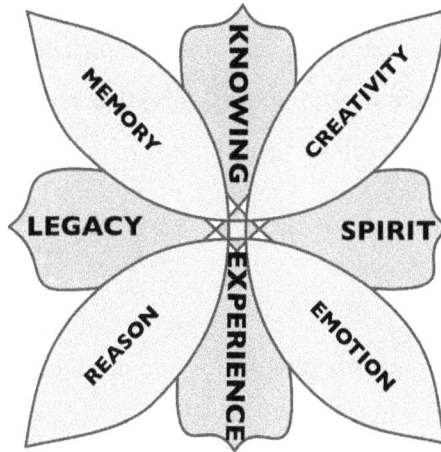

Figure 34: Dichotomies, parallels, similarities, and reflections.

They are not questions being asked by politicians or doctors, although, to give credit where it's due, doctors would like to know all they can. The same can't be said for politicians struggling for power, using the virus as a weapon.

Science

Science emerged from centuries of conflict between reason and emotion. Science advertises reason over emotion, but there is no such thing. Truth, confidence, certitude, and trust are foundational to science and emotional in nature. Science is an alternative use of emotional reasoning, not a replacement of it (Fleck 1979).

A battle for hegemony between untrusting allied superpowers has erupted in the virus's theatre of war. These same acquisitive efforts pulled the virus into the cities and infected the world. Similar to how oil is a positive resource for all nations, the virus is a negative resource all nations want to divest—like a hot potato. It's as if someone pushed the "mutually assured destruction" button and now all nations are fighting for the residuum.

A vaccine will be developed. It will hold the promise of crowning victorious the nation who possesses it. It will be a messenger RNA (mRNA)-based vaccine, similar to other RNA vaccines developed before, none of which have ever been successfully tested or approved (Wood 2020).

These are genetic modifying agents that rearrange your RNA and, perhaps, your DNA. They are not medicines. This new, accelerated vaccine effort, named "Operation Warp Speed," will skip many of the safety and all the long-term tests. It will be interesting to see who we're told should take it first (Boodman 2020), those people who are the most vulnerable, or those people who are the least profitable.

Ecology

To create ecological stability, deepen your positive engagement in each of the multiple levels of the ecology with which you're engaged. This leads to evolutionary options.

Things don't end well for a native species when its native ecology changes. And that's what we are, and this is what's happening to us. We can either adapt to the new ecology, work to restore the old ecology, or do nothing. Our search for pharmaceutical cures, preventative vaccines, and economic restoratives is the third choice: it does nothing to fix the ecological problem.

Solutions offered by conservationists are a combination of restoring the old ecology while doing nothing about the underlying forces that are upsetting it. Technology, which while innovative is largely reactive and weakly adaptive, does not address the ecological problem.

5G networks, electric vehicles, advanced weaponry, and other benefits of technology are not ecologically motivated. Adapting to our ecology would mean changing food production and consumption, and changing the global environmental impact on the land, sea, and air. Few nations can claim any progress. Globally, we can claim none.

The problem is that modern civilization is not designed for environmental sustainability. There have been some civilizations in the past that have done much better, but they had to because they didn't have any alternative. They also didn't have the environmentally destructive power we have now.

Hypnosis

The remarkable doctor, surgeon, and hypnotherapist Dabney Ewin said that "almost anything you can treat with cortisone or antihistamine will probably respond to hypnosis" (Shenefelt 2011). Cortisone is a type of steroid. Another steroid drug, dexamethasone, was recently found to reduce deaths by one-third for severely ill Covid-19 patients (RECOVERY trial 2020).

Over a half million people have died worldwide from Covid-19 as of late June 2020. This number continues to rise linearly, as it has for the last three months. I have heard no mention of the use of hypnotherapy to treat Covid-19 at any stage, despite its efficacy in emergency medicine (Iserson 2014). This was my motivation for writing my book *Covid-19: Illness & Illumination*.

The long-term environmental solution is to change people's awareness. Until people realize their ecological danger and grasp how it results from their actions, they won't change their actions.

Many argue for greater understanding, but understanding only changes when it's consistent with desire. Teaching people why they should want what they don't want—even if they understand what you're saying—is a fear-based strategy. It will not be effective.

People who love the Earth are already concerned with redressing environmental problems. People lacking this connection, or who don't want to address this problem, will only be motivated when their needs are threatened.

The hypnosis presented in each of these chapters is a taste of what might be done. These inductions aim to enhance your self-awareness, enhance your self-control, and expand your environmental awareness.

Like other forms of learning, hypnosis works by leading you beyond what you already know. You must immerse yourself in it to make new connections between old memories and sensations in order for it to create new feelings and levels of awareness. Once you have experienced these and their effect has been positive, you won't lose them.

> "The consilience of doing and being is essential. They must be balanced."
> — **Douglas B. Laney** (2021), Data & Analytics Strategist

Change

"As above, so below" has become a mystical buzzword, which is too bad, because it has a long history and a lot of practical meaning. Rejecting "as above, so below" is a rejection of the connection between opposites. This rejection has been a fundamental driving force in Western culture from before Christianity (Kingsley 1999) and has found its leading proponent in Christianity.

Ecology is the connection of opposites, as well as the connection between many disparate but related elements. The notion of balance is fundamental, and this is not "balance" as in moderation, but balance as in the bringing together of opposites.

It's no coincidence that sustainable cultures have been earth-based, or worshiped deities based on the Earth. They worshiped nature incarnate, rather than a dis-incarnated divine. Restoring ecological balance requires recognizing the ecosystem's importance as both fundamental and overarching. Humans have long fought over religion and gotten nowhere, but a conflict between all peoples and the environment—such as this virus and other ecological consequences present—is a conflict of a different order.

The rationalist in me would like to say that developing a sustainable ecology is a practical problem, but I suspect it's not. It's a spiritual problem, as it certainly is for those who revere the Earth. It certainly requires of people something more than a rational commitment. It is spiritual in the sense that spirit motivates action.

If a microscopic, ubiquitous, almost non-living thing can play a role in turning the minds, values, and behaviors of the Earth's dominant and disruptive species—which is us—then "as above, so below" is more than just a buzzword.

> "Religion and philosophy are to be preserved as distinct. We are not to introduce divine revelations into philosophy, nor philosophical opinions into religion."
> —**Isaac Newton**, physicist, alchemist, and theologian

References

Boodman, E. (2020 Mar 11). "Researchers Rush to Test Coronavirus Vaccine in People without Knowing How Well It Works in Animals." *STAT Health*.

https://www.statnews.com/2020/03/11/researchers-rush-to-start-moderna-coronavirus-vaccine-trial-without-usual-animal-testing/

Fleck, L. (1979). *The Genesis and Development of a Scientific Fact.* University of Chicago Press.

Gurova, L. (2010 May) "Fodor vs. Darwin: A Methodological Follow-up." *OAI.* https://www.researchgate.net/publication/44022043_Fodor_vs_Darwin_A_Methodological_Follow-Up

Iserson, K.V. (2014). "An Hypnotic Suggestion: Review of Hypnosis for Clinical Emergency Care." *Journal of Emergency Medicine*, **46**(4). https://www.researchgate.net/publication/259959216_An_Hypnotic_Suggestion_Review_of_Hypnosis_for_Clinical_Emergency_Care

Kingsley, P. (1999). *In the Dark Places of Wisdom*, The Golden Sufi Center Publishing.

Laland, K., et al. (2014 Oct 9). "Does Evolutionary Theory Need a Rethink?" Nature, 9 (14): 161-64. https://www.nature.com/articles/514161a

Laney, D. B. (2021 Oct. 5). "Digital Mindfulness: Being Digital Instead of Doing Digital." *Forbes.* https://www.forbes.com/sites/douglaslaney/2021/10/05/digital-mindfulness-being-digital-instead-of-doing-digital/

RECOVERY Trial (2020 Jun16). "Low-cost Dexamethasone Reduces Death By up to One Third in Hospitalized Patients with Severe Respiratory Complications of COVID-19." https://www.recoverytrial.net/files/recovery_dexamethasone_statement_160620_v2final.pdf

Shapiro, J. A. (2023 Jul 6). "Evolution without Accidents." *Aeon.* https://aeon.co/essays/why-did-darwins-20th-century-followers-get-evolution-so-wrong

Shenefelt, P.D. (2011). "Ideomotor Signaling: From Divining Spiritual Messages to Discerning Subconscious Answers during Hypnosis and Hypnoanalysis, A Historical Perspective." *American Journal of Clinical Hypnosis*, **53**(3):157-167.

Thomas, M. (2018 Mar 15). "To Control Your Life, Control What You Pay Attention To." *Harvard Business Review.* https://hbr.org/2018/03/to-control-your-life-control-what-you-pay-attention-to

Wood, G., and Spiegle, D.A. (2020 Mar 21). "COVID-19 Vaccines Are Coming, But They're Not What You Think," *The Atlantic.* https://www.theatlantic.com/ideas/archive/2020/03/two-extreme-long-shots-could-save-us-coronavirus/608539/

E7 – How Do You Feel?

September 8, 2020

Thoughts are the foundations of thinking. What are the foundations of feeling?

"You need to become fully conscious of your emotions and be able to feel them before you can feel that which lies beyond them." — **Eckhart Tolle**

Be Reasonable

We are designed to be reasonable. It seems that everything that anyone says either tries to be reasonable or tries to show the unreasonableness in something else. Academic studies are all reasonable. Representational art mixes reason with impression. Modern art attempts to provide different reasons. This presumption that reality is reasonable is a mind-box. We might be more critical of it if we knew how limiting it was.

I can think of three alternatives to reason-based reality—two that are human and one that is not. The human alternatives are feeling and impression. The nonhuman one is reflex, physical law, or some other interaction that doesn't require consciousness. To what extent do we consider these alternatives?

I would say that physical law is the domain of science. It is presumed to be reasonable, but reason is something that we add to it. The foundations of physical law are not reasonable— they just are. From them we build a theory to be tested against observation, but what is has the last word regardless of whether we can make any sense of it.

Our notion of what's reasonable is shortsighted, and I'll mention this in passing. I won't go into it, but, to the best of our knowledge, reality is not reasonable. It's recursive. The reality we experience defines itself as what we experience. We only see ourselves in another reality when we're in an altered state of consciousness. It is this recursive property that prevents us from defining our experience in terms of something fundamental. Our attempts to find something more real than what we experience lead us to the classic problems of logic: Russell's

Antinomy, Gödel's Theorem, and the Halting Problem. These logical dead ends tell us that reasonable theories are circular. We can't find a greater understanding than what we experience. I don't know how to add this to the current discussion, so I'll stick with our normal, flawed notion of the reasonable. In this flawed notion, we believe our understanding of ourselves is built on a reliable foundation: a series of logical steps that lead from cause to effect. This is logically impossible, and to tell the truth, we don't really care.

From our linear notion of what's reasonable, we create our objective point of view; and we've extended this to ourselves, viewing our identities as objects that exist. This is a dead end for a host of reasons. For one thing, we're never sure what we're looking at.

Feeling and Impression

Feeling and impression are more fundamental than theory and reason. Neither requires analysis in order for us to experience it; being reasonable is quite unnecessary. You might be tempted to throw all your chips in with feeling and impression, but things are not that simple. It turns out that both require a measure of thinking or, to put it another way, by thinking you can change your feelings and impressions.

This is the root of the paradox: You'd like to layer things in an orderly manner, and it's natural to put one's impressions at the bottom. Then put your feeling about your impressions as your next level of experience. After that, you'd be tempted to say that thinking arrives and you would start throwing concepts around. You might want to believe in these ideas, but this progression is not the way we develop our beliefs.

You have to perceive before you can have experience, as your perceptions exist in your mind. You have to have thought in order to feel. This applies to emotions but not to reflexes, so we must distinguish the two.

We make your lower leg move with the knee-jerk patellar reflex, and you don't need to be conscious for this to work. We can make a severed frog's leg jump with an electric current, and it doesn't even have to be alive. But we can't create an emotion in your conscious mind unless you are aware and minimally cogent.

It takes a lot of thinking to feel emotional about something. Even the simplest emotion, such as the startle reaction, requires knowing what you're seeing. People who were blind from birth and then have their sight restored cannot make sense of what they see. For them, a movie that you and I would find to be a tear-jerker or a thriller is just a lot of colors and shapes. This is not just a "fun fact"—we can make something useful out of this.

Visualize Things

Half of our brains are devoted to vision-related things. "Visualizing things" would be a better term, since external sight is not the issue. External sight is the province of the eye; visualizing is a mental process that operates independent of sight, and blind people "visualize" just as much as sighted people, as odd as that may sound.

Let's take this back to the question of how you feel. Impressions are not enough to make you feel, at least not with regard to the raw perceptions. I'm also talking about the higher feelings, not the reflexive ones. You feel by visualizing, in some general sense. I'm using the term "visualize" to mean that you recreate something in your mind that you've experienced before. This is not a simple process!

We know or think we know that the brain "understands" by recreating experiences it's had before. We're pretty sure of this regarding physical motion, as thoughts of motion involve the same neurons as the actual motions. This is called the "mirror neuron" structure of the brain. It is likely that this extends to thoughts and emotions. I suspect that thinking about an idea or feeling activates the same neurons that are activated when you experience thoughts or feelings. We have no proof of this because we can't locate the neurons where you experience thoughts or feelings in order to check what activates them.

The first insight this affords is that the way you feel is by re-experiencing how you felt before. This may sound obvious and simple, but it's not. The twist lies in appreciating the nuance of memory.

Memory

You don't really remember any "thing"—you build memories on-demand to represent experiences you've stored away in coded form. You may think you remember a red car on a dirt road or a friend's face on a summer evening, but you really don't. You remember the idea, and you recreate the images with whatever is at your disposal.

What you remember are assembled conceptual bits that are just enough to trigger your thoughts. If you've forgotten what kind of car it was, if you even ever knew, this won't stop you from remembering the red car. You'll just substitute any old car. If you've forgotten the details of your friend's face, you'll just airbrush in whatever you find in your memory.

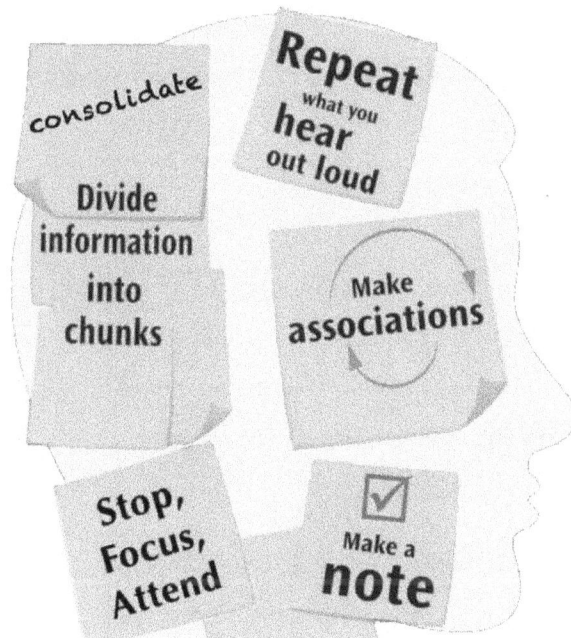

Figure 35: Some mechanisms of remembering.

If you were to focus with laser-like precision on that red car or your friend's face, you would "see" what you recall is your current notion of a red car. You think what your friend's face looks like. You will paste these into your construction of the dirt road or the summer evening. And this is just fine because it's sufficient. How often is your faulty memory ever tested, and so what if your and your friend's memories don't exactly agree? In fact, they never do and we never really care!

This is all cute and interesting. I think it's obvious, but it's rarely mentioned. We confront this in dreams every time we find ourselves holding a newspaper, but cannot read anything that's written on it. Or in a dream when we're holding a telephone but cannot see the numbers or cannot recall what we're supposed to dial.

Our memories of early childhood are often from a third person perspective: seeing ourselves playing or being walked. It depends on the context of the experience. If we're recalling a relationship, then we see ourselves in relationship. If we're recalling an experience, then we see it from a first-person point of view.

Neither of these visual recollections are what we saw in the past. They are reconstructions in the present. The important point that's overlooked is that we really don't have memories per se; we have collected bits and pieces that we reassemble like decoupage when we're asked to describe past events.

The Missing Bits

The reason this is important is that some of us are missing certain bits. We lack certain pieces that are essential for the reconstruction of certain feelings. It is as if we're lacking Lego pieces that are crucial for the construction of certain models. And the reason we're missing these pieces is that they are disturbing. They are like matches or firecrackers—we either lock them away or we dispose of them entirely.

And so it is that some of us, perhaps all of us, cannot feel things that others feel, or we cannot feel them in the same way. Why is it that some people are triggered so much more intensely than others? Why do some people flip out entirely when triggered by things that you think are minor? And why are some people so lacking in emotional affect that they can't love at all?

Here is the crux of the matter: there is much that you're missing. There is much more that you could feel. How do you feel, and what is the depth of your emotional repertoire? Can you expand to a broader range of feelings? You can. There are feelings you have not had or cannot remember having. Do you wonder why you have not yet reached the golden ring of life's contentment? This is why: you cannot remember it so you cannot recreate it.

I need to go one more step to make you see. We all have buried certain pains and frustrations, states of sorrow or anguish from our childhood that brought us to despair. These may have been so extreme that we've forgotten them entirely, or they may have been only extreme enough for us to forget parts of them—the sharpest edges.

But these bits and edges, like sharp pieces of colored glass, are essential in the reconstruction of the full stained-glass windows of our emotions. Without them, we're painting in soft earth tones and cannot recreate the blooms and bright sunrise.

Illumination

You may be able to recover, uncover, or release your pains and frustrations if the strongholds of your personality are willing to let them go. This is the fundamental question of your transformation: Are you ready for it? This is not a rational question because its answer is not to be given by your rational mind. The forgotten pieces are guarded by autonomous, subconscious aspects of yourself that will do what they think is right, regardless of what you want.

Psychotherapeutic methods such as rational emotive therapy, cognitive behavioral therapy, psychoanalysis, and other forms of talk therapy cannot make progress with those aspects of your personality that neither speak nor listen to you. These are effectively other personalities who have been shut out of the conversation or have set up shop outside your consciousness. It is because of them and your separation from them that you go around in circles, looking for a path you cannot find and a doorway that doesn't exist.

There are paths forward and there are doors, but they are in other dimensions. Here are four ways that you can find them.

1. Crisis: the most common way.
2. Reason: a long and repetitive road, like digging out of prison with a spoon.
3. Hypnosis: a direct jump into another dimension.
4. Psychedelics: the human cannonball approach to opening the doors of perception.

I do hypnosis.

E8 – Empathy I – Learn Empathy

December 30, 2020

The basic features of empathy. Why you need it, and what it does for you.

"Normal people have an incredible lack of empathy."
— **Temple Grandin**, animal behaviorist

I've been trying to think about empathy, but nothing happens, so I've been reading about it, hoping I would learn. Now I'm ready to talk about it because I've learned. I've learned that no one knows anything about it, so my ignorance need not hold me back.

There's a colloquial definition of empathy as feeling what other people feel. That might get you somewhere if you knew what other people feel, but how could you? What if I say that I feel what you feel and you say you feel what I feel? Are we empathizing? What if you're feeling blue and I'm feeling green and we describe them both the same way? And what is "feeling" anyway?

A step closer is to say that when I act like you feel, then I'm empathizing. When a person is acting fully and honestly, then that is good enough, but now our experience is based on being authentic and honest, and how well defined are those? As it turns out, authenticity and honesty are poorly defined. Empathy is poorly understood.

Two Sides of the Same Coin?

They say there are two kinds of empathy: emotional and cognitive. Emotional empathy is the feeling part. Having emotional empathy will lead you to act like another person. You will feel their pain, elation, or indifference.

Cognitive empathy is the understanding part. Having cognitive empathy will lead you to understand the thoughts, meanings, and implications that are in another person's mind. They even tell us that these two kinds of emotions can be seen in the brain's structure.

I would like to say that a bigger crock of poo there never was, but that's not true either. Most of the claims of states of mind being visible in structures of the brain are equally nonsense. I'll accept that certain fundamental aspects of fear are managed by the amygdala, and emotional activity connects the frontal cortex to the limbic system, but emotions themselves appear to be distributed throughout the brain. I see no reason to believe thoughts or feelings exist at distinct structural locations.

If we ignore the confused theories and misunderstood pictures of the brain, we can focus on more useful things. Why is it that some aspects of thoughts can be verbalized, while most aspects of feelings cannot be?

There is a discernible difference between similarity in thinking and similarity in feeling. It is possible that sometimes, under some conditions, if you think the thoughts of another long and hard enough, then you might have a glimmer of how they feel. Most of the time, this doesn't work.

You can as easily create a picture in your mind that represents the picture in another person's mind as you can take a photograph. A poor photograph will not capture the essence of what there is to see, but a good one might. And if you can feel what another person feels, then you'll be more likely to create an accurate picture of it.

But you also can learn to take accurate pictures using a formula, just the way you can learn to paint a good landscape using a formula. It won't be a great picture, but it will be good enough to get the job done. And that brings us to the bottom line: face-to-face with what empathy is really about. It's about getting the job done.

The job is the communication of shared experience. If you're 100% empathetic, then you are the other person. You are there and you will act like them, feel what they feel, and think what they think. You must have all three: actions, feelings, and thoughts.

Heroes

People who put themselves at risk to display what we hold to be the best aspects of character are called heroes. Are these people really thinking along the same lines as you and me? Probably not. Probably, they're not thinking clearly at all, they're simply acting in the way they've been trained: to act heroically.

Firefighters, soldiers, and emergency responders can do heroic things. They won't have a good explanation for their actions aside from saying that what they did was the right thing to do. These people are acting as we would like to act, but they're not thinking as we would think. They're probably not thinking about their safety.

When other people act to support our feelings without consideration of their own, it's heroic. If you considered doing this yourself, you'd probably consider yourself stupid. These people share our feelings but not our thoughts. They don't act out of emotion; they act out of training, reflex, or intellect. They are not motivated by empathy.

The Anti-Hero

Psychopaths are, almost by definition, experts at empathetic thoughts. If they're not, then they don't deserve to wear the badge of psychopathy and they're just confused. A psychopath appears to know what you think, and that skill enables them to both survive, manipulate the situation, and avoid detection.

Psychopaths are eventually exposed because they don't follow through with all the actions that are expected. Instead, they go off at right angles, do something completely incongruous, and blow their cover. At least, they would blow their cover if people understood their aberrant behavior was not an accident. This doesn't mean they understand, it just means they have their reasons.

Psychopaths are chameleons. We'd like to believe what we see, and we're easily misled by excuses. We cannot believe that another person would be so disingenuous or malicious as to say the right thing and do the wrong thing, so we believe the excuses.

Many people are disingenuous, and some are very much so. Excuses hide many dysfunctions. We should smarten up to the prevalence of psychopathy. Understanding empathy is a good place to start.

Alexithymia

This funny word refers to someone who doesn't have feelings. Psychopaths don't have feelings, so they're alexithymic, but they know how to seem like they do. That's what distinguishes the psychopath from the alexithymic. The alexithymic has neither. They don't get it and they don't appear to get it.

You know you're in the presence of an alexithymic because they'll give you a blank stare and they won't move, inflect, or attend in the right manner. You argue, cajole, and explain your feelings to an alexithymic, but if your thoughts are based on how you feel, they will not understand you. They'll only appreciate, understand, and agree with reasoning that is congruent with their own. A lot of judges are probably alexithymic. Of course, a good combat soldier should be as well.

Sympathy

Empathy remains difficult to define, but sympathy is much more tractable. Sympathy is when a person shares part of the thoughts and feelings of another, but not all of them and not the same ones. Feeling and thinking are present. There is overlap but not congruence.

In my Canadian town, white folks believe in reconciliation between Indigenous cultures and White culture: the European invaders. They think reconciliation can be achieved by allaying their sense of guilt, and that this will compensate for some of the destruction of indigenous culture.

This is sympathy: the projection of your feelings and ideas onto another person or group. Sympathy carries an element of discomfort and a motivation for relief. It's not enough to see a problem that needs to be solved, there's got to be some feeling in it.

The feelings of the sympathizer may not match those with whom they sympathize. Their thoughts might not either, but the actions have a measure of consonance, at least they appear so. Sympathy is sincere. If it's not sincere, then it's not really sympathy, it's pretension or condescension.

Those who seek to make the situation better have authentic feelings. Their thoughts and actions are consonant with their feelings. It's just that their mindset has a self-centered point of view. The sympathetic person understands the part of the situation that makes them feel ill at ease, but they don't understand the whole situation from the other person's point of view.

The sympathy that underlies reconciliation is not empathy. It's a desire to restore balance and relief from guilt. It is a component of empathy—a one-sided component—but it is not and does not paint the entire picture. Sympathy avoids the full, empathetic experience. The sympathetic person says they want to remove poverty, racism, and injustice, but they'll be satisfied when these problems are removed from view.

A person who has sympathy for your plight does not understand you and they'll be no help in resolving your feelings. They would like to take the thorn out of your foot, but they will not understand the trauma left behind. People are sympathetic to their vision of your problem as it affects them, not your vision of your problem as it affects you.

What It's Good For

Empathy is the glue for collective action and the foundation for synergy. It coordinates cooperation and sharing. Without empathy, there is no feeling of cooperation. There can be a reason and strategy for cooperation, but without the underlying motive, such blueprints are not stable. They would veer away from cooperation at the first splitting of the paths.

Empathy is required to be a therapist. It's also required to be a good parent or partner. In fact, empathy is required to be a good teacher or leader. A measure of a society's dysfunction can be seen in the lack of empathy of its leaders. On this basis, most of today's societies are dysfunctional.

It has been an epiphany for me to realize that I am extremely empathetic. I've only come to understand this recently because my family and social environment did not teach me to be empathetic and, as a result, I was hard-pressed to recognize it. I always wondered why I seemed to care so much more than others.

This seems to set me apart from almost everyone. Recognizing it feels empowering. I can now understand how I'm different and how I might be less different if I so choose.

Too Much Empathy

Can you have too much empathy? Would you like to be less empathetic? If you felt that you deeply understood other people or could, would you like to have less of this?

The question breaks into two parts: Do you want more control over the feelings you share with others? And second, do you want more control over how much you share other's feelings?

One can certainly imagine having too much of certain feelings. One could feel overwhelmed by an amplified version of what other people feel. This is subtle because feelings are subtle. A person becomes anesthetized to unremitting powerful feelings. To succeed under duress, a person can dissociate crushing feelings from their sense of self and, in that way, better cope with the situation. Coping is not a long-term solution, it is a tactic that can provide a bridge to a long-term solution.

As an empathetic person, should you detach yourself using the anesthesia that trauma can induce? Should you exercise a greater discernment so that you can experience only the clarifying feelings and not the disorienting ones? Should you be more resilient? And if you are more resilient and regain your equanimity sooner, have you lost your empathy?

These are interesting questions. I'm going to save them for another time.

What's Next

There are more installments in this series on empathy. The next part explores empathy as the root of emotional intelligence.

E9 – Empathy II – Empathy and Emotional Intelligence

March 31, 2021

Concerning the social role of empathy that's at the root of emotional intelligence.

"You can only understand people if you feel them in yourself."
— **John Steinbeck**, author

In the essay titled Empathy I, I referred to the unreal difference between cognitive and emotional empathy. Some think intellect and emotion are distinct because they involve different parts of the brain. These are two experiences of the same thing.

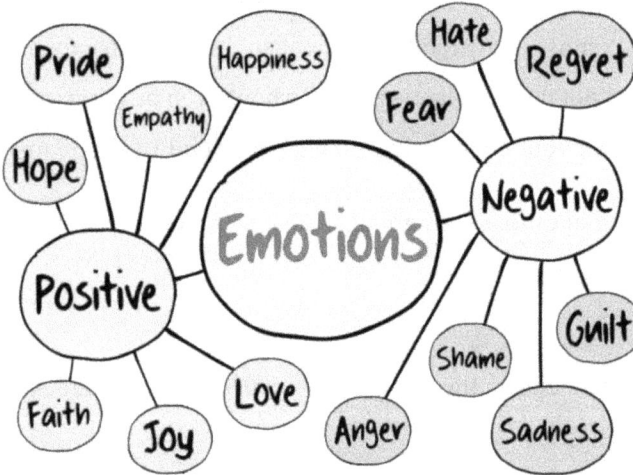

Figure 36: Emotions tend to be either positive or negative. Few are in between.

When I act like you feel but don't really feel it, am I empathizing? We accept many shades of authenticity, and it's difficult to judge another person's sincerity. Since insincerity is seen as betrayal, we rarely admit to being insincere even when we're misunderstood.

Emotion

Emotion emerges from integrating all that you know. It represents a visceral experience of what you think. Similarly, what your eyes perceive and what you think you see are complementary aspects of the same thing. Apperception is the combination of perception and cognition. What we call comprehension combines what you feel and what you think, emotion and intellect. One shapes the other. Without both your thinking is defective.

The two experiences of empathy are different aspects of comprehension. From an intellectual perspective, you use reason to build understanding. This is built on language, memories, and associations. With this, you build a story which is your understanding of what you see.

Your emotional perspective is a form of perception. Unlike vision, it is not generated by a sensory organ but by your limbic system. Your limbic system, a more central brain structure, receives signals from your peripheral nervous system, your gut, and other parts of your body. You feel and store emotions in your body.

We used to presume we rationalized first and developed emotional attitudes later. This is how things appear, since our feelings are unclear until they've been stated. In fact, we perceive and decide on a response first, based on preexisting reflexes, aptitudes, and attitudes. Then we build a rationalization after we've already decided what to do. This sounds exactly the opposite of what we experience, but we can see this happening in the brain. The person who you think of as "you" is not the master of these thoughts, but the product of them.

The emerging view is that emotion underlies cognition; emotions are things that pull thoughts together rather than things that hold us apart. The uncertainty that emotions make you feel accurately reflects your state of knowledge. The rationalizations you have concocted to explain your emotions are a crude approximation of them. When we investigate where thoughts happen, we find intellectual functions are localized. In contrast, emotions involve many brain regions.

Not all emotions are equal, and this is obvious. But we tend to give them equal weight, such as when we talk about the basic emotions of anger, happiness, sadness, fear, disgust, contempt, and surprise. It's as if we're trying to be democratic when, in fact, emotions are more like a layered ecosystem. Some grow out of others.

Discriminating emotions implies we can tell the feelings apart, but it does not mean that they exist as different. Telling one from the other doesn't mean they can be put into relation to one another. As with the experience of colors, their difference reflects experiences we create, not differences in what we perceive. Like color vision, it is likely that our different emotions are different mixtures of similar elements.

Names

Emotions are an example of the power of naming. The power of naming is our tendency to believe to be real those things that we can name. Seventy-five percent of people believe in the reality of God and the soul. But if God and the soul could not be named, forming a consensus would be difficult.

The fallacy of the reality of things that can be named is a cultural prejudice that has degraded our thought. It leads to our feeling entitled to what we want, which we can reinforce through discussion. We feel less obliged to those things that we should do or understand but don't discuss, because we are less able to form a consensus.

The power of naming is linked to the power of words, the development of the intellect, and the emergence of the ego. Once we can name ourselves, our feelings, and our needs, they become more real than those things we cannot name. This began with the first cave paintings, and it is still developing today. Integrating emotion and intellect is an essential task of our species. This leads to more integrated knowledge and a better chance of survival.

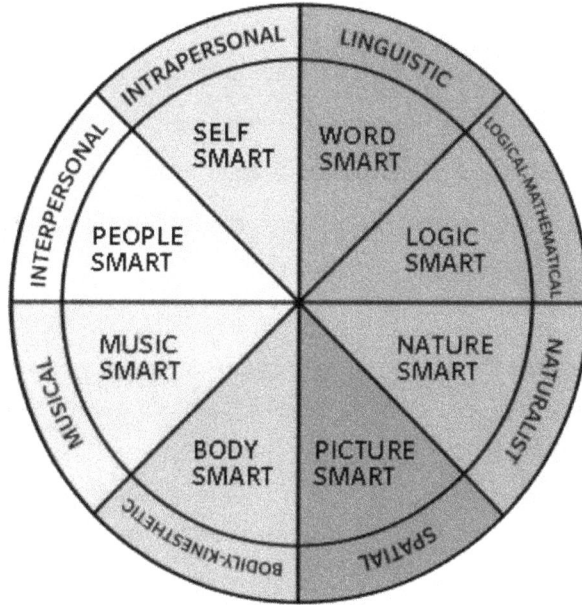

Figure 37: Aptitudes and the skills they support.

Intelligence

Think of empathy as a meta-emotion, something that integrates our emotional experience. It is the ability to understand emotion in others, similar to how intellect enables us to understand the thoughts of others. We are told to think of empathy as a reaction or reflex, something that just happens. Something that you have. It is likely much more than that.

Some people think intellect is measured by intelligence, and that intelligence exists on a single spectrum. We now recognize that intelligence comes in many forms, and some are more open to development than others. There are inherited abilities and built-in limitations. There are also different aptitudes required in expanding intelligence. For example, resilience, confidence, and extroversion may not help you find solutions, but they may help you find learning opportunities.

As intellectual intelligence changes, so does emotional intelligence. A person who learns to think better also learns to better manage their emotions. Similarly, people who do not learn intellectually do not learn emotionally. But let's be clear: learning intellectually does not mean learning facts or functions, it means learning to think and express oneself. Just as an engineer grows intellectually through the practice of engineering, so also does an abstract artist learn to think better through their practice.

The larger question is how to facilitate emotional learning. A slightly smaller question is how to facilitate empathic learning. We can ask smaller questions still about how to enhance learning of each of the emotions we identify as separate. But we don't ask these questions. It's only recently that anyone even phrased the question of emotional intelligence. There has been little attempt to understand emotional learning.

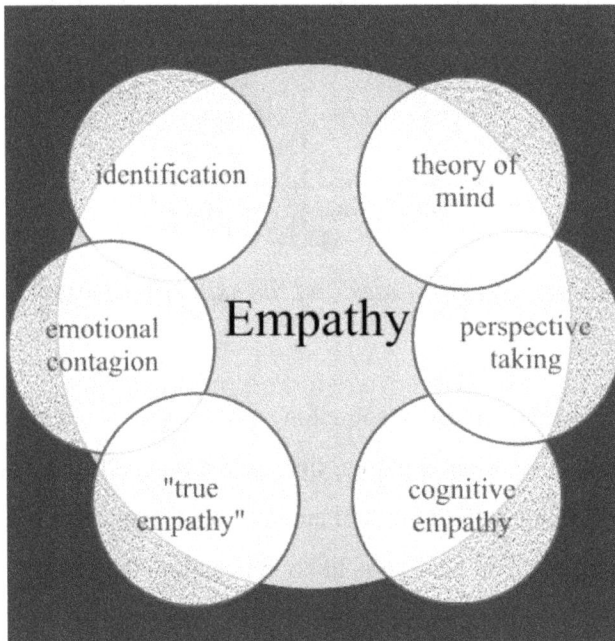

Figure 38: Skills and aptitudes that contribute to the development of empathy.

Empathy

Feeling is intelligence. Accept empathy as being able to understand the feelings of others. Focus on the learning of empathy. We must learn to understand the feelings of others before we can communicate our feelings.

As a species, we have only rudimentary abilities to communicate feelings. We are at a pre-language state in the realm of emotions. We are emotionally non-verbal. Think of learning empathy as how you would learn a new idea. It takes us back to the question of how we learn anything.

The question is not whether empathy is important; the question is not how much empathy should one have? Empathy is no more a "thing" than intellect is a thing. Empathy is an integral part of understanding, learning, and navigating emotional intelligence.

If you have ever wondered why human history has been such a disaster of conflict and suffering, the answer is that humans lack key components of emotional intelligence. In particular, they lack empathy. The last 10,000 years have been an instant in human evolution, an electrical short-circuit that has resulted in the abrupt emergence of intelligence before self-understanding. At this chaotic juncture, each person makes their own choice regarding whether to learn new skills or proceed forward blindly. The choice is between traditional structures or new abilities in a new field of risks and opportunities. This is the choice faced by many of my therapy clients.

Consider the situation of crossing a chasm, where, in this case, the chasm is your lack of empathy. There are several ways to approach the problem. You're familiar with the first two, and probably unfamiliar with the third.

1. The first approach is to view this as an impossible problem because you have no bridge. This is the materialist approach. From this viewpoint, you'll never understand yourself or others because you don't have this knowledge now and you never have. You proceed with what you already know and ignore the problem. This is what we usually do when confronted with an unsolvable problem. It's called denial, and the key to maintaining denial is rationalization. The image that comes to my mind is that of the caveman with a club over one shoulder and a woman over the other, returning to life in the cave.

2. The second approach is experimental. You recognize aspects of the problem, but not so much as to panic or despair. You shore up your defenses, arrange your priorities, and see what you can accomplish with the tools at your disposal. This can work for familiar problems and it yields incremental improvements, but it won't work for learning something qualitatively new because it maintains the status quo. This is the intelligent approach and you can compare it to building a huge cantilever. This might succeed if you were building a bridge, and the problem was a lack of engineering, but in this case, the span is too large. You can't reach a new destination by following existing paths.

3.   The third approach is exploratory, which means going beyond what you know. It's important to recognize that while this can feel dangerous, and it inevitably leads to certain kinds of loss, it does not have to be catastrophic. We're wired to fear novelty because of its destructive potential, but to explore successfully, you must gain some mastery of exploration. You must learn how to take risks, resolve loss, and incorporate useful novelty. These are exactly the skills institutions do not teach us and which we must learn ourselves.

Bondage

Start by freeing yourself from institutions. This is exactly counter to the institutional trend that we see in the world today. That is to be expected. Structures grow large and display their imbalance before they collapse. This happens both in the decay of concepts and the decay of structures. Sterile concepts like "the singularity," which is the complete control of consciousness by machines, go hand in hand with the failure of education to provide resources for independence.

Runaway growth often presages the need for change as the system reaches its extreme. We ignore the incremental destruction that we have isolated ourselves from, such as the destruction of the forests and the decimation of the insects, and we focus on the illusions that motivate us, such as prospects for new wealth, power, and exploitation.

Institutions try to maintain themselves by circling the wagons; forming alliances and excluding alternatives. Advertisements and inducements appear in crumbling institutions, encouraging support and extolling a bright future. The forces undermining these structures create opportunities that lie beyond these structures. Some form of reorganization is required to reach them. The choice is to give up one's autonomy and become an internal part of the system, or to move out of the system and expand outside the system's boundaries.

Freeing ourselves from institutions does not mean destroying institutions, it means creating possibilities beyond what they provide. For example, nationalism is emotionally constipating, while creativity can be emotionally releasing. Communities are constipating, but families can be empowering. At the root, your ego tends toward constipation, while expanding your sense of self allows for emotional release. Your ego internalizes the institutions around you.

Release

I work from the bottom up. I don't see intelligent change at the highest levels. The Covid-19 experience showed how politics moves to maintain its structure at the expense of people's lives. When confronted with a solution that threatens the system's built-in flaws, the system blocks those solutions.

I'm referring to the drug ivermectin, which could have ended the pandemic six months ago (see March 31, 2020 summary at TrialSiteNews). There have been four panels of expert doctors and epidemiologists. The study referenced here is the fourth. They have all come to the same conclusion, which is that ivermectin should be globally distributed to everyone now. The results of over 20 randomized clinical trials have established that ivermectin is effective in preventing infection by the SAR-COV-2 virus. This last meta-analysis concluded that this widely used medicine:

1. reduces the transmission of Covid-19 by 88%,

2. reduces the risk of death by 83%,

3. reduces by 50% the progression of the disease in those who are infected.

Instead of endorsing ivermectin, it was rejected because it threatened the power structure. Not only is its use not endorsed, but its supply is withheld. News about ivermectin has been censored by government and mainstream press.

The political structures are committed to supporting monetary investments and sacrificing human opportunities. They cannot sacrifice profit structures to support human opportunities. Repurposed drugs like ivermectin, from which profits have already been extracted, are not supported as they supplant the pharmaceutical equation that looks to continuity, control, and return on investment.

Politicians, industrialists, entrepreneurs, mainstream media, and invested leaders accept this equation. The beneficiaries of social control reject threats to social engineering. This is reflected in layers of preference for more conformity and less individuality.

Experimental vaccination and obedient group behavior are institutionally preferred because they are consistent with social control. The vaccination debate centers on the difference between institutional profit and individual benefit. This is not really a debate, it's a confusion. It could easily be clarified and people could be correctly informed, but institutions will not clarify this. The "vaccine debate" is a red herring that suggests independent thought is socially dangerous.

Medications, like ivermectin, are discouraged because they allow differences and encourage independence. Allopathic medicine is institutionally supported in order to constrain this independence, and most people accept this. Yet in the Covid-19 pandemic, we see doctors and frontline healthcare providers advocating for effective medicines while their controlling institutions—governments, hospitals, and public healthcare agencies—reject and suppress them. This institutional failure gave populists like Donald Trump the opportunity to rise to power and will do so again.

Personal empowerment involves building immunity and integrity through changes in diet, introspection, improvements in sleep and nutrition, and control of addictive patterns. These personal initiatives are institutionally unwelcome, as they encourage sensitivity at the personal, detailed, and socially uncontrolled levels of awareness.

We observe doctors advising improvements in these areas, but doctors are not trained and are not allowed to exceed their scope of practice. In the free market, such as it is, government agencies, medical colleges, and research and academic institutions fight to prevent unauthorized solutions such as herbal remedies, Indigenous healing, intuition, or unapproved innovation.

Personal empowerment threatens institutional power. Institutionally minded people are trained to deny it. We see this in the five-fold increase in psychopathy in people who are institutional leaders. These are antisocial people who have the power to control social change. The Covid-19 pandemic has exposed disorganization and accelerated change in political, economic, and social structures.

We won't solve the ecological crisis through institutional means. Instead, our large institutions will be destroyed by it. That may sound like a grim assessment, but that's only if you're attached to them; if you have built these institutional structures into your personality. If you're like most people, you have.

Learning empathy is related to the environmental crisis as the Covid-19 situation shows. If we had more empathy for the dying millions, we would not be as indifferent as we are to the role we play and the responsibility we have in policing our system. It is because we allow our institutions to define our thoughts and feelings that the pandemic continues, and this is similar to other structural crises.

E10 – Empathy III – Similarity and Differences

April 21, 2021

Empathy and sympathy are practically opposites. They move in different directions.

"If you made a sadist more empathic, it would just lead to a happier sadist."
— **Paul Bloom**, psychologist

In Empathy I, I asked, "Why [do] I seem to care so much more than others?" and answered that I'm more empathetic. But I need to further distinguish empathy from sympathy. You need this distinction if you're going to learn to be more empathetic.

We often see empathy and sympathy as similar or, for some people, indistinguishable. Not only are they different, they are practically opposites, and they move in different directions. This is the key to understanding empathy and learning how to have more of it.

"It can be very dangerous to see things from somebody else's point of view without the proper training."
— **Douglas Adams**, from *The Ultimate Hitchhiker's Guide*

Sympathy

Sympathy is an intellectual concept. It's based on a contrast of values. It leads to an opinion first and a feeling second, though feeling is unnecessary. Sympathy is an intellectual agreement that may or may not trigger a feeling. A person who has no feelings at all can still sympathize with others.

When you are sympathetic, you are seeing things from a blinkered point of view, a limited perspective that heightens some dichotomy. There is a tension in sympathy. It's not just "this or that," it's "this against that." If it was simply duality, then you'd be appreciative, but once you see one side as better than the other, you're sympathetic.

To become more sympathetic, you need to see alternatives, have some understanding of their difference or a belief that you do—it can be a thin and insincere belief—and you have to apply

388

a value judgment. Sympathy is shared ethics, not shared emotion.

Because sympathy is intellectual, it's often notable for its lack of genuine feeling. So it was with the Catholic inquisitors who sympathized with their victims, but murdered them anyway. You may sympathize with the impoverished or the criminal, but you do not share their trauma.

Sympathy is not a sharing of feelings, it is not a "coming together." Instead, sympathy is a setting apart. You can argue for sympathy, you can verbalize it. Hitler had sympathy. Dr. Spock had sympathy. Neither had empathy.

> "Empathy, he once had decided, must be limited to herbivores because, ultimately, the empathic gift blurred the boundaries between hunter and victim, between the successful and the defeated."
> — **Philip K. Dick**, from *Do Androids Dream of Electric Sheep?*

Empathy

It's said that there is an intellectual and an emotional component to empathy, but I think this is misleading. What passes for intellectual empathy is not empathy at all, it's simply a verbal means of communicating feeling, but if there is no feeling, then it's just verbiage. Lacking feeling, "intellectual empathy" is just a script, an act, and there is nothing empathetic about that.

There is only one kind of empathy, and that's emotional empathy. There are different ways of communicating empathy, and one way is intellectual. Empathy can also be shared artistically, physically, and demonstratively. A therapeutic demonstration of empathy is nonverbal and inactive and happens through a subtle mirroring of emotions.

Emotions are mostly communicated non-verbally and through non-conscious signals. That's what makes these signals emotional. You can't think them into existence, you must feel them into existence.

This isn't always true. A skilled actor can fake emotions. This is the primary distinctive feature of psychopaths. The difference between a psychopath and an actor is that an actor knows they're faking while a psychopath does not. An actor knows what it feels like to display emotions, but they've learned to make the demonstrations without having the feelings.

A psychopath doesn't have the feelings they display, and they don't understand that. They don't know what it is they're faking, but they still know how to play the role. An actor is cued by their feelings, a psychopath is cued by your reactions.

An actor mirrors; a psychopath manipulates. A good actor has a broad range of emotional displays, while a psychopath's skill set is narrow and consists only of what you and other people have shown them. Tell an actor to display emotion and they'll know what you mean. They're aware of the multiple emotions that are latent in any situation. Tell a psychopath to display emotion and they'll be confused. They won't know which emotion is appropriate and they'll need someone to tell them.

An actor can carry their display through emotional transitions. They might move between grief and sorrow to happiness and hope. These transitions will confuse a psychopath, as these transitions are displayed infrequently. They understand the display of emotion, but not the dynamics. They can fake the display, but it's unlikely that they can display the expected transitions.

Emotional empathy, which is the only empathy, is not intellectual. It requires no intellectual understanding and no explanation. To make the point more strongly, empathy cannot be generated by explanation or intellectual understanding. Explanation can only trigger a memory if you've had that memory, but it cannot create a memory of a feeling if you've never had it.

> "If you are irritated by every rub, how will your mirror be polished?"
> — **Jalāl al-Dīn Muḥammad Rūmī** (1207-1273), scholar and poet

Too Much Empathy

In Empathy I, I asked whether you can have too much empathy. It's clear that you can. There are two ways in which one can be too empathetic. One way is to be over-involved. Since empathy is a mirroring of emotion, one can have more than an appropriate amount. What's appropriate is whatever is appropriate for the situation. Being paralyzed may be appropriate in the moment, but being immobilized by empathy won't solve anything.

If the situation is one of sharing, then appropriate empathy is whatever it takes to facilitate sharing. Someone may experience sorrow and hope to emerge from it. Here, if you experience a similar sorrow to a level from which you can't emerge, then you'll end up leading them into deeper sorrow. You'll empathize too much with them, and then they'll empathize with you.

If someone is experiencing happiness and they'd like more of it, then by amplifying the empathic connection, they can be brought to a level of joy. Wise people can do this, they can empathize and they can amplify. They can foresee the dynamic of the emotion and they have some control over it. To use a poker analogy, they can match you and they can raise you.

The other way you can have too much empathy is to lose control of the dynamic. The dynamic is the natural progression of feelings. This is central to therapy in which many people's feelings have gotten stuck. They cannot feel and, because they cannot feel, they cannot move beyond feeling or their current level of feeling.

Trauma is an emotion that is stuck. It's stuck in the mind or the body. Because it's not being organically expressed, it cannot be resolved. Trauma is like a compost pile sprayed with an antibacterial: it cannot decay and so it persists and obstructs.

In this metaphor, the bacterium that decays trauma expands awareness and integrates understanding. But you cannot gain an awareness of what you cannot engage in, and you cannot fully understand what you forbid yourself from experiencing. These steps in the degradation of trauma both require energy and generate energy, and a traumatized person may not have the extra energy needed or the strength to endure the energy that will be released. The process of resolution must be delayed until each person is ready to experience it.

A traumatized person has repressed emotions and deep connections to their trauma that you likely do not have. If you're in a supporting position, then you need to know or infer more about the condition of the traumatized person than they are communicating to you. You need to know what's safe for them to engage in, and what you can safely experience and control in yourself.

If you don't know these limits, then you risk leading the traumatized person into greater trauma or harmful re-traumatization. You could also fall into your own emotional experience that is no longer a therapeutic mirror of the other person's, and in doing so, become a hindrance. Here are a few examples.

The Death of Esther

My mother and I were the first to arrive at my grandfather's apartment on the morning my grandmother died. He had awoken to find her dead in the adjoining bed and was in a state of shock. My mother and I were quiet, and we were present for him.

Other relatives arrived, and soon chaos ensued. People started unloading their coping strategies onto my grandfather, insisting that he listen to them, that he behave in a certain way, and that he take sedatives. Their empathy was out of control and it resulted in a total violation of respect and support. The crowd celebrated their fears and trampled my grandfather's grief.

Most people cannot empathize with death because most people are so avoidant of it. They cannot deal with the emotions of those people who come into direct contact with it. They encounter their own shock and impose their own avoidance. This is the wrong way to cope with the situation as it makes the other person's situation worse.

Helping the Victim

I've had many past life regression clients who were approaching the scene of their rape. It does not matter whether you "believe" in past lives. All you need to understand is that the regression experience feels real. It doesn't matter whether the trauma actually occurred, or occurred exactly as it's remembered, because the trauma is being created now, in the present.

Maybe it really happened in this life or another. Maybe something like it happened. Maybe there is the fear that it will happen in the future. In each case, the traumatic experience is a repository of energy emerging in current awareness. The question for the person leading the regression is whether it's appropriate and safe since, as the facilitator of the experience, you bear some responsibility for it.

There was a public outcry against false memory inductions, and the psychological community still believes this to be reprehensible. It is a Red Herring. There are no demonstrably "false memories" because all memories are false. It is the taking of memories literally that is unprofessional.

Memories are allegorical and can pertain to either the past or the future. When they're your own memories and you're in control, then your subconscious manages the emotional discharge. But when you're led in a trance or induced hallucination, you may be unable to control what's good for you.

As a facilitator in a hypnotic experience, or a sitter in a psychedelic experience, exercise cautious judgement for the person you're responsible for. Their protection is your responsibility. Being fully empathetic with their experience is irresponsible. Hold back, maintain perspective, make judgements, and control both their emotions and your own.

For people who are heading toward trauma or abuse in past or present life regressions, the only safe decision is to offer them protection. I don't deny the experience. I provide alternatives, power, safety, and protection. I work to arm them appropriately and give them various means of escape. The risk is of your being lost in their vision.

If they still choose to engage traumatic imagery after I have empowered them, then they can proceed with safety. They have the option and they have control. This may violate the helplessness and terror that they may need. I will not prevent that as long as they are insistent, are authentically directed to it, and I still have the power to extract them. There is no question as to the reality of these images. They are psychically real; physical reality is irrelevant.

Helping the Perpetrator

I had clients who were gangsters and accomplices to violence. Their situation held some attraction for them, but they were also ambivalent. There were issues of pride, power, autonomy, control, and money. Were I to fully empathize with them, I could not provide a new perspective. This was unfamiliar territory for me. There was a good deal of withholding on their part.

If I let my empathy run free, I would return to my own territory and have little guidance to offer them. Their conversation avoided emotions associated with anger and violence. Instead, it focused on peace and resolution. I did not want to explore what was bothering them because I didn't think I could handle it as well as they did.

My role—and this is what they were asking of me—was to help them navigate toward more peaceful lives. They were a couple, and they wanted to have a family. We only met once, and we did not work further, but I heard they were happy with our session. Their situation was delicate, and I hoped they found the support they needed.

> "When people are free to do as they please, they usually imitate each other."
> — **Eric Hoffer**, social philosopher

More on Empathy

So far, I've only clarified empathy. I next want to talk about creating and controlling empathy.

> "Before you criticize a man, walk a mile in his shoes. That way, when you do criticize him, you'll be a mile away and have his shoes."
> — **Steve Martin**, actor

E11 – Empathy IV – The White Man's Tongue

May 25, 2021

Healthy empathy is rooted in a healthy sense of self.

"It doesn't require many words to speak the truth."
— **Chief Joseph**, leader of the Nez Perce

Vicarious Introspection

This piece is about truth and empathy.

I'm told empathy is vicarious introspection, an experience of yourself that arises through your consideration of someone else's experience. This leaves room for both similar and dissimilar empathy, where similar empathy means you feel similar to how another person feels, and dissimilar empathy means you feel something different. Both feelings would be triggered by considering the same experience of another person. But how do you really know what the other person feels? It's reasonable to expect there is always a little of both.

Heinz Kohut was a Freudian analyst. The following statement comes from a video presentation on empathy. Kohut is famous for making simple things complicated. He's very sincere, but I find him to be completely opaque.

> "Introspection and empathy should be looked at as an informer of appropriate action."
> — **Heinz Kohut**, psychoanalyst

If that was all there was to empathy, then we could understand it in terms of what it makes you do. That's partly helpful, but it leaves a lot on the table. There is a fundamental part of empathy that's rooted in a shared sense of conflict, which reflects a lack of clear, appropriate action. There's a part of empathy that remains as thought and feeling and does not act.

I have to leave these psychologists and psychiatrists to their own imbroglio. I have little sympathy for them. (Sympathy: the feeling that another person deserves your attention.) I think empathy is fundamental and cannot be left as an impenetrable concept. We have to talk about our process of being reflective. Consider these two concepts that pertain to self-awareness.

Metacognition is an awareness of your thought processes and the patterns behind them. This allows you to recognize that thoughts and feelings are separate from who you feel yourself to be. As a result, you disconnect your identity from your thoughts and feelings.

Dissociation is an awareness of your thought processes and the patterns behind them. It allows you to recognize that you feel yourself defined by thoughts and feelings that are different from who you feel yourself to be. As a result, there is more than one of you.

Learning

Learning is life and is just as mysterious. Learning is change, growth, and evolution and is not programmed, mechanical, or reductive. All sustained change is some kind of learning and even temporary change is learning though it's lost.

The fundamental notion of determinism is that there is one predictable way forward. As long as things follow a predictable way forward, there is no learning. Changes of that sort are programmed. They are baked in the cake. That may look like change, but it isn't. It's just a new perspective on what was already there.

In empathy, there is a disruption, a branching of paths, a dissonance between your previous experience and the other person's experience that you're considering now.

You cannot experience exactly what another person experiences, there is always a difference. An essential part of empathy is combining the feelings of similarity and difference. That's where unpredictable things happen. Part of empathy depends on what you experience, and part of it depends on how you experience yourself.

Truth

In the stereotyped, potboiler Western adventure, the Indian proclaims, "White Man speaks with forked tongue." I saw these Western movies as a kid and I always wondered about this. It was obviously a Hollywood device, but there was something to it. On the one hand, it was obviously true because enemies always lie to each other. On the other hand, it seemed like more than just a complaint.

It's been said that the Western self is embedded in a culture of narcissism, and Kohut proposed that this was a coping strategy for our culture's effect of driving down our self-esteem. We become narcissistic and inflate our self-importance because we carry a degraded sense of ourselves. We see this in the worship of celebrities, people we see as smart, powerful, or attractive, and in our craving for money.

A drowning person will climb onto anything that floats, and a narcissistic person will take advantage of anything that provides them with advantage, including their morality. After all, morality rests on what feels right, and if you don't feel right, then the moral choice won't feel right either. Narcissism weighs morality toward what satisfies your personal need, and for the average Westerner, that is whatever makes them feel more secure.

As a culture, I don't think we Westerners know what healthy self-esteem feels like. I don't think we have a balanced sense of truth. This does something to the scales of justice and we see that everywhere and it's in our face. The fundamental disrespect our society shows for individuals is rooted in the self-respect that we don't have for ourselves.

We look outward to compensate, toward our social profile and as much authority as we can accumulate. We look to authority and institutions to give us "a little more porridge," in the words of Charles Dickens, and our morality is skewed toward our paterfamilias, the good father, God, society, and the government.

We speak to each other not as equals, but as contestants. We speak to foreigners as threats, runts of the litter, and those who are not entitled.

Of course, we cannot admit this to ourselves because that would undermine the value of what we strive for. You cannot lust after wealth at the same time that you recognize the poisonous effect of money. This is what makes narcissism a mental dysfunction: you cannot correct something as long as you are controlled by it.

Westerners hold out their hands to engage with the world, to be shepherds of our environment, and to build a sustainable culture, but our fists are closed. We can't see things as balanced because we're imbalanced. Even if you feel balanced—and how would you know if you were—you don't live in a balanced culture.

The playing field is not level. You maintain your sense of truth by maintaining your sense of identity. For the white man, this is always slipping. We're always reaching for more because we cannot find balance no matter how much we have.

Consider this: my description does not describe you. You know that if you just had a little more, then you would have enough. You know your needs are reasonable and that if you got what you needed, you wouldn't take more. You know this because it's happened before. You had what you needed occasionally, but it didn't last because something took it away.

To overcome narcissism in yourself, you must pass through a crisis of dissociation. You must find another you, and grow that you to a state that is strong enough to form an identity, and then disengage from the person you used to be. You cannot simply supply what's missing because the narcissistic self cannot hold it.

Because no one wants to disable a part of themselves, at least not while they still believe in themselves, the force to change oneself often originates from outside. It creates conflict that you either fight against or internalize as disease or dysfunction. When circumstances conspire to kill the narcissistic in you, it becomes a crisis.

Empathy

I'm heading toward empathy, which is what this is all about. I want a program to become more empathic, but something is blocking it. This is not simply a puzzle with a clean solution or a detective story in which we follow the clues. In this story, we are the detective and we are the culprit, and we're constantly running away from the clues.

I've not yet encountered a program for developing empathy that's worth a damn. I've encountered a few cognitive behavioral prescriptions that provide instructions for how to appear more empathic. This happy family whitewash is the staple of office etiquette and management training with the goal of making people more productive.

Psychologists talk about the need for a deeper feeling of connection with ourselves. Social reformers talk about our need to find a deeper connection with each other. Environmentalists talk about our need for a deeper connection with the Earth. The need is everywhere, and it's obvious, so why doesn't it happen?

It doesn't happen because we can't let it happen. We are not at liberty to become more empathic; we protect ourselves. This is another meme of Western culture, the meme of the savage unconscious alien or monster motivated by no reason other than to destroy us. Depending on the story, this force is portrayed as separated, attached, or an internal part of us.

We project this self-destructive part onto an external threat and marshal our forces in order to defeat it. When it's attached to us, we work to expose and then remove the spy or parasite. But when it's an internal part of us, it's insanity, and we flee.

The white man speaks with a forked tongue because the White culture has compromised our loyalty. We love our culture like a traumatized child loves his or her abusive parent. It's the only one we know. Whatever we say to the outsider, we have a different story for ourselves. In a compromised culture, we take it for granted that everyone is always looking out for number one. There are not enough of the essentials to go around, and the first essential that's at auction is truth.

The forked tongue is healed by shared truth, which is also the foundation for empathy. The forked tongue separates factions fighting for what they can't get enough of, whether that be self-respect, political power, or natural resources.

We could build an empathy training program on how to listen and commiserate, but if our presence is unbalanced or preoccupied, then our empathy will be too. The first order of business is to strengthen our personality so that it is strong enough to imagine an equal and collaborative role. To collaborate as equals, we need the ability to mirror in a balanced way, which requires a fairly intact self that is not narcissistic.

This seems impossible, but that's not acceptable. I will propose that we try to achieve this incrementally by becoming more metacognitive and more dissociated. By becoming more aware and detached, empathy and self-confidence can inform each other. If we can become more aware of what we lack in understanding others, we can see what we lack in ourselves.

I believe the key is imagination in the same way that imagination is the key to learning. My rule Number 7 in my book *Becoming Supergenius* is, "measure how well you learn not by what you can remember, but by what you can imagine." There must be a way to imagine empathy.

> "Empathy is not merely the basic principle of artistic creation. It is also the only path by which one can reach the truth about life and society."
> — **Kafū Nagai**, author

E12 – Empathy V – Ways of Knowing

June 2, 2021

Empathy is more than emotional following along, it's a transmission.

"Unexamined beliefs are not worth having."— **Socrates**

Transcendent Knowing

Thomas Ray is an ethnobotanist interested in the transcendent effects of psychedelics. He proposes that the landscape of transcendent experience does not just have one peak, but several. That these different peaks represent deeper insight into human nature than is normally accessible to us.

Rays says that our intellect has evolved away from this understanding because our intellect breaks things down and linearizes things, rather than building things up and appreciating their connected nature. He maps these peaks according to our emotional landscape, but the peaks are not simply extreme emotions, they are more than that. They are transcendent experiences that are reached through a combination and refinement of emotions. They are neural pathways that are opened by certain neurotransmitters and their associated psychedelic substances.

> "It appears that children are dominated by the affective domain, while adults are largely dominated by the cognitive mind, at the expense of emotions, feelings, and intuition. When we mature into adults, we find ourselves knowing the world largely through language, logic, and reason. We tend to lose touch with the way we knew the world as children, the archaic way of knowing, through feelings, through our heart."
> — **Thomas Ray** (2016)

Rational thinking is our first recourse. We're trained to believe that a reasoned approach is the most effective. Compulsory education is directed entirely toward shaping our reasoning skills. There is no emotional training aside from suppressing it.

Even the stereotyped advice of couples counseling, embedded in the admonition, "Do you want to be right or do you want to be happy?" is a subtle direction to do what's reasonable, as if you can feel happy without regard to what you think. What if this is all wrong?

Emotional balance is not a reasonable thing. One can balance one's resources reasonably, and one can get one's basic needs met reasonably, but is love or freedom reasonable? Can you measure them or put them in an equation? Does it help to know how to describe or use them in a sentence?

Ways of Learning

I want to address the question of how to learn empathy. I don't think that question can be answered reasonably. I don't think there is one answer, but there may be several.

If empathy is something you can have or not have, then it's a skill or a trait. If it's a skill, then you can develop it. If it's a trait, then you can express it, unless you don't have it, in which case you might regain it. If it's a trait you don't have, it may not be available to you.

Empathy is built on mirroring. It taps the elements fundamental to all sharing. Empathy is like a column resting on our basic social ability and supporting all aspects of caring for one another. If we can teach empathy more broadly, then we can improve the human species. Where is empathy in us, and what does it require of us?

You don't need to reason in order to empathize. We share feelings with dogs and other domesticated or domesticable animals. Rats can laugh, and maybe octopi can too. My naturalist friend Walter used to assert alligators had a sense of humor because they would taunt him, but I don't believe him.

Empathy is a sense of shared emotion that you either trigger or evoke. You don't reason it into existence, but you might remember it. If you've never had it before in your life, you may still genetically remember it in the same way that some people have genetically remembered balance, musical ability, or facility with language.

Learning empathy is a special learning. It is not a conceptual process, it's a recovery or invocation, both of which rely on memory. You won't gain the same feeling through reasoning. Real empathy is a combination of resonant feelings for which words are secondary. If memories are the roots, empathy is the trunk, the situation emerges as branches, and thoughts are the leaves on the tree.

You can only empathize if you can recover and re-experience the emotions that comprise another person's experience. And you can only do this if you can re-experience each of these emotions in yourself. You're presented with two tasks: to discern the emotions involved and the amount of each.

Ways of Hearing

A shadow that looks black beside the glaring sunlight of a white wall will look white against a pitch-dark hole. An ice cube against the skin will raise goose bumps on one occasion, while the same ice cube on the same skin will raise a burn blister on another. The only difference is your expectation. So it is with all perceptions. All perceptions are filtered through consciousness, and this is even more so with emotions.

We can't know if we're experiencing the same emotion as another. Since emotion is a nest of feelings, consequences, and associations, it's fairly certain that we are not. We believe that there are general aspects of shareable emotion even if these are not available to everyone. We mix these similarities to recreate the recipe for another person's state of mind.

We share some sensations, but sensations are not the same as perceptions. Chemistry and physiology determine sensation, but contrast and association determine perception. The key to having similar emotions lies in what you imagine them to mean. We don't all have the same imagination and we don't all have the same associations.

The key to empathy with another is both sharing the same breadth and depth of emotion and also sharing associations and imagination. The magic "chemistry" that happens between people results from this, and the less you share, the less chemistry there is between you.

Words are the deceptive filter. You can share the same vocabulary and body language, but if you don't share the same emotion, then these presentations are superficial. Learning empathy is then a question of not acting but of being. Do you have an emotional range to match another's, and do you have the insight, intuition, and control to follow their recipe? Some of these recipes are quite delicate, such as happiness. Others, like resentment, are easy to whip up and have a long shelf life.

Ways of Knowing

Building empathy is a second order of business. The first order of business is to expand the range and depth of one's emotions. However, regarding a specific sort of empathy, there is a specific recipe of emotions such that you may have what's required for one situation but not the next.

The project of learning empathy grows larger as it presumes emotional skills, and there are ranges of emotion whose access varies from person to person. I believe that with greater emotional aptitude, empathy comes naturally. Intention and attention are required, but empathy results from the emotional resonance.

Consider the piano as a metaphor. Emotional chords are those played by another person. You are the sounding board and if you have the proper resonance and bracing, designed to respond to the emotional strings of your combined sensibilities, then naturally, you will resonate.

We can go another step and envision more nuanced perceptions. These might be built from combinations of emotions and perceptions, such as connection to nature or feelings of transcendence. Thomas Ray describes these as "Mental Organs," which we'll consider in another post.

Gaining Access

Childhood is the realm of emotion. It was when emotion was flowering and after which your emotion was shackled by right-thinking and behavior. To reconnect to your emotion, to release or reshape it, that's where you should return.

Several things keep you from regaining your childhood mind. First, your brain's rhythms have increased, and this has led to a shorter emotional attention span and more distant access to childhood memories. Second, you've internalized vigilance, incessant thinking, and the belief that you are the single social persona that has been polished into being. And third, your ego has created a protective shell around your vulnerability that projects your image to the world and dulls expression.

You can reconnect with your older and more primary self through dreams and hallucinations, and to some extent through meditation, relaxation, and recreation, though these means are still filtered through your ego. It's not until the ego steps aside to allow what social behavior does not allow that you can reconnect with wider and wilder feelings and imagination.

Dreamwork is a doorway to a deeper emotional connection, but dreamwork is work and not casual dreaming. It must be directed, solicited, engaged, and recalled because otherwise, it will not interfere with the ego.

Psychedelics can be a doorway, but they also require work. This is not entertainment because the ego, in its role as protector of your fabricated self, will filter your psychedelic experience to protect itself. Those psychedelics termed entheogens can lift a person above the fences of the ego and enlarge one's vision. Preparing oneself properly is like getting in the center of the road, straightening out the steering, focusing straight ahead, and being able to navigate without running off the pavement.

Opening A Door

Hypnosis is a third doorway. Hypnosis invites emotion, provides a safe environment, and directs your focus. Of these three doorways, hypnosis is the only one that keeps you in the driver's seat. In hypnosis, you plan your experience and experience your plan. You can bring yourself to any time past, any emotion, or any place. You cannot command your past to present itself to you, but you can present yourself to your past and invite it to emerge.

This is self-hypnosis, regressing yourself with or without the aid of a hypnotist. Actually, few hypnotists would know what you wanted to accomplish outside of a regression into your past. I can lead this sort of regression and I will offer to teach other hypnotists how it can be done.

Hypnotists are taught regression to cause, where the cause that's referred to is some watershed event that has become ingrained in your unconscious and now underpins an unwanted behavior. Regression to reconnect with an earlier self or a more powerful emotion is not a standard protocol.

I believe work of this sort better prepares a person for dream and psychedelic work. By accessing, engaging, and directing the subconscious before exploring subconscious associations, one is better able to focus and address these emotions and the skills needed to manage them.

For example, if you aim to strengthen your connection with creativity and vulnerability of the heart, then you should build an intentional dialog with those characters who guard and mediate these experiences. These could be characters who you associate with early periods in your life who existed in real life or in your imagination. They could be real or imaginary caregivers you relied upon in your youth or that you rely upon now.

For example, if you conduct dreamwork in search of security, then you'll encounter characters who seem to know more about your situation than you do. These characters are creations of your mind built from people you've known, situations you've experienced, and unexpressed abilities you contain. These characters exist outside your conscious mind. They are separate from your ego identity. You can build a bridge from your ego identity to them through focus and intention. Building such bridges sculpts them into greater resolution as emergent aspects of yourself.

If you don't build these bridges in the subconscious, then your conscious intent will be weakly attached, such that your subconscious will pursue its agenda in the realm of dreams and hallucinations. What you want to forge is a kind of steering linkage that connects conscious direction with the traction of subconscious thought in the terrain of forgotten associations.

References

Jatinder, H. (2021 Jan). "Artificial Empathy? Humanity is Not Yet Ready." *Journal of the Royal Society, 114* (1): 4. https://doi.org/10.1177/0141076820975753

Ray, T. S. (2016). Mental Organs and the Origins of Mind. In *Origins of Mind.* Edited by Liz Swan: 301-26.

E13 – Empathy VI – Security

June 9, 2021

Empathy building is self-building. It starts with security.

"It is easier to build strong children than to repair broken adults."
— **Fredrick Douglas**, statesman

We seem to have basic emotions, but emotions are poorly defined. There's no way to know if we experience the same emotions. It is strange that we simply assume we share similar emotions when we clearly do not. We say we do, and at a superficial level, we act like we do, but that's mostly because we've been trained to react similarly. We copy each other relentlessly.

Culture is based on the fiction of like-mindedness. The unbridgeable gulf that separates each of our senses of self is disregarded because we think we have the same feelings. In managing feelings and social presentations, the easiest thing to do is follow the simplest, most common feelings. In our society, that feeling is selfishness built on fear, need, and isolation. Built, in fact, on our deep feeling that we are not recognized or understood. We tell ourselves that we understand each other but we know that we often don't. Social sharing does not remedy our alienation, it makes it worse.

If we actually knew our feelings, could communicate our feelings, and could share our feelings, then not only would we feel less isolated, but we would have a basis of understanding. We could trust each other beyond the simple world of "this is mine, and that is yours." If we understood our emotions, then we could control, apply, compare, rely on, and come to a common understanding. We could become allies. Right now, our allegiances are thin to very thin.

We communicate our emotions using stories, and we understand each other based on the stories we agree on. The stories are built of words, pictures, and associations. Some are built on deities, others on celebrities. These stories elicit the emotional pictures we're communicating. We use words to label the result and the underlying emotions. We give names to the stories and we put those stories in the dictionary or on the front page.

How to Learn Emotion

If you want to change, whether because something is pushing you or pulling you, you'll need something in you to change. You'll need to change your story. You'll have to let something go. Feeling secure is the place to start. It's a place from which you can judge what you can let go.

We approach our stories intellectually, investing in what makes sense. But not much does make sense when you know the full details, so we simplify. Reinforcing our emotions is how we simplify because it allows us to go right to how we feel. Once you've decided how you're going to feel, then you can interpret any story in a way that takes you to the destination of how you feel.

Emotions are memories of how you felt. You can use words to recall or create a situation that triggers a feeling, but words alone are not emotions and can't substitute for them. It is not the story that's emotional, it's the emotions triggered by the story.

In order to learn emotions, you must experience them, or you must recall your experience of them. It's possible, but unlikely, that you'll create experiences that you never had, but it's worth considering.

It is possible that we do this naturally in a less obvious form. That we amplify and recombine feelings to arrive at new feelings. I'm uncertain if this results in a new emotion or just a more complex combination. It's like our perception of flavors: how many do we perceive, and can we create new ones?

There is this thing called "Theory of Mind," which refers to your ability to understand how you see yourself and others. There is no one Theory of Mind that describes us all, as our abilities differ. Not all of us will be equally adept at learning emotions, nor will there be any common baseline for what we understand to be the emotions of others.

One thing seems clear: to arrive at a new emotion or to amplify an existing emotion, you must dig into memory and re-experience feelings and associations. To do this and remain intact, you must have some stability. When you stop thinking—if you do or can stop thinking

—you need to be in a stable and familiar state of mind to which you can return.

Trance

Trance is an alternate state of reality. In a trance state, you can be out of touch with the normal and in touch with the abnormal. Normal is not the same as real, and what's abnormal is not false. It's only different from what we expect. A trance state is a state of personal reality that can be, and often is, more real than what others experience or what you normally experience yourself.

Trance is the ideal state in which to explore emotions. That's probably why we do most of our emotional explorations while dreaming. Dreams are where we put together what we feel about what we've experienced in a holistic and atemporal way. We conglomerate feelings from distantly related times, and we disassemble recent and distant memories into new categories. We may even create new categories and arrive at a new understanding.

We remember little about our dreams, but we can learn to remember more. If you do, then you will find dreams affect your emotions. You become moody at some times and emotionally robust at others. Working with dreams is emotionally taxing work that people find difficult. You must go beyond being a witness and return to being a participant.

We do the work in our sleep where emotions are recast and manipulated. It's done subconsciously, and what we remember is only a small part of it. Our conscious mind is like a patron at a library who only knows what's in the collection when we take dream fragments into the waking world. The dream has been ravaging the stacks for hours before we awake. Afterwards, most of our dreams are gone without a trace.

Here, we'll use self-hypnosis in a program to become more empathetic. The exercise is to become more adept at managing, exploring, and exposing emotions. I've created the audio piece called Security as an exploration of stability. To clean off the emotional stage. To put down the tape like actors use in order to know where to stand. To give ourselves a place to work from.

Security (An Induction)

This is a guided visualization that directs you to step out of your conscious mind and disconnect from the world around you.

> *Security* is a hypnotic induction. **DO NOT** listen to this recording while you're driving a car, operating machinery, or doing anything that requires your attention.

I am going to ask you to return to a time of sensitive feelings. I'm going to create one scene and ask you to construct one of your own. Memory is a funny thing. It's not really a record of what happened, it's what you recall, and what you recall has as much to do with where you're going as it does with where you've been.

We're going back to feeling secure, so what I'm asking you to remember is what you know security can be.

Settle back. Lay your hands in your lap, over your stomach, on your chest, or at your sides. Take a breath and close your eyes. Place your focus at the top of your head.

Relax.

Imagine wrapping yourself with a large roll of gauze, as if you were making yourself into a mummy. Imagine yourself laid out on a board with your hands at your sides and your legs together, or you can sense yourself exactly as you are, seated or reclining with hands folded and your elbows sticking out.

Take this roll of gauze in an extra and detached pair of hands and roll it across the crown of your head and begin making wraps around your head, first covering your temples and your forehead, then your ears and loosely across your eyes. You can open your eyes and you can see through this gauze, but it makes things fuzzy, so relax and close your eyes. You can open them at any time, but the more interesting things to see are inside you.

The gauze goes around and around, secure under your chin, loosely around your neck. Now it covers your face, open for your mouth and nose so you can breathe. It feels protective, warm, and comfortable. Over your shoulders and around one arm, across your chest, and then the other arm, and it wraps around your chest. Close as a skin, soft, and flexible. Around your stomach and waist. Around your hips, butt, and groin like a diaper.

Your skin relaxes, your tissues relax, your muscles relax. Each leg is wrapped. The gauze settles the skin on your thighs, your knees, your shins, your calves. Carefully wrap each foot, first the left and then the right, feeling the ankles protected, around the arch, the top, the heel, the bones of your foot, and each of your toes.

All wrapped. All contained. All settled. And now that you're all protected, you can drift down into your imagination.

Imagine you're on a beach in the sun. You're lying on a blanket and the sun is warm, the sand is hot, and the air is cool. You feel the heat and the cool and all the textures all at once. You take it all in; you figure it out, relax, and forget. Let yourself drift.

Release.

There is the sound of waves, a slow shushing that grows and fades. A white noise made by the tumbling sand. A wave rolls in, and then a wave drains out.

A second wave rolls in and for a moment it is louder than the wind, and the wave drains out, ebbing to silence. The rolling starts again. The next wave draws back and then stumbles up the beach until it's spent and then slides back.

A third wave approaches, advances, throws itself down, and sinks into the sand.

Breathing with each wave, the waves count on, each wave the same, all the same, a train of waves, the ocean and the air. All one wave, back to the start of the waves, all the way back to the still dawn and the flat surface of the sea.

Think back to the first story you remember, that was read to you, or told to you, or you read yourself and that interested you when you were young. Maybe you don't remember the story, just the circumstances of where you were and who was near you. And maybe you can't recall too much, but just the feeling of that time. Slow yourself down, let yourself sink into that time now long past.

That was when you saw the world as bigger, its boundaries farther away, and maybe unknown and hard to imagine. And use that opportunity to recall what your world was then. A smaller and more contained world, a world within your house, your neighborhood, defined by your parents. Who were the people most important to you then? How well did you know them?

Did you have brothers, sisters, schoolmates, playmates, real or imagined? Can you remember a scene? There were many scenes. Can you remember your parents? There are many memories of your parents. Remember how slowly time passed? How much time did you spend around your mother or around your father?

Remember.

The memories are a stew and all the flavors mix together. An old stew simmered for years in your mind, mixing colors and flavors. You find some pieces, some memories; separating things into pieces, like old clay, like Play Dough.

The memories aren't separate, pictures aren't clear. Some lack sounds and some sounds lack pictures. You can hear them altogether, like a box of old knick knacks, items long since gone from your shelf, swept into storage along with pencils, paperclips, and old stamps. Lots of boxes. Lots of small boxes.

Take a breath, inhale... exhale. Slow down. Dropping down through layers of memory: three, and then two, and then one.

You're younger now, before clear memory, before a recollection of time passing. Snapshots, isolated images. Seeing yourself in the bathroom mirror.

Opening the cabinet. Your toothbrush. Towels. The shower curtain. The bathtub.

Your mother helped you dress. Picking out your clothes and putting on your clothes. The feeling of safety and security. Maybe you were waking up, or going to bed. Maybe you had a bath. Can you remember when you were bathed? The bathroom, the bathtub, and the warm water.

Imagine your mother's attention; how she felt about you. How much can you remember? How much can you feel in yourself? How much can you feel directed toward you? What emotions did you have when you were comfortable, safe, and complete?

Remember the stairs. The height of the stairs, the height of the banister, and how you negotiated each step. Look down the stairs, you stepped off from the top step. The bottom of the stairs approach as you move down step by step. How many stairs were there, do you remember? Fourteen, thirteen, or twelve?

Down the stairs: eleven, ten, nine, and you found your rhythm. Eight, seven, six. You feel grown up as you can go down the stairs by yourself. Move, balance, negotiate.

Five, four, and three. You're almost in the room at the bottom, the landing opening into choices. Two, one, and you're in a home with a front door and a world outside.

Was there a pet your family had, or was there a pet you knew? A kitten or a puppy that you had or you wanted? What was it like seeing something smaller than yourself, and what did you think about it?

Remember discomfort and dissatisfaction? Do you remember anyone's objections or frustrations? Maybe the harried look of your mother, or the hurry of your father getting ready to go somewhere. They exited the house or your room. They disappeared around the corner, or the door closed and they descended stairs toward the street, the path, or the sidewalk?

What did you feel for yourself? Were you concerned? Were you aware? Did you know what it was to feel compassion, presence, or security? What were your concerns? Can you recall them?

You wonder about the size of things, the extent, the distance, the time. Days roll by like waves. The seasons, the months of the year, the days of the week, the hours of the day. The sun, the dawn, afternoon, evening, and the night.

Imagine yourself thoughtful as a child. What did you have in mind? Maybe you remember the room and the sunlight through the window, the view out the window, or your room and the things you had. Imagine the shelf where you kept things and the things you kept there.

Imagine putting your toys in a box, in a chest, or in a basket. Let each toy pass through your hands, whatever you remember them to be. One was a stuffed animal. One was a model of a house, or a car, or a person. Did you have dolls or did you have soldiers? What were they to you who knew about homemaking and soldiering? Did they have life or were they just things?

Clean up your room. Put things away. Each thing, each object, each memory, maybe from the same time or from different times. Objects you used as far back as you can remember, as well as objects from later times, maybe a dollhouse, a toy car, a skateboard, socks under the bed, and a pair of sneakers.

Putting five things in the box. Watching each item, fascinated by the movements of your hands, placing one, two, three. Putting in the fourth in the box, and the fifth. And take a breath, inhale… and exhale.

Layering, stacking, arranging, placing one atop the next, remembering each item, disappearing and dissolving in your mind. Old memories turned to oil, to mud, to slate, to diamond. All now bedrock of the past. Still there like old, worn words etched in weathered stone.

Relax. Take a breath. Inhale… exhale.

You are younger still, but you're also yourself looking back, remembering what you saw and imagining what could be, what might be, what would be.

Imagine yourself as a toddler living in a family next to a quiet woods, or maybe near the seashore or a lake. Imagine a small home with a warm kitchen and a soft area just for you. Imagine your perfect parents, who love and understand you perfectly, who always know where you are and what you need, who meet your every need. Parents who are always busy but never gone, always building, making, or doing something and always there for you, having what you need when you need it.

They are always with you, and they feel what you feel. You don't have to think, or wonder, or worry, and you are not anxious. Let all your anxieties go. You are calm, and you have no worry because there are no unknowns to affect you.

All the wonder and the mysteries are puzzles to be explored and you are fearless, satisfied, and content. You are loved and secure. You are yourself, but you are not separate. Your parents are with you always. They are there outside you and you feel them inside you, like arms and legs. They are attached to you, and you love them and you love yourself. You are contained.

With this sense of love and protection, focus on your breathing. Letting these senses settle like sensations, become aware of your breath and let your breath take all of your attention. Feeling content, feeling love for yourself and your family, breathing with the gentle changes in your chest, in your blood, throughout your body. Sensations you combine with memories you recall and situations you imagine.

Take a breath, inhale… and exhale… and let relaxation spread throughout your tissues. The relaxation and security in your mind percolates throughout your lungs, bubbling, and your heart, and your blood. Let this move as a chemical, a vitamin, a hormone, something familiar and natural—like your immune system, like oxygen, like glucose—into the chemistry of your tissues, into your cells.

With each breath, you feel more centered and secure—inhale… and exhale—to the memories and imaginations of how it feels to be in that place of mind. Make that real and to keep it safe, it's in your bones. It is the world, the reality that's around you, that only you can know. No need to say or tell, and you can't explain. It can't be explained because it's inside you.

Far in the distance, the thin, real world rattles like a loose shutter in the wind, banging on the house of the world, dissonant, insistent. It's just the wind that rises and falls. You can tune it in or tune it out.

Rising up out of old memories into new ones, separated by time, measured only in memories, plastic and shapeable. Bring what's old and dear close, and what's new and uncertain far away. Unconcerned with annoyances like grass seeds on your pants cuff. Brush them off and breathe with the body in yourself. Breathing the comfort. Secure in the body's balance, knowing itself as secure, balanced, strong, resilient, and relaxed.

Coming back, counting back, breathing back, counting sheep, counting breaths, counting blood cells passing through capillaries, like a wind of life. We'll count to three: breathing once... and exhale. Breathing twice... and exhale. Breathing three times... and exhale, and relax, and be back.

Security is a hypnotic induction. **DO NOT** listen to this recording while you're driving a car, operating machinery, or doing anything that requires your attention.

Listen to a streaming MP3 audio reading of *Security*:
https://www.mindstrengthbalance.com/mindwp/wp-content/uploads/2021/06/Security.mp3

E14 – Empathy VII – Thought and Feeling

August 4, 2021

We have different emotions and different kinds of empathy.

"Empathy is the ability to step outside of your own bubble and into the bubbles of other people." — **C. Joybell**, author

I want to create empathy. Empathy is the key to collaboration and understanding. There are different understandings, so there must be different empathies.

The notion of intellectual empathy—called cognitive empathy—complements emotional empathy as a kind of scaffolding. Intellectual empathy lacks content. We think about empathy in order to give it space, but it's the feelings that make up empathy, not the thoughts.

Discussions of emotion are ineffective because most people are emotionally compromised. This is both a reflection of our incompleteness and our dysfunction. Our emotional range is built through experience and one can never have all experiences. Many emotions are so intense as to both enlighten and damage us. Full emotional function, across all emotions, is unachievable.

Reasoned discussion undermines emotion. We cannot reason our way to any emotional state. This presents a problem; why talk about it?

Unreasonable discussion can create emotional states. This is how I use hypnosis. When we unhitch the reasoning mind, we can lose our sense of time, place, and reality. We can—some more than others—slip into a state of feeling we really are in an unreal state. Hypnosis, like psychedelics, can take you to strange and foreign worlds.

Emotion

Consider this as a working definition of emotion: a family of thoughts and associations that generates feelings other people understand. This is quite relative. It refers to anything that fosters consensus. Emotional levels are also relative. What's appropriate in one situation may not be in another.

If empathy is sharing another person's feeling—not knowing but sharing—then both people recognize a common feeling, generate this feeling in themselves, and communicate the feeling. These three emotional things have to happen for empathy to manifest: recognition, generation, and communication.

Communication

Contrary to what some believe, empathy is not a one-person thing. You cannot "have empathy" for a situation that does not exist. You may feel empathetic toward a memory or an imaginary situation, but there's got to be something to empathize with. Empathy is not a solipsistic state.

Some situations that call for empathy may involve several emotions. If your emotional range does not include what the situation demands, then you won't fully empathize. In complicated situations, we can't be sure we're fully empathizing.

There are situations where being unsure of your emotions is empathetic. You're empathizing with another's confusion. The point is, there is not just one thing called empathy. You cannot "have empathy" as if it was "the thing." Empathy is resonating with other emotional states.

There are interesting situations where one person feels they are empathizing but they are misunderstanding the situation. This can be embarrassing when it happens in real life, leaving you to feel your actions were manipulated or inappropriate, but it is a standard dramatic ploy. Mystery plots typically throw you off the trail by fostering misplaced empathy for characters who are not as they appear.

In real life, there is feedback, and we strive to "get in touch" with the situation. We look for common ground that ensures that everyone agrees. This is the communication part of empathy.

Recognition

One of the greatest mistakes we make repeatedly is assuming that we understand other people. Naturally, we usually see in other people what we understand, so that we tend not to see what we don't. If you are suspicious, then you will question what you see. If you are trusting, then you will consider what you see as true. And if you're manipulative, you will evoke feelings in others that lead them to give you what you want.

One of the first steps in helping another person enlarge their understanding is helping them understand how much of each of these they normally engage in. This is meta-thinking; you are thinking about how you're thinking. You might start this by considering the idea that you're impervious to suspicion, trust, and manipulation. Then, ask yourself how things would develop if you were more suspicious, trusting, and manipulative.

If you're suspicious, then you'll find flaws in other people and their intentions. If you're trusting, then you'll share other people's plans without discernment. And if you're manipulative, then you will achieve your objectives but feel denied of other rewards.

Generation

I believe the greatest problem in becoming more empathic is being able to create emotional states in yourself. If you can't direct, amplify, and apply a feeling to a situation, then you will neither empathize nor understand the situation.

Love may not be a good example because it's complicated, but I believe many people cannot generate love in themselves. Because of that, they cannot love another person and they cannot empathize with the love others might feel toward anything.

If you cannot feel fear, then you cannot appreciate fear in others. This may sound beneficial, but it isn't. If you cannot empathize with fear, then you cannot share with others on the level of their basic needs. If you can't understand fear, then you become indifferent. Psychopaths typically cannot appreciate fear in others, but psychopaths are emotionally disabled.

Consider the connections between these words:

Creativity	—	Reason
Significance	—	Isolation
Body	—	Exposure
Comfort	—	Protection

These word pairs—those in the left and right columns—create contrasts that generate feelings.

I have created the audio titled Empathy-Contrasts I. It is a self-hypnosis induction that asks you to build feelings around these ideas. I believe that the greater your skill at calling for feelings to populate situations, the greater will be your ability to empathize in situations of these kinds.

Empathy, Contrasts I (An Induction)

This is the first in a series of guided visualizations designed to foster greater space for empathetic feelings.

> *Empathy, Contrasts I* is a hypnotic induction. **DO NOT** listen to this recording while you're driving a car, operating machinery, or doing anything that requires your attention.

Find a comfortable position where you can relax. Let your neck and your back settle into your chair, or couch, or bed. Find a position that takes some weight off your spine all the way from the top of your neck to your tailbone. Take a smooth, slow breath that fills your lungs down to the edges at your ribs. Inhale... exhale.

See yourself descending a staircase, taking one step at a time. One step down, two steps down, and with each step getting looser and more comfortable. Feel the horizon rising above you and you moving into the sheltering earth. Get a sense of the energies flowing through your body and let them settle like the spreading waves on a pond. Get a sense of the thoughts floating around in your head. The bits and pieces of the issues that are waiting for your attention. Inhale... exhale.

Imagine that your spine is the trunk of a tall and straight pine tree and that all the activity of the butterflies and the birds takes place at the ends of your branches. These are all the busy thoughts that live like little knots of tension in your joints and muscles where they flitter and chatter and vigilantly insist on taking up your mental space.

Imagine a strong, warm wind rising, sweeping in from all sides and rising up your trunk and up through your branches. As you inhale, the air gathers all around you and sweeps in from below. And as you exhale, the air percolates through the branches, twigs, and needles and flushes out all these little thoughts, chirping birds, knotty ideas, and fluttering issues. Like a leaf blower that shoots the loose litter into the air to be taken up by a vortex updraft and lifted into the sky.

The space it leaves, leaves you feeling like you're on vacation, a relief from the weight of the everyday, the absence of distraction and a warm clarity where there was before a mental itching and emotional pressure.

Take a breath and feel the comfort of no feeling and not having to plug up the holes in the world. There are no holes. There are no issues of concern. They've all been risen into the sky to be carried downwind to other parts of the woods and fields. Some high into the clouds to be carried into other valleys and forests, other watersheds.

In that space of having no sensation, there is a great relief in feeling your natural self, unfettered and unexpressed. More able to feel with care and quiet attention because all is quiet and you can hear, and feel, and see much better.

Remember when you were young and inventive, when you created little things in all the time when you had nothing to do? Maybe little things like simply going around the house to look for anything new, or walking to a friend's house and being aware of changes in the neighborhood.

Without expectations, you create everything you perceive, and you feel the subtle power to imbue what you see with the negative or the positive, to see what is there or what isn't, what might happen and what might not. This is creativity at the basic level, being open to change and recognizing the choices you have and the ones you make.

Consider reasoning, which you will apply like paint to the choices you choose to make real. Reasons are the colors that you paint by number, and as you paint in the reasons, the picture you've chosen takes form. Everyone has their reasons and everyone can be allowed to paint with different colors: green sky, purple grass, yellow air, and white rocks. Let go of your preferences and preconceptions and let someone else call out the colors: red ocean, purple rain, black leaves, and blue sun.

Escape to dream-reasons, just for a moment. No one will know and you don't care. How different might your feelings be if you had reasons different from your instincts? What if you didn't fall into your familiar lines at the first suggestion? Like a dream where things didn't look right. Could you simply relax and let it be a different world?

What is significant? What makes a difference? Are you sure? What if you're wrong? What are you afraid of? You have no fear. You have no worry. Nothing here need make a difference. You're free to think anything.

There are needs we have that we're not aware of, so ever present that they're overlooked. We have to take up space, we have to have a world to interact with. You need a place and you need to find yourself in it. Isolation is a nightmare, and it's not natural, and you can't accept it, but it's your choice and you can make different choices.

How connected are you to other people, and which other people are you connected to, and why these people? There are some connections that feel essential while others are passing or incidental. The essential ones give you something. The incidental ones feel tepid, like warm tea.

Pick one and put it on like it was a bubble or a story, a relationship whose premise you don't remember and whose conclusion you forgot. Essential relations have a feeling. You don't need the reasons and you don't need the details, and you'd have to make them up anyway.

Take a breath and inflate the bubble of consequences and situations. This is a picture of who other people are and how you see yourself. Look at yourself in these situations. You invent these situations or accept what others have invented, things that come from the feelings of the moment. Exhale and let them all escape to leave you with just the feelings. Inhale... and exhale.

Now take these feelings and step to one side of them. See yourself again as creative and attentive and these feelings as things that come up. Set them aside and return to that state of watching and listening without the distraction of feelings, without the colored perspective. Return to a white sheet of paper with black lines.

Those lines will be somewhat annoying in their demand for your attention. Erase the lines, the distinctions, the dichotomies so that you can again relax with all your space to yourself, separate from attachments, comfortable in an isolation that's full in any direction or connection you choose, and free from any of the requirements and demands you've learned.

Your body is separate, limber, flexible, and disconnected. Imagine you are both naked and comfortable. Why are we never comfortable when we're naked? Why have we learned to never show ourselves unclothed? What a sad thing to be ashamed and frightened of exposure, always needing to be covered.

Try to imagine, hard as it might be, that no one wore clothes, and no one cared because whatever anyone thought was okay. If you think skin is ugly, vulnerable, or seductive, or you think your skin is ugly, vulnerable, or seductive, then imagine you have fur that you can grow and shed like a deer or a rabbit has a summer and winter coat.

If that's too far-fetched, then imagine you're a Neanderthal and you wear one skin for summer and one skin for winter in a sort of Tarzan and Jane world, and that's all you need, and that's all anyone needs, and everyone agrees that's all that anyone needs, and you cannot imagine why anyone would want or need any more. Let this be so obvious and sensible that you cannot even waste any more time to think about it. Of the things that matter, clothes don't, and that's just how you feel, and can relax into the feeling that your body is so entirely capable that it needs nothing else.

But this is not how it is for other people. Imagine the depth of the shame and doubt that other people have about being seen naked, even the most brash and confident people. Imagine the sense of vulnerability and the fear. Imagine that kind of vulnerability regarding other things, like behavior, expectation, performance, or presentation. Other things for which we clothe ourselves.

Remember how you still feel in the real world of being judged and visible. Other people feel as worried and exposed as you would about so many things. They worry all the time about exposure. Maybe you worry all the time about it too, but it's become so natural that it no longer forms thoughts in your head, it just guards your thoughts and sets the boundaries.

Feel compassion for the sense of vulnerability others have and that you have, too. How this lingers always on the sidelines, quick to alert you, anxious and vigilant. Do you really need to worry? Could you not have greater faith in yourself? Does it really matter if others see superficial things about you? How much more would you know if you saw or sensed these superficial things about other people?

Look deeper, and below the skin, even though you cannot see the skin. Imagine what other people are in all of their bodies, and imagine what you are beyond what you see of yourself. Do you really know yourself well enough to know your real vulnerabilities? Would you like, or could you benefit from, seeing, knowing, and understanding the vulnerabilities of other people? What if you could share and help them? Would they align with you, and could you both benefit from deeper understanding?

Settle deeper. Feel your arms and how they extend from your shoulders. Sensation flows across your shoulders, down your upper arms, around your elbows, along your forearms, through your wrists, and spreads across your hands, warming the back of your hands and filling your palms. Feel your fingers, both pinkies, both ring fingers, both middle fingers, both index fingers, and both thumbs.

Imagine your arms are your branches that extend from your spine like from the trunk of a tree. A tree is naturally balanced as it grows to bear its weight, and you are naturally balanced when you grow in such a way as to balance the issues and forces in your life. Picture yourself as that tree and its branches, and the warm wind that has washed away all chattering thoughts.

You are left with the low frequencies, the hum of your body and the earth. From your core there is a rumble like the turning of gears, the distant sound of wind across a forest or waves on the coast. This is the base note that synchronizes the others, the fundamental frequency, all your thoughts and actions are harmonics. You are a resonant system, a musical instrument tuned to respond and vibrate in tune.

You cannot hear it, but you create a kind of pink noise, warm and rich. You cannot hear it because it's too many small things and not enough of the big things that we pay attention to. The low hum of the wind and the rustling of leaves, these are natural sounds like those you make but no longer hear. Imagine that you can hear them just beyond the edge of hearing.

When next your ears ring, imagine you can briefly hear your body's hum and a small few, just a few, of the resonances that ring above it. And if you listen, and if you stretch, you'll feel your body fold, extend, open, and return. Stretch and breathe. Extend your spine, arch your back. Broaden your shoulders and press down your arms.

Like a tree flexing its roots, you wiggle your toes and fingers. If not to move, then only just to sense their place and presence. Toes that connect you to place and direction, fingers that expand you to grasp and place. A spine with all of its energies to create feelings and emotions.

Come back to the present space of thoughts and boundaries. Recognize their edge but don't listen to their each and every word. Just remember their role as colorizers, texturizers, and taste buds. You pay a disconnected attention. But to them, like Chicken Little, the sky is always falling.

You don't need to enforce your own imperative. You can watch those of other peoples and, when you do, you might understand their vigilance and obsession.

You might entertain their ideas and suggest your own. You might help yourself and help others to disconnect from the mantra of discomfort. Be more attuned and in harmony with yourself, with the others, and with the earth.

Take a breath, inhale... exhale. Recognize you are okay now and you will be okay in the next moment, too. You have your issues, patterns, and habits. Some feel necessary and some feel comfortable, and you don't need to change anything yet. Just check in with each, clothe them for the day's weather, comb their hair, and send them out to play. In the evening they'll all come back and you can sing them to sleep. Take a breath, inhale... and exhale.

Empathy-Contrasts I is a hypnotic induction — **DO NOT** listen to it while driving a car, operating machinery, or doing anything that requires your attention.

Listen to a streaming MP3 audio reading of *Empathy, Contrasts I*:
https://www.mindstrengthbalance.com/mindwp/wp-content/uploads/2021/10/Empathy-Contrasts-I.mp3

E15 – Sex and Emotion

April 15, 2021

Do we really communicate in realms where we are not fully aware?

"Sex is emotion in motion." — **Mae West**, actress

We control the conscious mind with our thoughts. The unconscious mind rewards us with instant attraction, repulsion, and gratification. The subconscious mind reacts with a complex brew of memories that bathes us in associations. Sex, like a few other activities, involves a conglomeration of conscious and subconscious feelings. We communicate poorly on these topics.

Sex

I expect some of you have sexual thoughts at least once a minute, while others have them less than once a day. This is based on habit, circumstance, and personality. This makes for people who live in different worlds. Yet we rarely recognize, consider, or discuss this.

Death

We often refer to death and sex in counterpoint. I'm not sure why. Perhaps they seem to float at similar levels in our subconscious. One emerges as a fear, the other as a hunger. Superficially, they have little in common. I suggest it is because fear and lust are our biggest boundary issues.

Non-consciousness

Let's clarify what is not conscious. The unconscious comprises our instinctive reactions. Consider these to be chemical pathways below consciousness. All living things are attracted to food, sex, and security when they're in a state of need. They don't need to think about it. It seems like some chemical is doing it, though it could be hard-wired through some other means.

The subconscious is the realm of emotions molded by life experience, learned emotions triggered by circumstance. It runs its programs of its own accord, though we can reprogram the subconscious to varying degrees.

There is a trivial and a substantial level to the subconscious. The trivial level provides access to memories and associations that are under our conscious command. This level automatically retrieves memories and feelings upon our request. It is trivial and does not guide our personality.

Our substantial subconscious is the center of our being. It operates independently of us to support and define us. It feeds us the feelings, ideas, memories, and associations we consider acts of free will. We are its servants.

Most of our feelings have both unconscious and subconscious triggers. A hunger for food can come upon you unbidden, simply because your stomach tells you so. Also, the mention of food can set hunger off. The craving may be in the stomach or the mind, and it's the rhythm of the two together that builds to a crescendo. One without the other envelops us to a lesser extent than when we experience both together.

Fear operates similarly. You can feel fear in your body, as in a fear of heights, and you can feel fear in your mind, as when you ruminate on death. Fears in the mind can be allayed with reason. Fears in the body can be allayed with minor changes, such as backing away from a steep drop. You can feel the difference: one originates as tension in the body, the other as panic in the mind.

When we talk about fear and hunger, we understand each other. We share similar feelings. We may experience them to different degrees in varied circumstances, but we have common ground. And it is on this basis that coming together for a meal has an all-around salutary effect, as does a roller-coaster ride. This is communion through gratification and exaltation.

We feel the separate effects of hunger and fear on the mind and body. There is mixing and crossover, but we all seem to come out heading in the same direction in the end.

The Realm of Complications

It's not the same with sex. Sex does not affect each of us in the same way. We know this chemically, though the chemical measures are rather crude. Sex will stimulate different levels of the emotion-mediating chemicals oxytocin and vasopressin. It's difficult to untangle the effects. We try to understand their effects in the laboratory, but we have yet to succeed.

The effects of these hormones are staggeringly contradictory, interacting, genetically and epigenetically controlled. They trigger feelings of love, attachment, safety, and bonding, but also aggression, anxiety, defensiveness, and anger (Carter 2017). Sounds like your average sexual experience. Why is sex so complicated? No one knows.

Love can be accompanied by jealousy, erratic behavior, aggression, lack of awareness, irrationality, and other less-than-positive behaviors. Is chemical bonding a manifestation of dumbness? Is love a form of stupidity?

This may make sense. Bonding creates dependence. Implicit trust means that you are no longer thinking critically. When two entities merge, they dissolve the boundary between them and, one expects, that they reform that boundary around them. Sex is the closest we come to metamorphosis, but if an emotional metamorphosis is the goal, we mostly fail.

It is the dissolution and reformation of boundaries that gives some sense to this combination of seemingly contradictory emotions and behaviors. Lust is synonymous with the need for gratification. We often imply that lust is negative while sex is positive, but I see no difference. Both seem to be a potential trigger for boundary reformation when they work correctly.

Attraction versus Attachment

"Attraction appears to be a distinct, though closely related, phenomenon [to lust]. While we can certainly lust for someone we are attracted to, and vice versa, they can occur independently of one another. Attraction involves the brain pathways that control 'reward' behavior, which partly explains why the beginning of a romantic relationship can feel so exhilarating. People 'in love' experience a range of intense feelings, such as intrusive thoughts, emotional dependency, and increased energy, especially in the early phases of the relationship...

"Attachment is the predominant factor in long-term relationships. While lust and attraction are pretty much exclusive to romantic relationships, attachment mediates friendships, parent-infant bonding, social cordiality, and many other

intimacies as well. Romantic love appears to be universal, but the extent to which romantic or sexual love forms an important part of long-term relationships may vary. For example, only 4.8% of Australian university students report they would marry without romantic love compared to over 50% of those in Pakistan."
— **Clinical Knowledge Network**, from *Cupid's chemical addiction–the science of love.*

Empathy Versus Understanding

You may not be attached to someone with whom you empathize, but you must empathize with someone with whom you are attached. We're told empathy comes in two forms, cognitive and emotional, but this is not sufficient. There is more than just one kind of cognitive empathy.

Because he is so cogent, you can understand Edmund Kemper's explanations of how and why he killed people, but you would not be guided by his logic. You certainly cannot emotionally empathize with him.

Well, that's not exactly true. There are human elements in Kemper's story that will find some resonance in most people, but not enough to create full empathy. It gets back to the twisted nature of sexuality, fear, and attachment. There are confused elements in all of us, but we hold it together. Kemper did not.

We lack a shared understanding of the unique emotions of sexuality because there aren't any. We explore this in our romantic relationships to some extent, though we do a poor job of it. We don't explore this therapeutically, to my knowledge. The emotions of sexuality are a dark area not only because we lack a theory, but because we lack a language.

We find some clarity from the perspective of multiple personalities. Multiple personalities can explain pathology, but dissociation exists on a spectrum. Dissociation is basic to hypnosis and, to a less recognized extent, in other modalities such as Internal Family Systems and Active Imagination. Dissociation is implicit in the concept of working to integrate your personality.

In these approaches, you create a space to allow separate and divergent aspects of yourself to organize and speak. You don't impose an understanding on them, and you don't reconcile them with who you feel yourself to be. These aspects of yourself lie outside of the belief system to which you subscribe, yet they have a right to exist.

Unity Versus Separateness

When you engage in this process, you are attempting to bring allies together, move antagonists apart, and untangle the conflicts within yourself. The great impediment to this process is a lack of honesty, as it is in any negotiation. There are various reasons for a lack of honesty and we will explore those at some other time.

The exploration and unfolding of the emotions of sexuality precedes our integration of them. Understanding and integration are different. There are some things that you may understand that you don't want to integrate. Some emotions exist in counterpoint to others, such as the ability to feel separate and the ability to feel united.

Your object is growth, health, and strength. You achieve these by engaging, empowering, and expressing those emotions that embrace your situation and enlarge your awareness. Release, reframe, or decompose those aspects of yourself that suffocate your growth. You can only do this with their permission. They must be recognized. Ultimately, they release themselves.

Following Wilhelm Reich, as I understand him, sexual health is emotional health, which is a combination of the most creative personal growth with the deepest interpersonal sharing. It is a metamorphosis.

References

Carter, C. S. (2017). "The Oxytocin–Vasopressin Pathway in the Context of Love and Fear." *Frontiers of Endocrinology (Lausanne), 8*: 356. https://www.ncbi.nlm.nih.gov/pmc/articles/PMC5743651/

E16 – Managing Your Emotions

Finding emotions in your body makes a deeper connection than through your mind.

"No one cares how much you know until they know how much you care."
— attributed to **Theodore Roosevelt**

I'm slowly recovering from Covid-19's assault on my lungs. I'm writing a book called *Instant Enlightenment*. There is a connection between growing in spirit and coming to know one's heart and lungs.

In allopathic medicine, the heart and lungs have no emotion, although there is a recognition of the effect emotion has on the heart. Stimulating emotions increases one's pulse, sedating emotions decreases one's pulse, and disturbed emotions can damage the heart. This is not what I'm talking about.

Traditional Chinese Medicine connects organs and emotions, not organs in the Western sense but organ energy systems. The emotions of Traditional Chinese Medicine are culturally specific. They are not the same emotions that Western cultures share. I'm not talking about these either.

Emotions are a holistic experience. Your emotions are whatever you feel them to be. They are not the same as other people's. Our emotions are roughly similar because they draw on similar energies and similar parts of our brains, but each of us feeds different ingredients into the emotions we assemble.

Our emotions are a combination of nature and nurture. We do have specific brain areas that dominate various emotions. Emotions are assembled from our life experience and unique aptitudes. This has been colorfully described as our emotional chemistry and physics.

Our emotional chemistry is said to be what makes us similar or sets us apart. The perfect mate is said to be a person with "the right chemistry." Our emotional physics is what we can do with what we've got.

Those who know better reject the "right chemistry" idea of compatibility and point out that it's not what you start with that makes or breaks a relationship, it's what you make of it. Managing your emotions is a prerequisite to building an enduring relationship.

Bodywork can release emotions. More than that, bodywork can release trauma. But accessing the body can be done without manipulation. There are some areas of the body that don't move voluntarily and can't be manipulated, yet they're full of nerves and connected to our brains. There are aspects of these systems that we can only access with our minds. It is the mental energy stored in these systems that I'm talking about.

What follows are the sections from *Instant Enlightenment* which explore the heart and lungs. While it's valuable to explore one's emotions through intellect, mood, and memory, it's essential to explore emotions in the body through sensation and imagination.

Lungs

Get to know your body from the inside out. Don't just think about it or rely on sensation or pain to remind you. Go inside and explore what you can perceive, locate, and influence through your muscles, movements, sensations, and intuitions. To be enlightened is to be aware, and the place to start is in yourself.

Our lungs are under our control, though perhaps not as much as we think. Our lungs ask so little of us and allow us our autonomy, but when our lungs have a need, we must serve our lungs.

When I was young, I felt emotionally unsupported and cut off from my mother. I would have tantrums in which I would cry and hyperventilate, trying to get her attention and demanding an emotional connection. It didn't work because she didn't have it in her, and I could not understand. This went on for years until I resigned myself to it. I needed to be heard, and she simply couldn't. Ever since then, my lungs have been the place I store disappointment and loss. This is a resigned form of grief.

Over the years, I have recognized my mother's dysfunctions. She never grew up and could never provide. She remained a child her whole life, playing by herself in a solitude of her own. She was an ever-present absentee mother, present but not providing. Since my siblings were over 10 years older than me, I was effectively an only child. Lacking a mother meant I was alone.

These were the years between 3 and 8. Now I am returning to my lungs. The connection is indirect and certainly nonverbal. My lungs are just a location. There is emotional energy I'm looking to heal, but now there is physical damage as well.

In Traditional Chinese Medicine, the lung system houses our emotions of grief and joy. But it's not the physical lung, it is the lung energy. It is a mistake to equate the material with the energetic, yet we can explore one to find the other. The insights we're looking for are stored in the energy fields of our systems, not as sensations, but as intuitions that emerge from them.

We explore our bodies using movement, perception, memory, and thought, but we're looking for a deeper connection. We would like to hear our organs speak as voices, but what they have to say cannot be fully said in our language. Perhaps they speak in some other language or something we don't recognize as language.

Our broadest language is what we experience in our dreams, a combination of everything: emotions, words, people, drama, memories, and sensations. This is what we want to invoke in communing with our body, to sensitize all our faculties and allow any response. To do this, we must loosen our ego, set aside our words, distance ourselves from judgment, and detach ourselves from reason.

Connect with the organs of your body in a meditation that's deeper than mindfulness. And it's not the organs per se, but the energies they store. Be open to whatever messages you get. What is aroused in you is your truth.

Explore your lungs in space, sensation, function, memory, and emotion. For some of us, there may be words, sounds, music, or nothing. You don't know where ideas come from, but if you're focusing on the energy of your lungs and your lungs have something to tell you, then whatever currents are flowing through your mind may contain the message.

As in the cocktail party's noise, you may not distinguish separate voices. Let your imagination lead you. Let your imaginary ears and eyes find their focus. We exert ourselves to see faces in the foliage, but the shamans say they see these forest spirits everywhere. The difference is being open and receptive.

You are entering shamanic territory, a state of bridging different worlds. In this, you will never settle and you don't want to. It is a dynamic realm, and it is temporary. You must ground yourself before you enter, and you will return to being grounded after you exit.

Your journey is to an energy world that's different from your mind or the physical world around you. You are visiting to retrieve a message. Like a space traveler or an ocean diver, you are out of your realm. You are holding a lifeline back to the familiar, sensible, conscious, and grounded world. Back to a world that we believe is sane.

Don't expect it to make sense. Your lungs don't live in your world and you can't expect them to understand you. You must be gentle, attentive, and accepting. Most of all, you must be honest, and to be honest, you must be fearless.

Place your hands on your chest and breathe. After a few breaths, move your hands to your sides, back, and abdomen. Feel the skin and bones. Only a thin membrane holds in the blood the heart pumps through your lungs.

Simply attend. Use your imagination. Imagine a balloon, a sponge, a train, or a pendulum. If you've seen pictures of lung tissue, then imagine it is around you. Attend to the responses of your muscles as they expand and contract.

Is there tension? Are your actions smooth and controlled? Are you fully relaxed? Look into your memory; watch the images. Don't strain, don't try, just witness and support. Invite the history and the present to fully come forward. Accept both and make a comfortable space they both can occupy. Integration is about acceptance, not resolution. There can be a resolution, but you cannot make it happen. You can only invite it.

Heart

We think of the brain as the seat of intellect and the heart as the seat of emotions. The structure of the brain exceeds our understanding while the heart seems relatively simple: just a muscle with a lot of coordinated parts. It's more than that.

The heart is a partner to the lung and is connected directly to it. Most of the heart's energy is directed not to pumping blood through the body, but through the lungs. The muscles around the capillaries throughout the body push blood through your tissues. There is too much territory and far too much resistance for all your blood to be cycled every minute by the power of your heart alone.

Your heart synchronizes with your lungs, your breath, and all the tissues of your body. Your heart generates a magnetic field that permeates your tissues and extends beyond your body. You can't set your pulse, but you can stimulate or sedate your heart, and tension can interfere with your heart's coordinated function. With practice, you can gain greater control over your pulse.

In Traditional Chinese Medicine your heart's energy relates to your enthusiasm, vitality, joy, and restfulness. A lack of heart energy is associated with torpor, restlessness, depression, and insomnia. We feel heartbreak in our chest and we're asked to place our hand over our heart when stating our commitments.

> "If you have any type of heart disease, any strong emotion such as anger may also cause severe and fatal irregular heart rhythms. Expressions like 'died from fright' and 'worried to death' are not just hyperbole — they are physiologic possibilities. Furthermore, when patients with newly diagnosed heart disease become depressed, that depression increases the risk that a harmful heart-related event will occur within that year… Even in people with no prior heart disease, major depression doubles the risk of dying from heart-related causes."
> — **Srini Pillay**, MD (2016)

Emotions affect your heart, and debilitating emotions harm your heart. People feel in reaction to their experience with little control over their feelings. For most people, emotional expression is disparaged as immature. Being emotional is considered childish while emotional control is considered to be mature. This prejudice affects men more than women.

Aside from repression, we have few tools for regulating our emotions. Easily overwhelmed, most people seek to return to normal. But "normal" is normally dysfunctional, and returning to it puts us back where we started, only to begin the cycle again. Emotions are at the heart of our health and spirit.

Emotions affect the heart and your heart will affect your emotions; it works both ways. The question is whether we're talking about a simple muscle or an energetic system. The answer is that no one really knows because the two cannot be defined in even remotely equal terms. Allopathic medicine is entirely mechanical, Traditional Chinese Medicine is entirely energetic, and psychology is entirely uninformed.

Part of the answer to the question of how to deal with one's emotions is to recognize that emotions are difficult to understand. They summarize many things and often express our basic conflicts. Dealing with one's emotions is not a reasonable task. Emotions are not understood, they are experienced.

I am not telling you what to feel, though you should recognize the physical consequences of your feelings. I am asking you to investigate what you feel.

To be enlightened is not to have pure emotions or simple emotions, but to fully embrace your emotions. This naturally leads to some resolution, but it also leads to greater expression. Of all the features I've felt in the presence of enlightened people, the most palpable was their emotional presence. These people listened to me emotionally and spoke authentic, emotional truth.

When you embrace your emotions, some aspects of your conflicts will resolve. Difficult feelings may neutralize each other as their opposition may cause you to disconnect from them. Other feelings might lose their foundation, erode, and be washed away. A person with many conflicted emotions who embraces his or her conflicts will move toward resolution. If they don't, their search for resolution will at least become a priority.

Here is the key: You want to both be in control and allow your emotions to be beyond your control. It's a question of what emotions you project onto the world. Engage your conflicts without injuring others. Recognize how easily your struggles can manifest in the world that you create for yourself. Recognize that it is your choice to engage in struggle and take responsibility for it.

This is what it means to love your enemy. It means your enemy is not your real enemy, but your realization of the energetic enemy. You do not love your enemy in a personal sense, but in a spiritual sense. The enemy you see in the world is the manifestation of a deeper, broader conflict that affects many more people than yourself.

If you imagine yourself as a cell in the immune system of human culture, then your enemy is one of a million infected cells. Your task is not to heal or convert them, it is to dispatch the conflict, which may mean dispatching them. You have greater power over the negative when you appreciate and understand it. Demonizing the negative is to project your illusions and, in doing so, you lose sight of your adversary's vulnerability and need, as well as your own.

Emotion has its good and bad sides, its strengths and weaknesses. Emotional purity is yours to recognize and become fortified with. Emotional pollution is yours to clean up, repair, dissolve, or discard. In moving into the heart realm, you will encounter conflict. Proceed carefully and be prepared.

Your heart is a gateway to purgatory and, as many gnostic teachings will tell you, do not enter without a guide. Even if you've lived a perfect life—and perhaps more so if you've led a perfect life—you will encounter the generational conflicts and trauma carried in your lineage and your species. Many of the most sanctified people take on the most heinous conflicts. Your work does not get easier as you become more enlightened, it becomes more consequential.

In opening to your emotional truth, you are looking for two things: strength and guidance. You find strength in cleaning your history and resolving your trauma. You find guidance by dropping your defenses and asking for it. Guidance comes from somewhere else. It is not something you fabricate.

My role as a therapist—at least what I call being a therapist—is to evoke my clients' sense of strength and their connection with guidance. Without these, there will be little progress. With these, they can make positive, permanent changes.

You can map part of your emotional territory, but not the deeper and stranger places, at least not in any form you've mapped before. The mysterious territory will not make sense to you until you exit from it and gain an appreciation of the whole.

You need a guide, and the guide cannot be anyone outside you: no doctor, therapist, coach, or teacher will know your territory. Some people are too proud to admit their ignorance, and these people will not find their guide. The guide must emerge from inside you. They can only emerge once you've set your needs and preconceptions aside.

In putting ourselves aside, we confront our limits. We will not set our family aside and many of us will not set our job, authority, power, or privilege aside. The more of your preconceived structures you keep, the more your travel through the landscape of your emotions is delayed.

I'm not saying you have to abandon your family and culture, but you have to separate from your familial and cultural preconceptions. In your search for your emotional authenticity, you may find yourself resisted by those in your family and community for whom you are playing a useful role. You may also have to accept and repair relationships with people you've rejected or harmed. You can do this with humility, but you cannot do it with a sense of privilege or entitlement. Discovering your emotional truth requires leaving your ego behind.

More Than Mindfulness

The connection is to your heart; you are becoming heartful rather than mindful. The goal is to fully surround yourself with the energy of your heart.

The exercise of mindfulness focuses you both on what's in your mind and what's left when your mind is empty. Becoming heartful means focusing on the being and doing of your heart. This may start with the experience of your pulse in whatever part of your body you can sense it. It goes beyond the pulse to currents of energy and resonances in your body.

Go beyond the pulse as a verb and look for the energetic state of circulation. This exists as a rhythm in your brain and a sense of coherence in your body. Coherence means the symbiotic attachment of different parts of your body. Sense your pulse at various parts of your body.

You'll find the pulse is not synchronized in different parts, but it is coherent. Your pulse peaks at different times in different parts of your body. The beats are not synchronized, but they are coherent. Their duration is the same.

Explore your pulse in these different locations. Notice how your pulse feels different in these locations. You can hear your pulse in the waves of white noise in your ears. You can see your pulse in the scintillations behind your eyelids.

Your first task is simply to receive as much and as many sensations of your pulse as you can attend to. You may feel your pulse in several places at once, or you may cycle through focusing on different places. Discard your mind, your thoughts, and your emotions. You are just moving to the rhythms with attention but without a sense of the present, like dancing. This is a meditation and there is a next step.

The next step is to bring in an empty mind and let the beats flow through it. To invite and allow whatever memories and associations come while you are engaged with your heart's rhythm. You are not looking for sense or story; you are looking to dream without lucidity, letting conflict and chaos build your landscape.

Look, but do not look too carefully. Take what's shown without demanding more. As in a dream, you cannot examine the images without tearing the fabric. It's not until the meditation is over that the message is complete. Don't interrupt.

There may be no message or no apparent message. Remember what you can, and revisit the memory on occasions throughout the day. It could well be that the meaning is only clear when your mind is focused elsewhere.

The body meditation is unlike other meditations. It extends beyond the time over which you're engaged in it. Unlike a key that opens a lock, heartful meditation matures as your body responds. You are calling in your body's voices and some of them speak through other means, through the modulation of energies that appear only when you're in other states.

Stay relaxed as you go through your day. Remain attentive and thoughtful. Some memories are like drifting bubbles that take time to emerge. In the same way that it can take minutes to remember a word or a name, recalling the body's memories may take hours.

References

Pillay, S. (2016 May 9). "*Managing Your Emotions Can Save Your Heart.*" Harvard Health Publishing, Harvard Medical School. https://www.health.harvard.edu/blog/managing-emotions-can-save-heart-201605099541

E17 – Communicating With Honesty

Understanding thoughts and emotions in relationships.

"A lie gets halfway around the world before the truth has a chance to get its pants on." — **Winston Churchill**

Speaking and Feeling

What if you spoke to yourself and yourself answered in a different language?

Feelings and intellect are different ways of engaging with the world, and we poorly translate between them. Everyone knows this, yet hardly anyone works to reconcile the differences. Perhaps we don't understand the differences ourselves.

Our solution is to celebrate the intellect and denigrate our emotions. We keep our emotions in check and we tell ourselves they're under control. This is recognized to be a fallacy; our intellect rides on our emotions. The intellect keeps emotions out of the front office, but your emotions have a key to the back door.

We like to think that we have reasonable mastery over our behavior, and we pretend this means our behavior is reasonable. But reason is a foot soldier to our emotions, and emotions are higher up the chain of command. The same emotions we dismiss as crass and brutish guide our thoughts more than they're guided by our thoughts.

We communicate in words and profess commitment to our presentations. Yet, so often, people's actions do not live up to our expectations and, to be fair, we don't live up to other people's. We write this off as miscommunication, evasion, and sometimes dishonesty. What we don't recognize is that we communicate in two languages, one verbal and the other nonverbal, and we communicate two intentions, one intellectual and the other emotional.

If we're really skilled, honest, and maybe lucky, our intellectual and emotional intentions coincide. When this happens, we'll give the same verbal and nonverbal messages. But when they don't align, our verbal message is dominated by our intellect, while our nonverbal

441

message is emotional.

Disagreement

Disagreement is the source of much of our frustration, and I believe most of our miscommunication is intentional. Not intellectually intentional, but more along the lines of emotionally noncommittal. Call it ambivalence, confusion, dishonesty, or betrayal. Whatever we call it, the result causes much suffering.

We take little responsibility for our communication. Rarely do we reopen past issues to rebuild understanding. This is partly because we're not sure what other people think, and partly because we hope misunderstandings have been resolved. Good relationships require constant reworking at their foundations, and few of us do this work. That's why many of our relationships are in trouble.

Disagreements go unresolved because bridges have been burned or the misunderstandings are too great. We skirt around our communication failures, trying to shore up broken resolutions. Leaky boats rarely fix themselves, they get worse, and the same is true with relationships.

Our preference to avoid recognizing problems lets those people who make a habit of betrayal slip by unrecognized. As long as we don't call them out, they continue to believe they're acting reasonably. The problem is more one of failing to be proactive than failing to react. Once everyone's intellects and emotions are in conflict, the relationship boat is not only leaking, it's on fire.

Words have a life of their own, and most of what we say we don't really mean. It's just all we can think of. If you learned to speak what you felt, if you really could communicate your emotions, then not only would you be better understood, but you would raise everyone's communication to a higher level.

Emotions are not word-based, and when we try to convey emotions verbally, we're on shaky ground. When we verbalize, we know what we're saying, but we're not sure of what we mean. When we communicate from our emotions, we know what we mean, but we can't really put it into words, or we refuse to.

Relationships

My most serious misunderstandings have come from my domestic relationships. In each of the two relationships that failed, I didn't see it coming. I consider myself a victim, but I also consider it my fault.

It was my mistake to have accepted emotional debts based on credit I should never have granted. I believed in good faith. I believed in that ultimate of intellectual delusions: that love will find a way.

I suspect this would describe many of those of you who are reading this. I would not be surprised if, after all your experiences, you're not doing much better at what you're doing now than you were before. It is a mistake to blame yourself for being misunderstood—unless you knew you were lying and did it anyway—but it's correct to blame yourself for accepting without question what you wanted to believe.

If you were lying and knew you were, then your future is bright and your path to improvement is clear: stop lying. Your mistakes are plain and all you have to do is reform. Once you do, then you'll be in the same boat as the rest of us: trying to achieve honest communication. At least you'll have a chance.

You are to blame for believing what you were told, not for accepting the facts, but for accepting the implications. It's your error for emotionally believing what you were intellectually told. Not only were you foolish then, but you'd be foolish now if you did it again. In fact, giving emotional credence to intellectual statements is almost a contradiction.

More likely, you did the best you could in expressing yourself, but what you did not do was take responsibility for believing what you heard. And what you heard was more what you wanted to hear, and less of what was authentically meant by whoever said it. When these errors of trust pervade work and friendship, they are tolerated, but they can be fatal in intimate relationships.

Commitment

We make statements intellectually, but we make commitments emotionally. The intellect sees the world as a puzzle and fits jigsaw puzzle pieces together. It's always open to making adjustments.

The emotions represent the complete picture, the whole puzzle. Changing one's commitment changes everything; it creates a new picture. It's like tossing out one jigsaw puzzle in favor of another. So, what happens to the partner who is still trying to fit together the pieces from the old puzzle?

We are poor at reconciling our intellectual and emotional presentations because we don't know what they mean ourselves. Our left brain's reasoning is not fully informed of our right brain's emotions. I may be more uncoordinated than most, but that also enables me to see the two parts separately. I've learned to see the shape of the individual pieces, and I've learned to appreciate the whole.

One of my partners was great at making commitments with absolutely no emotional foundation. She did not know what a commitment was, and I could not understand how one could entirely lack integrity. I cannot blame her for her lack—she never experienced integrity—but I failed to understand. I believed what I heard because I wanted to. That's only as good as it goes, which is a lovely example of an intellectually useless emotional truism.

Certainly, we all lean toward what we want, and it's our discernment that keeps us out of trouble. This is why people become more discerning and less impetuous with age. Older people have been around the block a few times. They've seen what younger people don't believe, which is that if you do what you did before, then what happened before will happen again.

It's your fault when you don't recognize a mistake the first time. That doesn't mean you can avoid it the next time. It means you're responsible for seeing it. Some mistakes are too costly to repeat, and your mistakes are the only faults that you can fix.

How does one fix these kinds of errors? One starts by recognizing the distance between intellectual constructs and emotional truths in oneself. Recognize that between what you do know and what you don't know lies a vast plain of ignorance. It looks small, like a puddle you can jump over, but that's because you see neither its contents nor its boundaries. When you try to jump over what you don't know, you'll flounder in a sea of ignorance.

By recognizing the disparity between intellect and emotion, you can build bridges between the two that have some foundation on both sides. It's our own responsibility to understand the contracts that we accept. "Read the fine print," they say, but the emotional terms are not written. You must find them in nonverbal form.

Judging from my own mistakes, and those I infer my clients make, it's clear that understanding the true feelings of another is not a simple matter. Our odds of success would be greatest if all parties were honest, and that's the problem: all parties are not honest. Honesty doesn't even exist where there is no insight. How does a person without integrity learn what it is, or appreciate the value of it?

Honesty

Truth is the brick and mortar of relationships, but it can get no farther than you are honest with yourself. Just as my previous partner did not know her feelings, she could not present herself truthfully. In most disagreements that I encounter, and in many of the misunderstandings I explore, there is a great lack of truth.

Distinguish what's true from what's fact. This will allow you to distinguish what's false from what's a lie. Facts and falsehoods have little to do with truth and lies. In matters of the heart, most people can be trusted to convey the facts, but few people will tell the truth.

The reason is simple: there is one kind of fact and two kinds of truth. The two truths are the intellectual and the emotional, and while the intellectual truth is closer to fact, the emotional truth is more significant. And just as intellect and emotion don't speak the same language, the two kinds of truth don't share the same universe. This means that when you're assessing another person's truth, you really have two separate truths to consider.

When treading on intimate territory, people won't tell the truth because they don't know it, and they don't know it because the truth is emotional and they cannot understand it themselves. Instead of telling the truth and disadvantaging themselves—since all presentations seem equally false—they reinterpret your questions and give you the facts. Do you love me? Yes. Can I depend on you? Yes. Are we best friends forever? Yes. Gone in a year.

If you're like me and many others, you'll take the facts as truths that justify your hopes. You'll dismiss the fears of others because you don't want to hear them. You are practiced in using rational arguments to overlook emotional feelings in yourself.

Emotional truth means seeing your emotional ignorance. This is not a factual truth. It is not absolute. It is the truth about how much you don't know. It takes a lot of self-respect to see and to accept your ignorance.

Goals and Means

I approached relationship partners in the same way that I approached mountaineering partners: two people trusting their lives to each other in order to reach a goal. Mountaineering partnerships are a beautiful thing, but romantic relationships are more like two thieves robbing a bank, both looking after their own interests.

What else would you expect when people have a common goal but no common means? That is the difference. In physical or financial pursuits, we share and understand the means to the goal, but in relationships, we don't share a common means.

Maybe I was just too naïve; I'm inclined to feel that way now. But I know what commitment means, and I know when I can offer it. In contrast, most of the "smarter" people with relationship problems don't know this.

I was certainly wrong in assuming both honesty and commitment from others, and I was wrong in equating facts with truth, but I can now distinguish the two. That's a skill many people need to learn.

Encouragement

How do I communicate these distinctions to you? I can talk about it as I'm doing here. I can model it. It's much more subtle than you might think. Finally, you have to be ready to hear it, and most people are not there yet.

Being ready is the most important ingredient. If you're not ready, you won't hear what I say, you won't appreciate what I model, and you won't care. You might take honesty as a sign of weakness. Some of my clients have done that, and I recognize it when it happens. They're looking for a "Dr. Goodbar," an official version of Mr. Goodbar. Someone who knows all, sees all, and affirms what they believe in. Doctor Goodbar does not exist.

When you're ready for full honesty from others—which means you're ready to see what you don't understand about yourself—then there is not much more that I can do for you. My task is really just to get you to that point. Once you cross the threshold of honesty, the world changes. You then see the uncertainty, dishonesty, parasitism, and betrayal in others and, possibly, in yourself.

Maybe you want a better relationship or job, or to improve your finances or your family situation. You'll feel the need, express it sensibly, and form a plan. We're marginally competent at each of these things, which means we'll come up with a plan that might work.

But the most important thing is to be honest about all that you don't know. To recognize all the things that violate your hopes and preconceptions. Until you do that, your plan is going to go the same way as your previous plan.

These days, when things have gotten increasingly confusing because of how interrelated they are, honesty is confused with pessimism. Optimism is popular. Pessimism is a lack of faith.

The Law of Attraction is believing reality is attracted to your wishes. It's a faith that circumstances will arrange themselves, which they do under the right conditions. But in more chaotic times, circumstances are whatever is flushed out of the bushes. Those circumstances don't tend to line up.

The function of a counselor is not to advise you. It's to help you find emotional truth, see the line between truth and falsehood, and cheer you across it. They can't force you, but they can continue to hold you to the line, and they might refuse to work with you if you won't cross it.

E18 – Why We Fight (Because We Don't Connect)

March 3, 2023

The origin of conflict in relationships and the importance of establishing resonance.

"When you find yourself stuck in an oversimplified polarized conflict, a useful first step is to try to become more aware of the system as a whole."
— **Peter T. Coleman** (2011), psychologist

Speaking from Here, Hearing from There

The emergence of psychedelic-assisted therapy is making the importance of understanding altered states clear to some people. We experience altered states frequently but rarely pay any more attention to them than we do to the clouds. Despite psychedelic states being obviously altered, those who work with psychedelics therapeutically are still not taking altered states seriously.

I speak to therapists and clients, and these are two distinct groups. Clients and prospects are more in touch with their emotions than most people. Perhaps I should say they are in conflict with their emotions, but whatever the case, they're aware of conflict from a first-person point of view. They are aware of their investment in their states of mind.

Therapists, psychologists, and people in general are out of touch with their emotions. They are practitioners, not adepts, and their job is nine to five. There is both a preference for and a professional bias toward being emotionally disconnected. Emotions are hard to control voluntarily, and intentional control of emotions is short-lived and incomplete.

The intellect creates rules and boundaries and, by themselves, these offer the illusion of control. Rules and boundaries are good for maintaining order, but bad for resolving chaos. The profession of therapy, and the institutions that fund and endorse therapy, are all about control. You won't find an emotionally reactive therapist or an emotionally governed institution, at least not under normal circumstances.

Speaking to intellectuals about emotions is like speaking to teachers about learning, physicists about reality, or priests about agnostics. You are only heard from the mindset of the person you're speaking with.

If someone has a narrow view of reality, then that is how you'll be heard. If you're trying to communicate something outside another person's worldview, then you're probably wasting your time. Encourage a selfish person to be open-hearted, and they'll listen to you with self-interest.

> "A person can be reached only at his own level and only to the extent of his capacity. When there is no capacity to understand, you cannot force even the greatest and most wonderful treasures on a person."
> —**Saint Germain**, fictional character in Maria Szepes', *The Red Lion* (1997, 272)

Fleeing, Freezing, and Fighting

We focus on the three modes of reaction: fighting, fleeing, and freezing. We could alternatively focus on various modes of engaging: intellectually, emotionally, and physically. There are other modes as well, such as instinct, spirit, and the subconscious.

Just as there are various ways to intellectualize—scientifically, therapeutically, and religiously—there are various ways to approach conflict. If we want to react more effectively, then we'll have to consider these other modes and levels.

I want to focus on fighting, but I suspect fighting can't be fully understood outside the other modes of action. The trichotomy of fight, fly, or freeze appears to be exclusive to other animals —they behave in one or another of these modes exclusively—but this is not the case with humans. Humans see these as alternatives on a pallet from which we create hybrid mixtures.

Animals that don't intellectualize or dispute may react in one or the other of these three ways. But even with other animals, these are more symbolic acts rather than committed states. The decision to fight, flee, or freeze is quickly reevaluated when the situation changes. We may only see these three reactions in the behavior of animals, but we should not assume that these other animals think as we do.

We react by mixing our modes of action. While advance, retreat, and surrender are intellectual categories, our emotions do not reduce in this way. We normally engage in multifold strategies, fleeing from some issues, engaging in others, and refusing to react to certain circumstances. What we identify as a true fighting mode is an obdurate commitment to a combative state of mind, regardless of circumstance.

People Don't Play a Zero-Sum Game

When people reflect on conflict, they focus on the cause and overlook the purpose. People assume we fight in order to win a contest or prevail in a disagreement, but we fight for dominance. We need dominance because we're insecure.

We hear this state of mind in the rationalizations of pugnacious generals who focus on complete destruction rather than immediate goals. This is what wiser animals do not do, it is also what wiser investors do not do. The intellectual locked in an emotionally altered state, unable to extricate themselves from an emotional reaction, becomes obsessed.

> "You've got to kill people, and when you've killed enough, they stop fighting."
> — **Curtis LeMay** (Rhode 1986), General, US Air Force

I'm not interested in what triggers a dispute, I'm interested in why we engage in it. Most fights between people start over incidental issues. The fights seem overblown when we only look at the trigger. Triggers don't cause disagreements, they set them off. Disagreements are more about how a person thinks, and less about what a person thinks. They're more about why you acted and less about how you acted.

We fight over things that are unclear. When you witness a conflict, it may look like the sides are drawn and the rewards are clear, but they're usually not. It's more common that a conflict has been triggered by an insignificant issue. The argument develops to clarify larger issues, grievances, and goals.

We rarely fight battles over material possessions or simple solutions. If we don't know how to fight incremental battles, we can only aim for a one-sided victory. In this, we cannot achieve balance. If we don't know what we're fighting for, then we're drawn into a conflict of emotions.

Emotions Don't Reach Conclusions

This is a failure of emotional understanding, becoming captive to one emotion and locking out others. It is an inability of our intellect to play a balancing role in facilitating our shift between emotions. This is the origin of family violence and political abuse.

This failure to connect intellect with emotions results in one dominant emotion keeping control until it undermines itself or the situation, and this is what emotions do. Emotions represent dominant points of view that are one-sided summaries. If you cannot engage an emotion intellectually, then it will control your thinking until it loses its reason to exist.

An emotional argument does not end when the aim is achieved because there is no aim. The only emotional conclusion is emotional exhaustion.

Intellectualizing Emotions is Not Engaging

Psychotherapy fails when it disengages from emotion. We see this in what's offered as emotional or behavioral therapy, which combines sophistry and intellectual manipulation. We see this in psychedelic-assisted therapy, in which clients enter an entirely emotional state and therapists emotionally disengage from them. There is a useful place for manipulation—it's called reframing—but it's combined with emotional engagement.

In the current model of psychedelic-assisted therapy, emotions are addressed in the integration phase that occurs after the experience. This is sleight of hand that hides a practitioner's lack of knowing how to engage in the psychedelic space. Therapists who are no better at handling emotions during a psychedelic experience will not be any better at handling emotions afterward. Intellectualizing emotions does not work, it only seems better when you're in an intellectual state of mind.

You engage emotions by being intellectually present in an emotional state. This is not the denial that we've been taught at home and in school. It means talking in tears, sorrow, shame, or anger, not talking over tears or repressing one's feelings. Emotions have their own voice, separate from yours, and it is engaged and demonstrative. Emotions are not interested in intellectual projections. They are interested in immediate, perceptible results.

Awareness Leads to Self-Awareness

In order to manage grief, anger, or psychedelic states of mind, you must become self-aware while you are in those states. Attempts to recover a "normal" state of mind, a nonemotional state of mind, will not lead to a balanced emotional state. It leads to a repressed emotional state.

Rather than leaving the emotion and retreating into a state of anesthesia and disconnection, go into emotion and gain connection. This is the aim of regression, somatic, and Eye Movement Desensitization and Reprocessing (EMDR) therapy. In each of these, the approach is a balanced combination of intellectual and emotional engagement. Each of these therapies aims to help you learn a higher level of insight and control.

Navigate States of Mind

Learning to navigate states of mind requires going outside established psychology, psychotherapy, and psychiatry. Those practitioners are not trained to teach others or master their own altered states. Compare our academic training to a shamanic initiation in which one passes through states of horror, transfiguration, and psychic death.

Western health professionals are trained to enforce consensus reality, avoid professional burn-out, and continue to deliver measured doses of academic therapies. Western therapists are taught a simulated form of empathy, which they're instructed to use along with emotional disengagement.

True engagement happens when you share the same emotion. It's only when you resonate with another person that you understand them, and you don't understand them because you share similar concepts. You understand them because you share similar emotions. The reason we fight with each other is to get the other person to share our emotional state.

We make the mistake of thinking that by telling someone how we feel, they'll share our feeling, but this only works if we are in touch with our own feeling. It does not work if we are detached from it.

To project our feeling onto who we imagine another person to be does not result in inclusion, it furthers separation. As long as you maintain a dichotomy between your thinking and feeling selves, you will not invite inclusion and you will not find a balance.

Balance occurs when the antagonism within yourself stops. This does not mean resolution, it means acceptance. It does not mean compromise; it means recognition.

This balance may not be stable—a new state of balance rarely is—but it can be explored and expanded. This is the time to engage your intellect. It happens when you can speak from your emotions without being overwhelmed by them.

In order to navigate your states of mind, you must be in those states both intellectually and emotionally. That means you must be able to speak, think, connect your thoughts, and act with clarity while you're in an emotional or otherwise altered state of mind.

This is what we are not doing when in conflict with another person. We are not yet doing it in psychedelic-assisted therapy. We're starting to do with the regression, somatic, EMDR, and other state-altering therapies. If you're interested in gaining emotional control, if you're interested in overcoming strife and struggle, then this is what you'll need to do.

E19 – The States We Make

March 30, 2022

We don't just make waves, we are waves.

"When we wake up from our confused state of mind, that is enlightenment."
— **Dzogchen Ponlop Rinpoche**, Tibetan Buddhist scholar

Home

Consider us to be architectural beings. There is a vision that begets a design, construction that creates a container, and a variety of living entities that consider us their home. The whole affair represents the experience of being. The quality of life for the entities depends on the success of the accommodation and the original design.

This is a metaphor for our state of being. There is a design, but it's a design of memories and associations, not blueprints and mechanical specifications. A structure is built in the realm of neurology, behavior, and environment. This is a structure of psyche and spirit, not structural engineering.

Living entities inhabit this structure. They are parts of yourself, persistent but not always clear. Your personality comprises whatever crowd shows up, made from your familiar cast of characters. Your being is the family home represented by whatever parts of yourself are awake at the moment.

The container you create is the mental house that you inhabit. It can be pleasing and tastefully adorned. It can be average and uninspired, or it can be a total wreck on the verge of collapse. As your wide range of moods shows, you are not particularly unified.

Family

Your mental inhabitants are the people who are at home in your mind. Some talk to you a lot and others are silent. Some have a "take charge" attitude, while others are so hidden or lost you may have forgotten about them. They are the relationships between your memories entered

454

through experience and the ideas hosted or banished by popular vote among your attitudes, enhanced or retarded by genetic aptitudes, learned skills, and luck.

You can exercise intention in creating your personality at any one moment, but it's unclear how much effect you have and it isn't necessary. After all, you are the self that you're presenting, and you have a personality even without trying. Your ability to control yourself depends on how much distance you can achieve. You can refine yourself.

It's a good idea to reflect on who you are and how you're coming across. If you have no distance, then when you reflect, everything seems just fine. Your attitudes are justified and your jokes are funny. The more distance you can bring to bear while still seeing yourself in context, the more you'll appreciate how you're seen by people with a different point of view.

I once joined a group of six young Mongolians—men and women—who shared a taxi that only fit four comfortably. We crammed five of us into the back seat. My friend was in the front seat and I was unacquainted with those layered on top and beneath me in the back.

This humorous violation of personal space was interesting because, as an American in Mongolia, I was not familiar with the culture and our communication was poor. I knew the others thought it was funny, but not why, and I was unsure of where to put my hands. I didn't know how my expressions were read or my comments interpreted. I had lots of ideas and they were probably wrong.

Creation

We build our state; we design, construct, and inhabit it. This will happen automatically if we don't think about it, and even when we do think about it, a lot happens without our being aware of it. The more we are aware of it, the better our creations turn out. At least we're more likely to take responsibility for them.

The design is emotionally based on what we want at the moment. With a dash of reflection and a dollop of rationalization, we construct our state by pulling the equipment that we think will be useful from memory: caution, courage, stillness, silliness, love, along with a few unwashed feelings. We are the herd and the shepherd, the fox, the hounds, and the hens.

Be self-confident, trust your intuition, and question everything you do. You can do both without sacrificing either if you can hold two points of view at the same time.

One point of view is your thinking mind. The other is an arm's length connection to your higher self. The connection is at arm's length because your higher self has little tolerance for your ego. They are of different dimensions. Your higher self will not fit beside your ego. It does not speak the language of your mind, and it is not interested in most of the chatter with which we busy ourselves.

Your thinking mind shifts among your different perceptions with the rhythm of your attention. You are alternately automatic, intellectual, emotional, and sensory. Behind this calliope of thought forms, your higher self presides, but it only presides if you're humble and without pretension. Your higher self is aware of a larger world than you are.

Most of the time, we're too busy. We take ourselves too seriously for our higher self to take much interest. We're not listening and we're not open to suggestions of a deeper nature. Your higher self doesn't involve itself in most of your affairs, primarily because you don't invite it. Inspiration doesn't come unless you ask for it.

I frequently invite the advice of my higher self. I can only do this when I slow myself down. My higher self looks at the biggest picture. It looks for things that can obstruct my ability to get things done. I think slowly. That can get me into trouble unless I plan ahead. If you're in a rush or under pressure, then you're giving primacy to current forces and present needs. That may be required under the circumstances, but it prevents greater care. It limits the associations you can make with the past and future.

A weekend trip with my college outing club in the dead of winter brought us to the base of the largest mountain in New Hampshire. We'd been delayed, and it was after midnight. We had hiked through deep snow under a full moon, along an unbroken trail at a temperature well below zero. We couldn't see the trail. It then became clear that we were not on the trail. This was well before the days of GPS navigation, and we were lost.

We were not completely lost. You can't be completely lost unless you lose your memory, but most of the group didn't know where they were to start with. It was getting colder. They were tired, and they didn't know what to do.

If we followed our footsteps back to the cars, we'd have to abandon the trip and spend the night driving home. The followers relied on the leaders and the leaders were lost. Without the intuitional guidance systems that some of us have, people panicked. Have you ever felt like this?

There weren't a lot of choices and there wasn't a lot of pressure, so the situation had plenty of room for contemplation. For me, the wilderness is all about contemplation and the wilder it gets, the more thoughtful I become.

It must have been the contrast between the beautiful night, the wondrous woods, and the crying coeds that gives this old memory such staying power. I don't even remember how it all turned out except that we eventually found our way.

State

It takes a different attention to keep ourselves in balance. We build our states of mind in stages and we can get confused at any stage: their design, construction, and those aspects of our personality that we include. All our faculties can come into play at each stage. We do this automatically.

Be aware of what you design, the mind components out of which you frame it, and those parts of yourself that inhabit it. The chances are that you designed your state of mind to accommodate selective parts of your personality to begin with. The state of mind in which you would sit on a bed of nails is not the state of mind with which you prepare breakfast. We prepare our daily schedules, but how well do we prepare ourselves for them?

Your future depends on your state of mind, or the states of mind you create for yourself. Your state defines the world line on which you travel. This world line takes you into the future. While you cannot remake the past reality, you can choose the person you'll be and the perspective you'll see. You may or may not be fully "in the now," but would that tell you all you need to know to connect to the past and future?

Your state is your preparation for the future, an architecture across time. Realize that the farther you look ahead, the more paths exist and the more freedom you'll find if you can see it.

You can always change the design of your state of mind. The memories and associations from which it's built can and will change if you're open to new experiences. The population of your personality, the whole-cloth attitudes you accommodate, are yours to mold. You are not their servant; don't follow their orders. They don't have access to your higher self, only you do.

If there is any real magic in this world, it is your ability to conjure and dispel entities within yourself. You can change your state with a wave of your hand. You can manage the elements of personality that will inhabit the mind that you construct.

You cannot dictate the dominance of your moods or the hierarchy of your personalities. You must help them work together. There will be dominant voices you're attached to or subservient ones, and they will not all agree. Your best hope is to bring them together to resolve their differences. To do this fully requires releasing those who might otherwise frighten you, which is why we never do it.

Your higher self can guide your parts, but it can't control them by brute force. What your parts decide must be their decision. At least they must think so. Your creation of the proper state provides a home for the family of your parts. Your state of mind can be your higher self's vision of the future.

> "A leader is best when people barely know he exists, when his work is done, his
> aim fulfilled, they will say, 'We did it ourselves.'"
> — **Lau Tzu**, founder of Taoism

Postscript

To collect this dust of thoughts into a ball headed in some direction, I will summarize each essay. They follow an evolutionary progression from pre-cognizant: sensory, through protohuman: emotional, to primate: thoughtful. My purpose is to weld together three disparate modes of thinking without elevating any one mode to dominance.

These modes of experience are complementary and distinct. More than distinct, they are different and the development of one does not develop another. All are separately necessary, and all can be synthesized at a higher level in an integrated awareness.

An integrated human mind recognizes, respects, and draws upon these three in collaboration, though not in equal measures or simultaneously. It's at this higher level where we find stability. The sane person steps back and lets all their voices speak.

There is no single measure of sanity. Sanity juggles modes of experience that need not agree and often don't. These three modes are three legs resting on each person's unique geography. Your stability depends on your maintaining cohesion within a society of mind.

Sensations

S1 – How Wise is the Body?

Our bodies are perceptual filters and contribute to many of our memories and associations. Getting in greater touch with your body results in a deeper connection with your mind.

S2 – Cultivating Mind–Body Health

Your body works to maintain balance while your mind strives for growth. Their shared interest in longevity and their different opinions about risk lead to different programs for health.

S3 – You Are the Echo of Memories You've Forgotten

Memories are present reconstructions of the emotional fragments that form our character. We mistake impact for accuracy and memories are not accurate; they define our present state of mind.

S4 – The Origin of Chronic Illness and the Nonsense of Medical Hypnosis

Chronic illnesses can persist because of their emotional components and some illnesses originate from them. Issues of denial, depression, anxiety, anger, and fear can grow into illogical symptoms.

S5 – How the Placebo Effect Implies Learning, and Learning is Hypnotic

Your subconscious is the engine of your awareness, and your emotions are the fuel. The placebo effect is an action of your body generated by your mind. It motivates learning.

S6 – Attachment, Resistance, and Secondary Gain

Your life flows like water through emotional terrain. You change the course of your life by terraforming this landscape, working both with and against yourself.

S7 – Trauma and Healing

Current trauma is fueled by distorted memory, while ancestral trauma is culturally informed. Reconstruction is detective work. You are the only person who can create a recovery frame of mind.

S8 – Memory, Amnesia, and Your Self

We don't question memory because what we remember is essential. To doubt it threatens our hold on reality. But what really happened, and why do you remember so little of it?

S9 – Imagination

We make up everything that we know and think, but some of us are more creative than others. Are the rest of us lacking in our abilities, or do we just not use our imaginations?

S10 – Interoception

Learn to better control your body's functions if you want to live better and longer. Start by being more attentive, sensitive, and responsive to your body's subtle cues.

S11 – Interoception, the Colon

Take an incredible journey through your bowels. Reintroduce yourself to your colon, and how you might play a more conscious role in its many functions.

S12 - Conversations with My Anus

Our first contact with a non-human intelligence will not be extraterrestrial but with an intelligence within our bodies. It will speak using thought forms we know. Listen carefully.

S13 - Liver and the Lack of Sleep

I take you into your liver to explore its effects on sleep and consciousness. If you were as aware of your liver as you are of your heart, how would you relate to it?

S14 - Sex Addiction

The sexuality of Western culture is misguided and conflicted. Sexual dissatisfaction is a leading cause of frustration and hostility. Sex addiction reflects our blindness to dysregulation.

S15 - The Worlds Inside You

You are rivers of energy, creating oceans of awareness. Your consciousness has more structure than the surface of a map. Most of us remain in a valley of comfort and obligation, but we can discover new worlds.

Thoughts

T1 - How Smart Are You, and How Would You Know?

Within your limits, you are less, and beyond your limits, you are more competent than you presume. Beware of endorsements and welcome self-doubt. Learn about your limits by crossing them.

T2 - Why It's Dangerous to Believe What You Think

Those best informed see more risks and options, while the least informed see what they're told. The least trustworthy people are often the most confident. In an uncertain world, be cautious.

T3 - Black Magic and the Millionaire Mind

Affinity fraud is a deception in which trust is fabricated and then violated. Here I describe one of many schemes that combine deception, distraction, and manipulation.

T4 – Learn to Think

Thinking is the capstone of human experience. We question whether other animals think, but hardly question whether we do. We exercise little skill because we rarely consider how we build our minds.

T5 – The Reality of Illusion

Substance takes up space. Everything else is processes we represent in our imagination. The essential human project is not distinguishing what's true, it's imagining what's possible.

T6 – How I Seem to Be (Different)

I believe nothing I'm told. This is a good policy for therapy and science and is essential in the pseudosciences. My goal in speaking with you is to leave you knowing less and asking more.

T7 – Who's Conscious?

If we consider ourselves to be the agglomeration of many skills, attributes, memories, and situations, then all the prep time that's gone into getting us here—centuries of it—is part of our personality.

T8 – The Fundamental Question

Fundamental answers make little sense, and the questions they're supposed to answer make no sense at all. The notion that wisdom is built on a pyramid of ever more focused insights is a self-serving fallacy.

T9 – The Time of Your Life

Time is the ordering of our experience in and reactions to the world. We speak of time as if it's a thing, but it has no substance. Time does not progress at the same rate for any two people.

T10 – It Comes from Space

Our sense of reality derives from our sense of space and time, but what we perceive is an assembly of networks. The most important networks are in our minds, and they are the source of our reality.

T11 – Independent Thinkers

Independent thinkers are portrayed as saviors and terrorists, but mostly they're ignored. Most people don't recognize the mediocrity and incompetence that's plentiful all around us.

T12 – Where Thoughts Come From – I

Asking about the origin of thoughts is a different question from asking about their contents. It's a question of how they're put together, not what they're made of.

T13 – Where Thoughts Come From – II

I suggest thoughts are built from conceptually smaller things called oughts. Oughts are not thoughts, they are ineffable. They're seeds of memory, feeling, and association that are triggered by experience.

T14 – Where Thoughts Come From – III

A constructive theory of thought enables us to speak more precisely about the emergence of ideas. We can refine our questions about identity, free will, and determinism.

T15 – Where Thoughts Come From – IV

The theory of oughts is built on ideas of network ecologies that are fundamental to the natural world. It allows a measure of mathematical precision. That precision will be worth the effort.

T16 – Beyond Sight and Feeling

We don't understand ourselves because we don't experience our full reality. That includes perceptions we can't describe, ideas we cannot understand, and forces we cannot measure.

T17 – Thinking

Consciousness comes down to thinking. If your experience doesn't emerge as thought, then is not recognized as being fully conscious. While there are different kinds of experience, it's thinking that ties them together.

T18 – Kinds of Thinking

If we don't think about thinking, our thinking becomes stale, flat, and lacking in breadth. Our subconscious sits like a huge library, which we won't think to enter unless we ask deeper questions.

T19 – Reality of Craziness

Many of the ideas we need lie off the reasonable path and some are outside the domain of sanity. To traverse these crazy, dark lands requires strength, courage, and resilience. Your mental health lies in and beyond these territories.

T20 – To Be Confused I – Physics

The doors of transformation are labeled with confusion. Physics offers a good place to start to learn confusion because all of its trails lead to nonsense: to things you cannot understand because they make no sense.

T21 – To Be Confused II – Awareness

I like games for the organized confusion they can create. I'm attracted to those games that are the most confusing, games in which I understand the goals but not the means.

T22 – To Be Confused III – Music

Because music is not spatial, it introduces us to alternative structures, presenting us with cacophony, repetition, expectation, and emptiness. Confusion is something we can create and destroy.

T23 – To Be Confused IV – Facts and Feelings

As much as we like order, it is a fiction we construct. Nothing new ever comes from order, and there is little creative potential in it. If order is all that makes you comfortable, then you'll never be happy creating anything.

T24 – News, Memory, and Truth

We sift through the news, consider as true those ideas that might help us, but what results is unreliable. Your skills and knowledge are the only tools you can rely on.

Emotions

E1 – Emotion

Emotions are not things, they are reactions to things that summarize feelings. They are things you can have, but which are not healthy to be. Separate having from being before growing.

E2 – Emotional Thinking

We use intellect to navigate the landscape of our separateness. Emotion is the geography of our connectedness, and emotional thinking makes that landscape meaningful.

E3 – Emotional Ignorance

We have a bias to see the negative and try to separate ourselves from it. We have become adversarial because we're forced to depend on others. We need to overcome this emotional ignorance.

E4 – An Unusual Awareness

We lose holistic awareness as the world is compressed, and we lose control as we expand into a network of relationships. Better understanding requires both making sense and understanding what doesn't make sense.

E5 – Thinking, Time, and Identity

What we think of the world and what the world "thinks" are entirely different. We'd like to defend our thoughts as reasonable, but they are not really. Learn to think beyond the reasonable.

E6 – Consilience: Reason and Emotion

Reason and emotion are more than different ways of thinking, they are different ways of filtering our experience. Reason is linear, while emotion builds a holistic network. To establish balance, you must be free of the dichotomy of success and failure.

E7 – How Do You Feel?

We assume we're the architects of our thoughts and feelings, but the closer we look, the more we see that we don't know how we're put together, and we have little control over it.

E8 – Empathy I – Learn Empathy

Empathy is said to have a cognitive and an emotional part, the first leading to shared thoughts and the second to shared feelings. Empathy is the active ingredient of human culture.

E9 – Empathy II – Empathy and Emotional Intelligence
Feelings precede thoughts. It could not be any other way because feelings trigger thoughts. Without feelings, thoughts dissolve. Feelings both motivate and conclude our thoughts.

E10 – Empathy III – Similarity and Differences
Empathy is an essential skill. Sympathy is the toxic component of it. Keeping them apart is important. Without its empathetic component, sympathy becomes a weapon.

E11 – Empathy IV – The White Man's Tongue
Our faith in reason blinds us to the network of deeper truths. We're oblivious to the fork in the path between the understandings we create and the understandings coming from our senses.

E12 – Empathy V – Ways of Knowing
How do you learn empathy? It's one thing to mimic someone in learning to dance or play the guitar, but if you mimic an emotion that you don't have, then have you learned it?

E13 – Empathy VI – Security
To develop our emotions requires us to sacrifice a measure of our security. But if we have little security to start with, we'll be unwilling to sacrifice what we have, and we won't learn.

E14 – Empathy VII – Thought and Feeling
Your ability to empathize is determined by your ability to share another person's emotions. There are many emotions you may not have, many you may not want, and some that may actually be dangerous.

E15 – Sex and Emotion
Sexuality involves essential emotions. A healthy sexuality provides a pathway to meaningful, co-creative relationships. Lacking a healthy sexuality, these relationships are difficult or impossible to achieve.

E16 – Managing Your Emotions
The Western medical understanding of organs and the Eastern medical understanding of these same organs are entirely different. Until you understand this dichotomy, you won't understand your emotions.

E17 – Communicating with Honesty

There is a higher notion of honesty than telling the truth or stating the facts. This honesty is metaphysical, obscure, and full of contractions. It is not taught, rarely modeled, and if you don't learn it for yourself, then you'll be navigating in darkness.

E18 – Why We Fight (Because We Don't Connect)

Compromise is always a failure. Reconciliation through compromise fails because it condones destructive emotions. A co-creative solution can only be found in a shared, positive reality.

E19 – The States We Make

Your personality is like a bumper car ride in an amusement park, except in many more dimensions, and you're driving all the cars at once. It will always be confusing and that is as it should be. When managing your mind stops being a learning experience, your mind has no further role.

Thanks for considering these ideas. If you've found them useful, please post an encouraging reader review at this book's online site at any vendor, or on the book's GoodReads page at https://www.goodreads.com/book/show/204979265-sensations-thoughts-and-emotions. This will help the book and help others discover it!

= The End =

About the Author

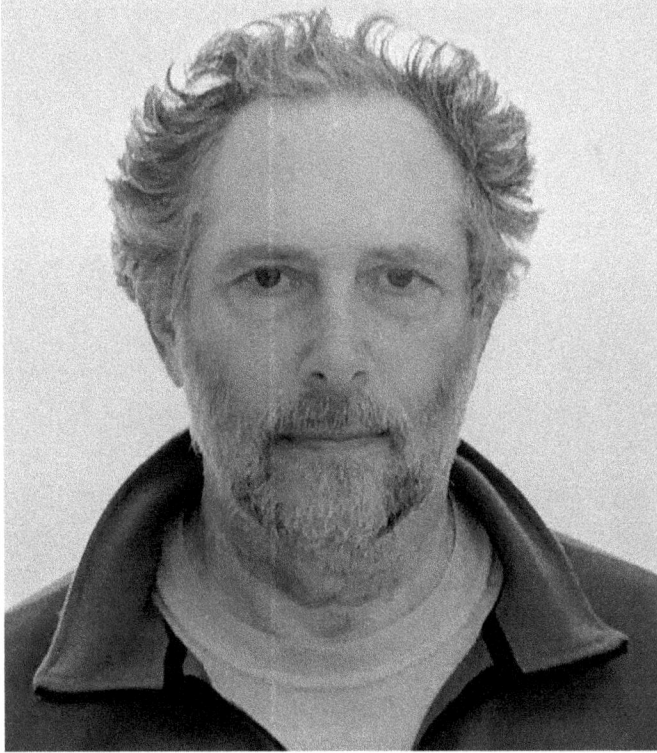

I was inspired to wonder about things before I started schooling. I can't identify what sparked this wondering, so it must be genetic. Included in my family's orbit were some of the world's great artist-engineers: Sandy Calder, Bucky Fully, Charles Eames, Frie Otto, Frank Lloyd Wright, and others. I don't really remember them, but they made an impression.

Curiosity has direction and consequence; my schooling offered neither. Before and while I was a teenager, I independently practiced diving, weight lifting, bicycle racing, classical guitar, slot car racing, archery, fly-fishing, rock climbing, and other hobbies. I attempted to learn science and to read the classics. My interests were tolerated, supported by no one, and I failed to realize every goal except rock climbing. They were interesting failures, and I wasn't disappointed. After each endeavor, I found myself pointed in another direction.

At Hampshire College, in Amherst, Massachusetts, I focused more seriously on physics, women, sex, guitar, esoteric spirituality, international travel, and foreign culture. I prodigiously pursued mountaineering and was disappointed in my professors, uninterested in drugs, and repelled by the college mindset. I studied philosophy but avoided psychology.

I learned that no serious effort should be seen as a failure, but it took graduate school and a PhD in physics to teach me that the seeds of the most meaningful success are sown in failing in conventional standards. I was a failure as a physicist, but now, after 40 more years of studying physics, I am succeeding by my own standards.

I am addicted to the endorphins of exploration and discovery. At 17, I somehow appeared in an in-flight magazine in an article titled "The Overachievers." When I was 22 and still an undergraduate, I worked as a research computer programmer in the astronomy group of Charles Townes at the University of California in Berkeley.

Completing my physics PhD and failing to find employment in the field, I started my company Braided Matrix, Inc. to design, patent, and produce a modular business accounting system. I had no experience with business or accounting before that, but, after 20 years, I gained much experience in both. I had hoped to sell the business for a large profit. Instead, I folded the business and moved into psychology.

In the 1990s, building on my studies in neurology, philosophy, culture, and religion, I began brain-biofeedback training both as a client and a student. The field of neurofeedback was only starting and lacked schools and certifications, so I attended conferences and mentored with leaders in the field.

The field of neurofeedback led, naturally and unnaturally, into psychedelics, shamanism, herbalism, scuba diving, soarplane piloting, and metaphysics. My background in esoteric Eastern and Western spirituality provided a strong fulcrum against which I moved into hypnosis and, finally, psychology. But it was all rooted in my years of experience with odd, extreme, and accomplished people across many disciplines and cultures.

I came from an art-focused family, moved through a society of obsessed mountaineers, then through what Thomas Mann called "the glass bead game" of physics, the new cultures of the Afro-Caribbean, and the old cultures of Indigenous Americans and traditional Mongolia. I gained and lost two families, but have kept the two sons and the image of my dysfunction mirrored in two ex wives.

As a psychotherapist, I am now dealing with the old problems of our new culture: dysregulation, chronic illness, and personal transformation. I work in the areas of psychology, neurology, personal growth, and culture. My work on the foundations of quantum mechanics and computational neuroscience are fruitful and more relevant to psychology than you might think. For more information, visit my website at www.mindstrengthbalance.com.

Alphabetical Index

476

www.ingramcontent.com/pod-product-compliance
Lightning Source LLC
Chambersburg PA
CBHW081142020426
42333CB00021B/2636